Fundamentals of Phonetics

A Practical Guide for Students

Second Edition

Larry H. Small

Bowling Green State University

PEARSON

Boston ■ New York ■ San Francisco
Mexico City ■ Montreal ■ London ■ Madrid ■ Munich ■ Paris
Hong Kong ■ Singapore ■ Tokyo ■ Cape Town ■ Sydney

for
my parents
and
dB

Executive Editor and Publisher: Stephen D. Dragin
Senior Editorial Assistant: Barbara Strickland
Production Supervisor: Joe Sweeney
Editorial-Production Services: Walsh & Associates, Inc.
Composition and Prepress Buyer: Linda Cox
Manufacturing Buyer: Andrew Turso
Cover Administrator: Joel Gendron
Electronic Composition: Publishers' Design and Production Services, Inc.

For related titles and support materials, visit our online catalog at www.ablongman.com.

Between the time Web site information is gathered and published, some cities may have closed. The publisher would appreciate notification where these occur so that they may be corrected in subsequent editions.

Library of Congress Cataloging-in-Publication Data
Small, Larry H., 1954–
    Fundamentals of phonetics : a practical guide for students / Larry H. Small.
  —2nd ed.
      p.   cm.
    Includes bibliographical references and index.
    ISBN 0-205-41912-7
    1. English language—Phonetics—Problems, exercises, etc. I. Title.

PE1135.S49   2005
421'.58—dc21

                                               2004047744

Printed in the United States of America

10 9 8   09 0 8 07

Contents

Preface to the Second Edition

As in the first edition, the major purpose of *Fundamentals of Phonetics: A Practical Guide for Students* is to provide students with sufficient practice to become efficient in the skill of phonetic transcription. Each chapter still provides students with an abundance of practice exercises in order to aid in the learning process. Some of the exercises have been edited, and several new exercises have been added. Many of the references have been updated to reflect current philosophy and best practice in our field.

The actual format of the second edition has not strayed much from the original. However, additional material has been added to several of the chapters. Several changes to Chapter 2, *The Phonetic Representation of English,* will help the reader more fully understand the concepts being presented.

In Chapter 7, *Clinical Phonetics,* an in-depth discussion has been added to address assessment options for children with phonological disorders. Also, several taped examples of children with phonological disorders have been added to the *Review Exercises* at the end of the chapter.

Due to the large increase in the foreign-born population in the United States, the complexion of our nation is always changing. In fact, since the publication of the first edition, the Hispanic population has become the largest minority group in the United States. After Spanish, Chinese has become the most common foreign language spoken in the home (displacing French as the number two foreign language spoken in America). Chapter 8, *Dialectal Variation,* has been updated in order to stay current with these latest demographic data. In addition, a section has been added on Arabic- and Russian-Influenced English (complete with recorded examples).

As with the first edition, supplemental recordings of many of the exercises are available on audio CD from Allyn and Bacon. These recordings are essential in helping students learn the subtleties of pronunciation, both with the segmental and suprasegmental characteristics of speech.

Acknowledgments

There are several individuals who deserve credit for their help in the creation of this second edition. I would like to express my appreciation to George Allen, who took the time to go through the first edition with great effort and care. His suggestions and corrections are invaluable. A thank you goes to Adele Miccio for her suggestions and feedback, and to my colleagues Lynne Hewitt and Tim Brackenbury for their comments and support.

The reviewers of the second edition deserve special praise. Thank you to Jessica Barlow, San Diego State University; Patricia Lohman-Hawk, New Mexico State University; W. Chad Nye, University of Central Florida; and Laura Snow, University of Washington. Also, I would like to express my utmost gratitude to Barbara Strickland and the editorial staff at Allyn and Bacon. A special thank you goes to Steve Dragin, Executive Editor, for his guidance and motivation.

Last, I would like to acknowledge all of the students and faculty members from around the country who have provided me with positive feedback on the first edition. Your support is both overwhelming and inspirational.

Preface to the First Edition

The major emphasis of a phonetics course for students in the hearing and speech fields is on learning to transcribe spoken language. Therefore, a phonetics textbook should heavily emphasize the *practice* of phonetic transcription. That is the purpose of *Fundamentals of Phonetics: A Practical Guide for Students*. The first time I taught phonetics, several years ago, I discovered that I was not particularly happy with any of the textbooks on the market. As I continued to teach phonetics over the years, I continued to try different textbooks. Still, I was not satisfied. Each available text had its own particular merits, but I could not find the "perfect" text that, in my opinion, could supplement my lectures. (This might explain why my first phonetics instructor never used a textbook.) I was particularly disappointed that most texts just did not provide enough practice exercises for students to become proficient with the skill of phonetic transcription. Therefore, the seed was planted for the creation of this book.

This text covers several topics, in an attempt to introduce students to the field of phonetics. In Chapter 1, *Phonetics: A "Sound" Science*, there is a brief overview of the study of phonetics, introducing the various branches of phonetic science. Chapter 2, *The Phonetic Representation of English*, introduces students to the particular problems associated with using the Roman alphabet to represent the sound system of English. This chapter introduces the IPA as the solution to the problem, as well as addressing several aspects of phonology. Chapter 3, *Anatomy and Physiology of the Speech Mechanism*, provides an overview of the anatomical structures involved in the processes of respiration, phonation, and articulation. The individual speech sounds of English are introduced in Chapter 4, *Vowel Transcription*, and Chapter 5, *Consonant Transcription*. These two chapters acquaint students with the production and transcription of all of the individual speech sounds of English. The characteristic differences between vowels and consonants are also discussed. Chapter 6, *Connected Speech*, focuses on how speech sound identity often changes when words are put together to form sentences and how those changes are transcribed. In addition, Chapter 6 examines the transcription of stress, intonation, and timing of words in sentences. In Chapter 7, *Clinical Phonetics*, you will be introduced to the process of typical speech development in children and also to methods of transcribing disordered speech patterns. Chapter 8,

Dialectal Variation, concentrates on transcription of dialects common to the many speech communities distributed throughout the United States.

I would like to acknowledge some individuals who served as the catalyst for the development of this book. First, I would like to acknowledge my parents for not only bringing me into this world, but also for their support and love. I would also like to thank the late Elliott Blinn who suggested to me that I travel away from my home university to work on this book during my faculty leave. Had I not taken his advice, you probably would not be reading this now.

The creation of this book would not have been possible without the help of several individuals. I especially would like to thank my mentor and friend, Zinny Bond, who sparked my interest in phonetics while I was still a doctoral student. She is a never-ending source of inspiration. Thank you also to Edwin Leach, Norman Garber, and the entire faculty and staff of Hearing and Speech Sciences at Ohio University for providing space, a computer, and continued camaraderie, all of which assisted me in the initial stages of this project.

My colleagues in the Department of Communication Disorders at Bowling Green State University deserve thanks for their continued support. A special thanks goes to Linda Petrosino for being not only a great department chair, but also a great friend.

The reviewers of this text provided valuable comments. Thank yous go to Raymond G. Daniloff, University of North Texas; Lauren K. Nelson, The University of Northern Iowa; and Robert A. Hull, Jr. Valdosta State University. Also, I would like to express my appreciation to Jeannene M. Ward-Lonergan, Ronald C. Scherer, and Diane L. Williams for their expertise, and for the time they spent making editorial comments on earlier versions of this work. A special mention goes to Cathy Bressert, Brent Marquart, Ruth Alexander, and Janielle Zinna, my graduate assistants, who were extremely helpful in the editing and revising process.

Other thank yous go to Donna Colcord, Chuck Hayden, and Sandy Michalski of St. Vincent Mercy Medical Center of Toledo for helping with the video fluoroscopy necessary for the creation of the X-ray tracings found in Chapters 4 and 5. I would like to acknowledge George P. Lonergan for his help in creating the drawings used in the text. The audio CD and supplemental cassette tapes were created with the help of Erik Trenty and Recording Services in the College of Musical Arts at Bowling Green State University. In addition, I would like to thank Steve Dragin, Liz McGuire, Kathy Whittier, and the rest of the editorial and production staff associated with Allyn and Bacon for their encouragement, support, and guidance during the creation of this text.

Finally, I would like to thank the hundreds of phonetics students I have taught over the years. Their invaluable comments and suggestions during the writing of earlier versions of this book gave me the drive necessary to persevere in its completion.

Phonetics:
A "Sound" Science

As college students, you are all familiar with the speaking process. Speaking is something you do every day. In fact, most people find speech to be quite automatic. It is safe to say that most of us are experts at speaking. We probably have been experts since the time we were 3 or 4 years old. Yet, we never really think about the process of speech. We do not, as a rule, sit around thinking about how ideas are formed and how their encoded forms are sent from the brain to the speech organs, such as the teeth, lips, and tongue. Nor do we think about how the speech organs can move in synchrony to form words. Think about the last party you attended. You probably did not debate the intricacies of the speech process while conversing with friends. Speaking is something we learned during infancy, and we take the entire process for granted. We are not aware of the speech process; it is involuntary. So involuntary that we often are not conscious of what we have said until after we have said it. Those of you who have "stuck your foot in your mouth" know exactly how automatic the speech process is. Often we have said things and we have no idea why we said them.

Phonetics is the study of the production and perception of speech sounds. During your study of phonetics, you will begin to think about the process of speech. You will learn how speech is formulated by the speech organs. You also will learn how individual speech sounds are created and how they are combined during the speech process to form syllables and words. You will need to learn to *listen* to the speech patterns of words and sentences to become familiar with the sounds of speech that comprise spoken language. A large part of any course in phonetics also involves how speech sounds are transcribed, or written. Therefore, you also will be learning a new alphabet that will enable you to transcribe speech sounds.

The idea of studying speech sounds may be an odd idea to understand at first. We generally think about words in terms of how they appear in print or how they are spelled. We usually do not take the time to stop and think about how words are spoken and how spoken words sound to a listener. Look at the

1

word "phone" for a moment. What comes to mind? You might consider the fact that it contains the five letters: p-h-o-n-e. Or you might think of its definition. You probably did not say to yourself that there are only three speech sounds in the word ("f"-"o"-"n"). The reason you do not consider the sound patterns of words when reading is simple—it is not something you do daily. Nor is it something you were taught to do. In fact, talking about the sound patterns of words and being able to transcribe them is an arduous task; it requires considerable practice.

As you soon will find out, the way you believe a word sounds may not be the way it sounds at all. First, it is difficult to forget our notions of how a word is spelled. Second, our conception of how a word sounds is usually wrong. Consider the greeting, "How are you doing?" We rarely ask this question with such formality. Most likely, we would say, "How ya doin'?" What happens to the word "are" in this informal version? It disappears! Now examine the pronunciation of the words "do" and "you" in "Whatcha want?" (The informal version of "What do you want?") Neither of these words is spoken in any recognizable form. Actually, these words become the non-English word "cha" in "whatcha." With these examples, you can begin to understand the importance of thinking about the sounds of speech in order to be able to discuss and transcribe speech patterns.

EXERCISE 1.1

The expressions below are written two separate ways: (1) formally and (2) casually. Examine the differences between the two versions. What happens to the production of the *individual* words in the casual version?

Formal	Casual
1. Are you going to eat now?	Ya' gonna eat now?
2. Can't you see her?	Cantcha see 'er?
3. Did you go?	Ja go?

Phonetics is a multifaceted field of study, containing several interrelated branches. **Historical phonetics** involves the study of sound changes in words. There is a constant mutation over time in the pronunciation of words in all languages. The way we pronounce words in English today is vastly different from the pronunciation of English from 300 to 1700 A.D. For instance, between the fourteenth and seventeenth centuries, there was a marked evolution in the pronunciation of English long vowels. This change in vowel pronunciation is known as the Great Vowel Shift. Due to this shift in vowel pronunciation, the words we know today as "bite," "beet," "bait," and "boot" were pronounced (prior to 1700 A.D.) as "beet," "bait," "bet," and "boat," respectively (Stevick, 1968).

When saying a word, such as "phonetics," there is an intricate interaction between the lips, the tongue, and the other speech organs. To more fully understand the process of speech production it is important to understand the individual role of each of the various speech organs. **Physiological phonetics** involves the study of the function of the speech organs during the process of speaking. The knowledge of the muscles and innervation of the speech organs is especially important in fully understanding their operation during the production of speech. **Acoustic phonetics**, on the other hand, focuses on the differences in the frequency, intensity, and duration of the various consonants and vowels. Differences in the acoustic attributes of speech sounds allow listeners to be able to perceive how sounds, syllables, and words differ from one another. For instance, it is the specific acoustic attributes of the initial consonants in the words "mug," "hug," "rug," and "thug" that allow listeners to tell them apart. **Perceptual phonetics** is the study of a listener's psychoacoustic response (perception) of speech sounds in terms of loudness, pitch, perceived length, and quality. **Experimental phonetics** involves the laboratory study of physiological, acoustic, and perceptual phonetics. Laboratory equipment is used to measure the various attributes of the speech organs during speech production as well as to measure the acoustic characteristics of speech.

The scope of **clinical phonetics** involves the study and transcription of aberrant speech behaviors, that is, those that vary from what is considered to be "normal" speech. Disordered speech may be found in either children or adults who might have experienced a hearing impairment, fluency disorder, head trauma, stroke, or a phonological (speech sound) disorder.

The study of phonetics also involves the study and transcription of individuals displaying differences in their speech patterns due to dialectal variation. For instance, in the United States, individuals from the southern states and from New England pronounce certain sounds differently when compared to individuals from the Midwest. Also, the forms of English spoken by African American and Spanish populations are characterized by dialectal variations when compared to Standard American English. Knowledge of dialects is extremely important when establishing a treatment plan for speech-impaired individuals whose speech patterns reflect regional or ethnic dialectal variation. Because a dialect should not be considered a substandard form of English, a speech therapist will be concerned with remediation of clients' speech disorders, not their dialects.

Another "sound" science related to phonetics is **phonology**. Phonology is the systematic organization of speech sounds in the production of language. The major distinction between the fields of phonetics and phonology is that *phonetics* focuses on the study of speech sounds, their acoustic and perceptual characteristics, and how they are produced by the speech organs, without reference to how speech sounds are combined and used in language. *Phonology* focuses on the linguistic (phonological) rules that are used to specify the manner in which speech sounds are organized and combined into meaningful units, which are then combined to form syllables, words, and sentences. Phonological rules, along with syntactic/morphological rules (for grammar), semantic rules (for utterance meaning), and pragmatic rules (for language use), are the major rule systems used in production of language.

Once you have mastered the concepts in this text, you will be able to transcribe the speech patterns of your clients using the **International Phonetic Alphabet (IPA)**. This alphabet is different from most alphabets because it is designed to represent the sounds of words, not their spellings. Without such a systematic phonetic alphabet, it would be virtually impossible to capture on paper an accurate representation of impaired speech patterns of individuals seeking professional remediation of their speech problems. Using the IPA also permits consistency among professionals in their transcription of typical or atypical speech.

Phonetics is a skill-based course much like courses you may take in keyboarding or sign language. In many ways, it is like learning a new language because you will be learning new symbols and new rules to represent spoken language. Yes, we are still talking about English. However, the new symbols you will be learning will be representative of the sounds of English, not their spelling. As with the learning of any new language, phonetics requires considerable practice in order for you to become proficient in its use when transcribing oral speech patterns.

This textbook is designed to promote practice of phonetic transcription principles. Many phonetics books provide readers with considerable technical information on the anatomy of the speech production mechanism as well as information related to speech acoustics. This information is essential for a complete understanding of the process of speech production. This material is usually covered in other courses in hearing science, speech science, and anatomy of the speech and hearing mechanism. Therefore, there is no attempt to replicate that information here.

Each of the chapters has exercises embedded in the text that will help emphasize particular points. At the end of each chapter, you will find Review Exercises so that you may gain expertise with the material presented. The answers to most of the exercises are located at the rear of the book. By providing answers to the exercises, you will gain immediate feedback, and you will be able to learn from your mistakes. There is no better way to learn! To aid in the learning process, all new terms will be in bold letters the first time they are used. In addition, all new terms can be found in the Glossary at the back of the book.

Study Questions at the end of each chapter also will help you explore the major concepts presented. Assignments at the end of most chapters were designed to be collected by instructors. The answers for Assignments are not given.

There are several conventions that will be adopted throughout the text. When there is a reference to a particular Roman alphabet letter, it will be enclosed with a set of quotation marks: for example, the letter "m." Likewise, references to a particular word will also be enclosed with quotation marks: for example, "mail." Individual speech sounds will be referenced with the traditional slash marks: for example, the /m/ sound.

A set of optional audio CDs provide listening exercises to accompany the text. Clinical practice generally requires phonetic transcription of recorded speech samples. Reading words on paper and transcribing them is not the same as transcribing spoken words. The audio CDs are designed to increase your listening skills and your ability to transcribe spoken English. Exercises requiring the audio CDs will be indicated with a CD icon in the margin of the text.

Variation in Phonetic Practice

As the IPA is introduced throughout this text, alternate methods of transcribing speech will be introduced. Students should become familiar with alternate transcription symbols. Although the IPA was developed for consistency, not everyone transcribes speech in the same manner. The IPA does allow for some flexibility in actual practice. If you were to pick up another phonetics textbook, you would probably find some minor differences in transcription symbols.

One reason for the difference in the selection of transcription symbols is that the typical computer (or typewriter) keyboard does not lend itself well to the IPA. For ease of typing, some keyboard symbols are substituted. For example, when transcribing the word "dot" it might be easier to type /dat/ than the correct IPA form /dɑt/ since the symbol /ɑ/ does not exist on a typical keyboard. (A specialized font was used to create this textbook.) Most of us, however, will not be using a keyboard when transcribing speech; we will be writing.

Another reason for differences in use of transcription symbols is simply ease of use. For example, the speech sound at the beginning of the word "red" has been traditionally transcribed with the IPA symbol /r/. According to the IPA, the initial sound in "red" should be transcribed with the symbol /ɹ/. The IPA symbol /r/ represents a *trill*, a sound not a part of the English speech sound system. Because /r/ and /ɹ/ do not both exist in English, the symbol /r/ has been routinely substituted; writing /r/ turned 180 degrees is difficult and cumbersome. Most speech-language pathologists and audiologists have customarily used the symbol /r/ instead of /ɹ/ in transcription. Therefore, the tradition will be continued in this textbook.

As future speech and hearing professionals, you will be using the IPA to transcribe the defective speech patterns of your clients. Because the IPA was not originally designed for this purpose, clinicians vary in their choice of symbols in transcription of disordered speech as well.

Transcription practice also differs from individual to individual due to personal habit or the method learned. For instance, the word "or" (or "oar") could be transcribed reliably in all of the following ways:

/ɔr/, /or/, /ɔɹ/, /ɔɚ/, /oɚ/

All of the above forms have appeared in other phonetics textbooks and have been adopted by professionals through the years.

Several years ago, I was assigned to a jury trial that lasted two weeks. Due to the length of the trial, the judge allowed us to take notes. So that no one could read my notes, I decided to use the IPA! Because I had to write quickly, my transcription habits changed. At the beginning of the trial, I transcribed the word "or" as /ɔɚ/ due to personal preference. By the middle of the trial, I had switched to /ɔr/ simply because it was more time efficient.

Is one method of transcription "better" or more correct than another? Some linguists and phoneticians might argue that one form is superior than another. The form of transcription you adopt is not important as long as you understand the underlying rationale for your choice of symbols. In addition, you need to make sure that you are consistent and accurate in the use of the symbols you adopt. Throughout this book, variant transcriptions will be introduced to increase your familiarity with the different symbols you may encounter in actual clinical practice in the future.

As you read this book, and as you attempt to answer the various exercises, please keep in mind that English pronunciation varies depending upon an individual's dialect. The pronunciations used in this book often reflect the author's Midwest pronunciation patterns. This does not mean that alternate pronunciations are wrong. The numerous text and recorded examples, as well as the answer key, may not be indicative of the way *you* pronounce a particular word or sentence. Always check with your instructor for alternate pronunciations of the materials found in this book.

2

The Phonetic Representation of English

As you begin your study of phonetics, it is extremely important to think about words in terms of how they sound and *not* in terms of how they are spelled. As you begin your study of phonetics, it is extremely important to think about words in terms of how they sound and *not* in terms of how they are spelled. *The repetition of this first sentence is not a typographical error.* The importance of this concept cannot be stressed enough. You *must* ignore the spelling of words and concentrate only on speech sounds. If you have been troubled in the past with your inability to spell, do not fear—phonetics is the one course where spelling is highly discouraged.

For many, ignoring spelling and focusing only on the sounds of words will be a difficult task. Most of us started to spell in kindergarten or in first grade as we learned to read. It was drilled into our heads that "cat" was spelled C-A-T and "dog" was spelled D-O-G. Consequently, we learned to connect the spoken (or printed) words with their respective spellings. Imagine the following fictitious scenario between a parent and a child reading alone together before bedtime:

> "O.K., Mary. Now, let's think about the word 'cat.' It's spelled C-A-T, but the first speech sound is a /k/ as in 'king,' the second sound is an /æ/ as in 'apple' and the third sound is a /t/ as in 'table.' Notice that the first sound is really a /k/ not a letter 'c.' Words that begin with the letter 'c' may sound like /k/ or may sound like /s/, as in the word 'city.' Actually, Mary, there is no phonetic symbol in English that uses the printed letter 'c' . . ."

Obviously, this type of interchange would cause children to lose any desire to read!

The Difference between Spelling and Sound

Examine the word "through." Although there are seven printed letters, or **graphemes**, in the word, there are only three speech sounds: "th," "r," and "oo."

Now examine the word "phlegm." How many sounds (not letters) do you think are in this word? If you answered four, you are correct—"f," "l," "e," and "m." Obviously, letters do not always adequately represent the number of sounds in a word. Letters only tell us about spelling; they give no clues as to the actual pronunciation of a word. It is imprecise to talk about a sound that may be associated with a particular alphabet letter (or letters) because the letters may not be an accurate reflection of the sound they represent. For instance, the grapheme "s" represents a different sound in the word "size" than it does in the word "vision." What do you think is the sound associated with the letter "g" in the word "phlegm"?

EXERCISE 2.1

Say each of the following words out loud to determine the number of sounds that comprise each one. Write your answer in the blank.

Example:

_3_	reed	_4_	frog	_4_	wince

____	lazy	____	smooth	____	cough
____	spilled	____	driven	____	oh
____	comb	____	why	____	raisin

An alphabet that contains a separate letter for each individual sound in a language is called a **phonetic alphabet**. A phonetic alphabet maintains a one-to-one relationship between a sound and a particular letter. Our (Roman) alphabet is not phonetic because it contains only 26 alphabet letters to represent approximately 42 English speech sounds. In elementary school we all learned that the English vowels were "a, e, i, o, u, and sometimes y." In actuality, there are approximately fourteen vowel sounds in our language. One reason that second language learners of English experience difficulty with pronunciation is due to the fact that the English sound system is not well represented by the Roman alphabet. By examining the spelling of the words "through," "cough," "bough," and "rough," it is immediately apparent why learning English as a second language is particularly difficult. These four words have completely different vowel sounds, yet they all share the letter sequence "ough."

Because the Roman alphabet contains fewer letters than the number of speech sounds in English, one alphabet letter often represents more than one speech sound. For instance, the grapheme "c," in the words "cent" and "car," represents two different sounds. Likewise, the grapheme "o" represents different sounds in the words "cod," "bone," "women," "bough," "through," and "above." These examples provide further evidence why it is inappropriate to discuss sounds in association with letters. After reading the information above, how would you answer the question, What is the sound of the letter "o"?

Another way sound and spelling differ is the fact that the same sound can be represented by more than one letter or sequence of letters. **Allographs** are different letter sequences or patterns that represent the same sound. The following groups of words contain allographs of a particular sound, represented by the underlined letters. You will see that the sound associated with some allographs is predictable, while the sound associated with others is not. Keep in mind that for each example, although the spelling is different, *the sounds they represent are the same.*

loop, through, threw, fruit, canoe
mail, convey, hate, steak
trite, try , tried, aisle, height
for, laugh, photo, muffin
shoe, Sean, caution, precious, tissue
eked, visa, heed, meat

Note in some of the examples that *pairs* of letters often represent one sound because there are simply not enough single alphabet letters to represent all of the sounds of English. These pairs of letters are called **digraphs**. Digraphs may be the same two letters (as in "hoot," heed," or "tissue") or two completely different letters (as in "shoe," "steak," or "tried").

EXERCISE 2.2

Examine the underlined sounds (letter combinations) in the words in each row. Place an "X" in front of the one word that does not share an allograph with the others.

Example:

____ raid	____ cake	____ hey	_X_ back
____ shoe	____ measure	____ ocean	____ sufficient
____ chord	____ liquor	____ biscuit	____ rag
____ moon	____ through	____ though	____ suit
____ wood	____ done	____ flood	____ rub
____ ice	____ was	____ press	____ scissors

Another oddity of the spelling of words involves "silent letters." Although the word "plumb" has five graphemes, the final letter has no connection to the pronunciation of the word. Consequently, "plumb" has only four speech sounds. These "silent" letters also can be found in the words "gnome," "psychosis," "rhombus," "khaki," and "pneumonia."

Many oddly spelled English words, and those that contain "silent letters," are often related to the origin of a word, and usually reflect a spelling common to the language from which it was borrowed. For example, words such as "pneumonia," "rhombus," and "cyst" are derived from the Greek language, helping to explain their particular spellings. In addition, we borrow entire words from other languages, keeping their spelling intact. This only adds to our spelling irregularities. Examples of some words borrowed from other languages include:

savoir-faire (French)   sushi (Japanese)
daiquiri (Cuban)   chutzpah (Yiddish)
kindergarten (German)   jodhpurs (Indian)
cacao (Spanish)   lasagna (Italian)

Morphemes

If our system of spelling is so irregular, how are we ever able to learn the complexities of the English language? How do we learn to read and write? Actually, our English spelling system is not as odd as it appears. In fact, only about 25 percent of the words in English have irregular spellings (Crystal, 1987). Unfortunately, many of the irregularly spelled words tend to be the ones used often in our language.

One key to the regularity of oddly spelled words can be found if we study the spelling patterns among words that share similar meaningful linguistic units, or morphemes. A **morpheme** is the smallest unit of language capable of carrying meaning. For instance, the word "book" is a morpheme. The word "book" carries meaning because it connotes an item that is composed of pages with print, binding, two covers, etc. The word "chair" is also a morpheme; it conveys meaning.

Now consider the word "books." It contains two morphemes, the morpheme "book" and the plural morpheme, represented by -s. The -s ending indicates the plural form of the word, that is, more than one book. Since -s carries meaning, it is a morpheme. Other examples of morphemes include regular verb endings (such as -ed and -ing as in the words "walk**ed**" and "call**ing**"), prefixes (such as pre- and re- as in "prepaid" and "reread") and suffixes (such as -tion in "constitution" and -ive as in "talkative"). Take a moment to examine the three pairs of words below. Notice that each word pair shares the same morpheme. Say each pair aloud. What do you notice?

*music music*ian   *phlegm phlegm*atic   *press press*ure

Hopefully, you noted that although each pair shares the same morpheme, the pronunciation of the morphemes in each pair is different. English morphemes tend to be spelled the same even though the words that share them are pronounced in a different manner. English spelling may not appear to be so odd if one considers the spelling of the morphemes that form the roots of many irregularly spelled English words (MacKay, 1987).

Morphemes that can stand alone and still carry meaning, such as "book," "phlegm," "music," or "press," are called **free morphemes**. Morphemes (bold) such as **pre**(date), **re**(tread), (book)**s**, (music)**ian**, and (press)**ure** are called **bound morphemes** because they are bound to other words and carry no meaning when they stand alone.

Knowledge of morphemes also is useful in the study of child language development. The average number of morphemes per utterance is a useful tool employed by speech-language pathologists in examining language behavior in children. This measure is commonly known as **mean length of utterance (MLU)**. By analyzing MLU, it is possible to determine whether a child is progressing through specific stages of language development, with respect to both the typical developmental sequence and the appropriate time frame.

EXERCISE 2.3

For each item below, think of another word that shares the same morpheme.

Example:

create   <u> creation </u>

1. deduce	_____		6. great	_____
2. protect	_____		7. honest	_____
3. potent	_____		8. decent	_____
4. scrutiny	_____		9. late	_____
5. labor	_____		10. magnet	_____

EXERCISE 2.4

Indicate the number of morphemes in each of the following words.

Examples:

__1__ cucumber   __2__ reading   __3__ reworked

____ caution   ____ running   ____ lived   ____ relistened

____ warmly   ____ finger   ____ talker   ____ kangaroo

____ prorated   ____ clarinetist   ____ sharply   ____ swarming

---

Phonemes

Because it is difficult to use the Roman alphabet to represent speech sounds, the IPA has been adopted by linguists, phoneticians, and speech and hearing professionals for the purpose of speech transcription. The IPA was created for adoption by languages worldwide by the International Phonetic Association, formed in 1886. The IPA symbols are consistent from language to language. For example, the English word "sit" and the German word "mit" (meaning "with") both have the same vowel. Therefore, we would use the same vowel symbol to transcribe these words (/sɪt/ and /mɪt/, respectively). If you were familiar with all of the IPA symbols, you would be capable of transcribing languages other than English. Keep in mind that you would need to know the IPA symbols for speech sounds that are not part of the English language. A list of all of the common IPA symbols used in English is located in Table 2.1. The complete IPA chart (revised to 1993, updated 1996) is located in Figure 2.1. Take some time to examine the IPA chart. There are several sections of the chart that need to be highlighted. The large area at the top, labeled "consonants (pulmonic)," shows all the consonants of the world's languages that are produced with an egressive, or outgoing, airstream from the lungs. All English consonants are pulmonic consonants. Many of these symbols may appear foreign to you. Compare the IPA pulmonic consonants with the English consonant symbols given in Table 2.1. You will see that many of the symbols in the IPA chart represent sounds not present in English. Also, call your attention to the section of "non-pulmonic" consonants that are produced with an ingressive, or incoming, airstream. Non-pulmonic consonants include the "clicks" often heard in some African languages.

A very important section of the IPA chart is labeled "vowels." You will note that the vowels are placed in various locations around a four-sided figure. This *quadrilateral* is a schematic drawing of a speaker's mouth, or oral cavity. The placement of the vowel symbols within the quadrilateral is roughly based on where the tongue is located during production of the various vowels. As with the consonants, many of the IPA vowel symbols are representative of speech sounds not found in English.

The area marked "diacritics" presents another array of symbols that are used in conjunction with the IPA consonant and vowel symbols. The use of diacritics indicates an alternate way of producing a certain sound. The use of diacritical markings is explained in more detail in Chapter 7.

The last section of the IPA chart most important for our purposes is labeled "suprasegmentals." The suprasegmental symbols are used to indicate the stress, intonation pattern, and tempo of any particular utterance in a language.

TABLE 2.1   The IPA Symbols for American English Phonemes

	Symbol	Key Word
Vowels	/i/	key
	/ɪ/	win
	/e/	reb<u>a</u>te
	/ɛ/	red
	/æ/	had
	/u/	moon
	/ʊ/	wood
	/o/	<u>o</u>kay
	/ɔ/	law
	/ɑ/	cod
	/ə/	<u>a</u>bout
	/ʌ/	bud
	/ɚ/	butt<u>er</u>
	/ɝ/	bird
Diphthongs	/aʊ/	how
	/aɪ/	tie
	/ɔɪ/	boy
	/eɪ/	bake
	/oʊ/	rose
Consonants	/p/	pork
	/b/	bug
	/t/	to
	/d/	dog
	/k/	king
	/g/	go
	/m/	mad
	/n/	name
	/v/	vote
	/ŋ/	ri<u>ng</u>
	/f/	for
	/θ/	<u>th</u>ink
	/ð/	<u>th</u>em
	/s/	say
	/z/	zoo
	/ʃ/	<u>sh</u>ip
	/ʒ/	beige
	/h/	hen
	/tʃ/	<u>ch</u>ew
	/dʒ/	join
	/w/	wise
	/j/	<u>y</u>et
	/r/	row
	/l/	let

THE INTERNATIONAL PHONETIC ALPHABET (revised to 1993, updated 1996)

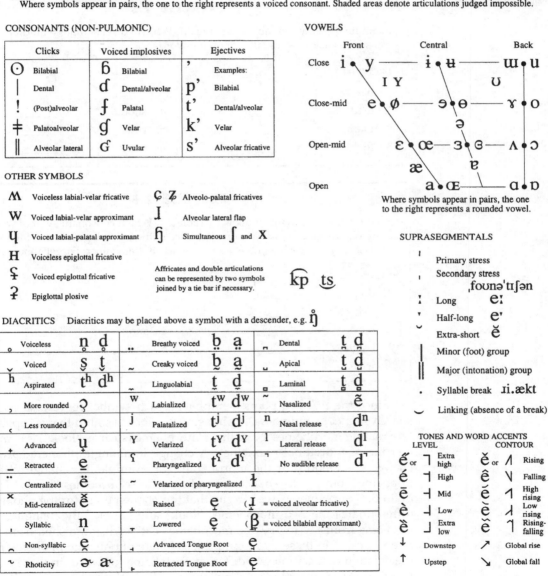

FIGURE 2.1 The International Phonetic Alphabet (revised to 1993, updated 1996). This chart first appeared in the *Journal of the International Phonetic Association* and is reproduced by permission of the International Phonetic Association.

13

As you look over the entire chart, you will notice that many of the unfamiliar symbols appear similar to the letters of the Roman alphabet. This was one of the guiding principles of the International Phonetic Association when creating the symbols for the IPA. That is, all symbols of the IPA were designed to blend in with the letters of the Roman alphabet (*Handbook of the International Phonetic Association*, 1999).

Initially, the IPA chart will be confusing to you. As you progress through this text, the IPA chart will become less confusing and more meaningful in your study of phonetics.

EXERCISE 2.5

Examine the vowel symbols in Table 2.1. Which vowel symbol would be used to transcribe each vowel in the following words?

Example:

beast   i

1. lend   _____   4. should   _____
2. man   _____   5. rude   _____
3. flick   _____   6. week   _____

EXERCISE 2.6

Examine the consonant symbols in Table 2.1. Which consonant symbol would be used to transcribe the *last* consonant in each of the following words? Hint: Listen to the last sound in each word as you say it aloud. Remember: Forget about spelling!

Examples:

dog   g
rich   tʃ

1. ram   _____   4. sung   _____
2. laugh   _____   5. bath   _____
3. wish   _____   6. leave   _____

Since the IPA is a phonetic alphabet, each symbol represents one specific speech sound, or **phoneme**. A phoneme is a speech sound that is capable of differentiating morphemes. Note that a morpheme (such as "look") is composed of a string of individual phonemes. A change in a single phoneme always will change the identity of the morpheme. For example, by changing the initial phoneme from /l/ to /b/, the morpheme "look" becomes "book." Using our definition of phoneme, we can say that the phoneme /l/ (or the phoneme /b/) differentiates the two morphemes "look" and "book." By changing the final phoneme from /t/ to /b/ the morpheme "cat" is distinguished from the morpheme "cab." In these two examples, a change of only one phoneme results in the creation of a completely different morpheme (or word, in these examples). Words that vary by only one phoneme are called **minimal pairs** or **minimal contrasts**. "Look"/"book" and "cat"/"cab" are examples of minimal pairs because they vary by only one phoneme. Other examples of minimal pairs include "hear"/"beer," "through"/"brew," "clip"/"click," and "brine"/bright." Notice that these words differ by only *one speech sound* even though spelling shows more than one letter change.

EXERCISE 2.7

For each word below, create a minimal pair by writing a word in the blank. The first five minimal pairs should reflect a change in the initial phoneme; the second five should involve a change in the final phoneme.

Examples: initial phoneme change   seal   <u>meal</u>

                 final phoneme change   card   <s>cart</s>

initial phoneme change		*final phoneme change*	
1. tame	_____	6. heart	_____
2. late	_____	7. tone	_____
3. call	_____	8. web	_____
4. could	_____	9. cheap	_____
5. boil	_____	10. rub	_____

Complete Assignment 2-1.

Distinctive Features

Although phonemes are minimal sound units that are capable of distinguishing morphemes, phonemes can be segmented into even smaller units. Phonemes are actually comprised of small parcels of information that characterize each phoneme in a language. These parcels of information, **distinctive features**, help in distinguishing one phoneme from another. Jakobson, Fant, and Halle (1952) first introduced the idea of a distinctive feature system to distinguish phonemes of all languages. This system often has been criticized by individuals interested in the *production of speech*, since the Jakobson, Fant, and Halle system did not attempt to address spoken language, per se. They were more interested in creating a system of features capable of categorizing uniquely all phonemes of any language (whether spoken or not). In addition, their classification system relied upon acoustic (auditory) features of phonemes that do not relate to how speech sounds are produced by the speech organs.

    In an attempt to improve upon this distinctive feature system, Chomsky and Halle (1968), in their now classic *The Sound Pattern of English*, described a distinctive feature system that relied more upon the articulatory characteristics of speech sounds (i.e., how they are spoken). This system was another attempt at categorizing and distinguishing phonemes in all languages, not just English. For this reason, it is somewhat burdensome to adopt this system when classifying the approximately 42 English phonemes.

    Both the Jakobson, Fant, and Halle and the Chomsky and Halle classification systems are binary, or two-dimensional. That is, there are two possible values for any one distinctive feature. If a phoneme possesses a particular feature, it is given a "+" value. If the phoneme does not contain that feature, it is given a "−" value. The Chomsky and Halle distinctive feature system for selected English consonants is given in Table 2.2, along with definitions of several of the features.

    Examine the features for the phonemes /p/ and /b/ in the first two columns of Table 2.2. A comparison of these phonemes indicates that the only feature that distinguishes them is "voice." Note that /p/ is classified as [−voice] and /b/ is classified as [+ voice].

TABLE 2.2   Distinctive Features for Selected English Phonemes

	p	b	t	d	k	g	f	v	s	z	θ	ð	ʃ	ʒ	m	n	ŋ	r	l
vocalic	−	−	−	−	−	−	−	−	−	−	−	−	−	−	−	−	−	+	+
consonantal	+	+	+	+	+	+	+	+	+	+	+	+	+	+	+	+	+	+	+
high	−	−	−	−	+	+	−	−	−	−	−	−	+	+	−	−	+	−	−
back	−	−	−	−	+	+	−	−	−	−	−	−	−	−	−	−	+	−	−
anterior	+	+	+	+	−	−	+	+	+	+	+	+	−	−	+	+	−	−	+
coronal	−	−	+	+	−	−	−	−	+	+	+	+	+	+	−	+	−	+	+
voice	−	+	−	+	−	+	−	+	−	+	−	+	−	+	+	+	+	+	+
continuant	−	−	−	−	−	−	+	+	+	+	+	+	+	+	−	−	−	+	+
nasal	−	−	−	−	−	−	−	−	−	−	−	−	−	−	+	+	+	−	−
strident	−	−	−	−	−	−	+	+	+	+	−	−	+	+	−	−	−	−	−

Vocalic	Phonemes that are produced with a vocal tract constriction no greater than that associated with the vowels /i/ and /u/, as in the words "beet" and "boot," respectively. In addition, the vocal cords are close enough to allow for spontaneous voicing.
Consonantal	Phonemes produced with a marked constriction along the midline of the vocal tract.
High	Phonemes produced with the tongue raised from its neutral position.
Back	Phonemes produced with the tongue retracted from the neutral position.
Anterior	Phonemes produced with a constriction in front of the palatoalveolar region.
Coronal	Phonemes produced with the blade of the tongue raised from the neutral position.
Voice	Phonemes produced with the vocal folds vibrating.
Continuant	Phonemes produced that do not result in a complete blockage of airflow through the constriction in the vocal tract.
Nasal	Phonemes produced with airflow through the nasal cavity (with a lowered velum).
Strident	Phonemes produced with a great amount of noise.

Note: After Chomsky & Halle, 1968.

Now examine the abbreviated distinctive feature classification scheme for the English liquid phonemes /r/ and /l/ (given below). /r/ and /l/ are the only English phonemes belonging to this classification.

	/r/	/l/
vocalic	+	+
consonantal	+	+
anterior	−	+
coronal	+	+
voice	+	+
continuant	+	+

After examining the classification for these two consonants, it is clear that they each have a *distinct classification* scheme, even though most features are shared. The more features any two phonemes share, the more alike they are in terms of speech production. In the case of the liquid consonants, the shared features include the following:

[+ vocalic]	The constriction in the vocal tract is not greater than that for the English vowels /i/ and /u/ as in the words "heat" and "hoot," respectively.
[+ consonantal]	/r/ and /l/ are produced with a constriction in the midline of the vocal tract (vowels are produced with virtually no constriction).
[+ coronal]	The blade of the tongue (the portion just behind the tip) is used in production of these phonemes.
[+ voice]	The vocal cords vibrate during production of both consonants.
[+ continuant]	/r/ and /l/ are produced without a complete blockage of airflow through the vocal tract constriction.

Notice that the only way in which these two consonants vary is in terms of **place of articulation**, that is, *where* the sound is produced in the mouth. The anterior feature is the only one that distinguishes these two phonemes:

	/r/	/l/
anterior	–	+

The consonant /l/ is [+ anterior], which means that it is produced by elevating the tongue in front of the hard palate in the mouth cavity. /r/ is [– anterior] because it is produced by raising the tongue close to the hard palate.

/r/ and /l/ are the only consonants in English that have both [+ consonantal] and [+ vocalic] features. (All other English consonants are [–vocalic].) Therefore, only two features, consonantal and vocalic, are necessary to identify the liquids as a group, and only one feature, anterior, is necessary to differentiate between them.

A group of phonemes (such as the liquids) that can be identified by fewer features than necessary to identify its constituent members is called a *natural class* (Ingram, 1976). In this case, the two features, [+ consonantal] and [+ vocalic], identify the liquids as a class. However, it takes a third feature, anterior, to be able to distinguish /r/ from /l/. One other example of a natural class of sounds is the English nasal consonants.

The notion of a natural class of phonemes is important to the assessment and treatment of individuals with phonological disorders. When describing the speech errors a client exhibits, distinctive feature analysis may reveal problems not only with individual phonemes, but also with the class of sounds to which they belong. This may provide useful information to the clinician when planning treatment.

EXERCISE 2.8

Using Table 2.2, respond to the following.

1. List the three English nasal consonants.
2. Which three phonemes are considered both [+ high and + back]?
3. Which phoneme is [+ strident, + voice, and – coronal]?
4. On which feature do the phonemes /t/ and /d/ differ?
5. Are there more voiced or voiceless phonemes in English?

Allophones: Members of a Phoneme Family

Up to this point, the term *phoneme* has been discussed as a speech sound that can distinguish one morpheme from another. However, there is another way to define *phoneme*. We could also say that a phoneme is a family of sounds. Speech sounds are not always produced the same way in every word. For example the /l/ in the word "lip" is different from the /l/ in the word "ball." You might say to yourself: "How are they different? They are both /l/s." You need to consider how these /l/ sounds are produced in the mouth when saying these two words. In "lip," the /l/ sound is produced with the tongue toward the front of the mouth, and in the word "ball" the tongue is retracted, causing the sound to be produced in the back of the mouth. Say them to yourself and you will discover that this is indeed true. These are but two examples of the /l/-family of sounds.

Members of a phoneme family are actually variant pronunciations of a particular phoneme. These variant pronunciations are called **allophones**. The front (or light)/l/ and the back (or dark)/l/ are allophones or variant productions of the phoneme /l/. These two variants both can be found in the word "little" (the first /l/ is light, the second is dark). Try saying "little" by using the dark /l/ at the beginning of the word. Although the word may sound funny to you, it is still recognizable as the word "little." For this reason, the variants of /l/ are not individual phonemes. Saying the word "little" with either the front or back /l/ at the beginning of the word *does not change the identity or meaning of the original word*. That is, it does not result in the creation of a minimal pair.

EXERCISE 2.9

Try saying the /p/ sound in the word "keep" two different ways:

1. exploding (or releasing) the /p/
2. not exploding the /p/

(These are two allophones of the /p/ phoneme.)

Certain allophones must be produced a particular way due to the constraints of the other sounds in a word. For instance, the dark /l/ in the word "ball" is usually produced in the back of the mouth because it is preceded by a back vowel (a vowel produced in the back of the mouth). Say the word out loud and you will see that this is true. Now try saying "ball" with the /l/ in the front of the mouth—it is hard, if not impossible. Now think about the light /l/ in the word "lip." This /l/ is produced in the front of the mouth due to the fact that the vowel in "lip" is a front vowel. These two allophones of /l/ are not interchangeable due to the phonetic constraints of their respective words. These allophones are said to be in **complementary distribution**.

Another example of complementary distribution involves the allophones of the phoneme /g/ in the words "get" and "got." The /g/ sound in "get" is produced closer to the front of the mouth and the /g/ in "got" is produced further back, again due to the vowel environment. These allophones are not free to vary in terms of where in the mouth the sounds are produced.

In English, when /p/ is produced at the beginning of a word, a small puff of air occurs after its release. The puff of air is called *aspiration*. Say the word "pit," holding your hand in front of your mouth. You should be able to feel the puff of air escaping from your lips following the production of /p/. Whenever the phoneme /p/ follows the phoneme /s/, as in the word "spit," it will always be *unaspirated*. Say the word "spit," holding your hand in front of your mouth. You should feel less air than when you said the word "pit." Hold your hand in front of your mouth, alternating the productions of these two words. You should be able to feel the variance in the airstream on your hand. These two allophones of /p/, aspirated and unaspirated, are in complementary distribution. Although in English the unaspirated allophone of /p/ never occurs at the beginning of a word, it is found to occur at the beginning of words in many other languages including Spanish, Mandarin Chinese, and Pilipino (the official language of the Philippines).

In contrast to the examples just given, some allophones are not linked to phonetic context and therefore can be exchanged for one another; they are free to vary. In Exercise 2.9 you were asked to say the word "keep" two different ways, either releasing the /p/ or not. In this case, it is up to the speaker to decide. The phonetic environment has no bearing on whether the /p/ will be exploded or not. In this case, the allophones of /p/ are said to be in **free variation**. Likewise, the final /t/ in the word "hit" may be released or unreleased, depending on the speaker's individual production of the word. These two variant productions (released or unreleased) are allophones of /t/ that are in free variation.

Systematic versus Impressionistic Transcription

Suppose a child has a speech disorder resulting in the production of all /l/ phonemes in the back of his mouth. Transcription of the word "slip" would yield the following: /slɪp/. This style of transcription is termed **systematic phonemic transcription**. Systematic phonemic transcription also is referred to as *broad transcription*, or simply *phonemic transcription*. Phonemic transcription makes no attempt at transcribing allophonic variation. Virgules (or slash marks) always are used with phonemic transcription. When using phonemic transcription, there would be no way to indicate whether the phoneme /l/ was produced in the front or the back of the mouth.

Specialized symbols, called **diacritics**, are used to indicate allophonic variation, such as the dark /l/ or unreleased /p/, when transcribing speech. Knowledge of the allophones associated with variations in speech production is necessary for what is called **systematic narrow transcription** or *allophonic transcription*. Allophonic transcription of the word "fall" with a dark /l/ would be [fɑɫ]. The curved line, or *tilde*, over the middle of the [ɫ] indicates production of the dark /l/. Notice that brackets, not virgules, are used with this style of transcription. By using allophonic transcription, we also can differentiate between the released (exploded) /p/ and the unreleased /p/ in production of the word "keep" ([kip] and [kip⁻], respectively).

Both systematic phonemic and systematic narrow (allophonic) transcription require knowledge of the sound system of a language prior to analysis of a speech sample. There are times, however, when transcription of an unknown sound system may be necessary. Suppose for a moment that you are a famous phonetician and that you are familiar with all of the symbols of the IPA (including the symbols not common to English). You have been recruited to transcribe speech samples taken from aliens who just landed on U.S. soil. Because you know nothing about the alien's speech or language patterns, you would need to listen very carefully and would need to put down on paper every phonemic and allophonic detail associated with their speech. Every detail would be important, because you would be interested in trying to understand the rules that explain how the speech sound system is structured. This type of transcription, where nothing is known about a particular speech sound system prior to analysis, is termed an **impressionistic transcription** (another form of narrow transcription). Impressionistic transcription also might be used when analyzing a speaker of a language with which you are not familiar. This form of transcription may be employed when working with a child who has severe speech deficits affecting the rules associated with typical speech development. Brackets are used when performing an impressionistic transcription.

EXERCISE 2.10

Match the terms that can be associated with phonemic, allophonic, or impressionistic transcription. There will be more than one correct answer for each term.

____ phonemic
____ allophonic
____ impressionistic

1. broad transcription
2. narrow transcription
3. use of virgules

4. use of brackets
5. systematic transcription

Syllables

In conversational speech, it is often difficult to determine where one phoneme ends and the next one begins. This is due to the fact that in connected speech, phonemes are not produced in a serial order, one after the other. Instead, phonemes are produced in an overlaid fashion due to overlapping movements of the articulators (speech organs) during speech production. Because there is considerable overlap in phonemes during the production of speech, many phoneticians suggest that the smallest unit of speech production is not the allophone or phoneme, but the **syllable**.

As you know, words are composed of one or more syllables. We all have a general idea of what a syllable is. If you were asked how many syllables were in the word "meatball," you would have little difficulty determining the correct answer—two. Even though you have a general idea of what a syllable is, in actuality it is quite difficult to answer the seemingly simple question, *What is a syllable?* The reason for this difficulty is that a syllable may be defined in more than one way. Also, phoneticians often do not agree on the actual definition of a syllable.

We will begin our definition by stating that a syllable is a basic building block of language that may be composed of either one or more vowels alone or a vowel in combination with one or more consonants. This is the definition typically found in a dictionary or in a junior high school language arts textbook. However, for our purposes, this definition is not adequate. This definition is based on vowel and consonant letters, not vowel and consonant phonemes.

In most cases, it is easy to identify the number of syllables in a word. For instance, we would agree that the words "control," "intend," and "downtown" all have two syllables. Likewise, it is easy to determine that the words "contagious," "alphabet," and "tremendous" each have three syllables. However, it is not always so easy to determine the number of syllables in a word. Using our simple dictionary definition, the words "feel" and "pool" would be one-syllable words. That is, they each contain a vowel in combination with one or more consonant letters. Many individuals, however, pronounce these words as two syllables. On the other hand, some people pronounce these words as one syllable depending on their individual speaking style and dialect. The word "pool" is pronounced by many as "pull," as in "swimming pull." Likewise, some southern speakers pronounce the word "feel" as "fill," as in "I fill fine."

Another example involves the words "prism" and "chasm." According to the basic definition, these words would be considered one syllable, because they contain only one vowel. However, most speakers would probably consider these words to consist of two syllables. One last example involves the pronunciation of words like "camera" or "chocolate." These words have three vowels, but can be pronounced as either two or three syllables, depending on whether the speaker pronounces the middle vowel or not (i.e., "camra" or "choclate"). Both pronunciations would be considered to be appropriate for either word.

Obviously, a better definition of "syllable" is necessary to help overcome these difficulties. One way to attempt to redefine the syllable might be to more fully describe its internal structure, using terms other than consonant and vowel. It is possible to divide syllables in English into two components: **onset** and **rhyme**. The onset of a syllable consists of all the consonants that precede a vowel, as in the words "**spl**it," "**tr**ied," and "**f**ast" (onset in bold letters). Note that the onset may consist of either a single consonant or a **consonant cluster** (two or three contiguous consonants in the same syllable).

In syllables with no initial consonant, there would be no onset. Examples of words with no onset would be "eat," "I," and the first syllable in the word "afraid." Note that the second syllable of "afraid" has an onset consisting of the consonants /f/ and /r/.

EXERCISE 2.11

Circle the syllables in the following one-syllable and two-syllable words containing an onset. (For the two-syllable words, circle *any* syllable with an onset.)

ouch	crab	hoe	oats	elm	your
react	cargo	beware	atone	courage	eating

The rhyme of a syllable is divided into two components, the **nucleus** and the **coda**. The nucleus is typically a vowel. The nuclei of the words "split," "tri**ed**," and "fa**st**" are indicated in bold letters. However, several consonants in English may be considered to be the nucleus of a syllable in certain instances. In the words "chasm" and "feel," the /m/ and /l/ phonemes would be considered to be the nucleus of the second syllable of each word (if "feel" is pronounced as a two-syllable word). In these words, the consonants /m/ and /l/ assume the role of the vowel in the second syllable. When consonants take on the role of vowels, they are called **syllabic consonants**.

The coda includes either single consonants or consonant clusters that follow the nucleus of a syllable, as in the words "spl**it**," "tri**ed**," and "fa**st**." In some instances, the coda may in fact have no elements at all, as in the words "me," "shoe," "oh," and "pry."

EXERCISE 2.12

Circle the letters that make up the nucleus in the following words. Some of the words have more than one nucleus.

shrine	scold	plea	produce	schism	away
elope	selfish	auto	biceps	flight	truce

EXERCISE 2.13

Circle the word(s) (or syllables) that have a coda.

through	spa	rough	bough	row	spray
lawful	funny	create	inverse	candy	reply

To further illustrate the nomenclature associated with syllables, the structure of the one-syllable words "scrub," "each," and "three" are detailed in "tree diagrams" (Figure 2.2). The onset, rhyme, nucleus, and coda of each word is labeled appropriately. The Greek letter sigma (σ) is used to indicate a syllable division. Note the null symbol (ϕ), which indicates the absence of the onset and coda in two of the examples. Diagrams of the two-syllable words "behave" and "prism" follow the diagrams of the one-syllable words (see Figure 2.3). Notice in Figure 2.3 that the consonant /m/ in "prism" forms the nucleus of the second syllable.

Syllables that end with a vowel phoneme (no coda) are called **open syllables**. Examples include "the" and both syllables of the word "maybe." Words that consist solely of a vowel nucleus, as in the words "I," "oh," and "a," also are considered to be open syllables. Syllables with a coda—that is, those that end with a consonant phoneme—are called **closed syllables**. Examples of closed syllables are "had," "keg," and both syllables in the word "contain." When determining whether a syllable is open or closed, you need to pay attention to the phonemic specification of the syllable, not its spelling. More examples of open and closed syllables are given below.

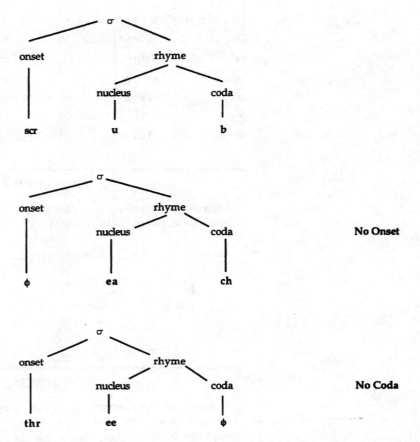

FIGURE 2.2   Syllable structure of the one-syllable words "scrub," "each," and "three."

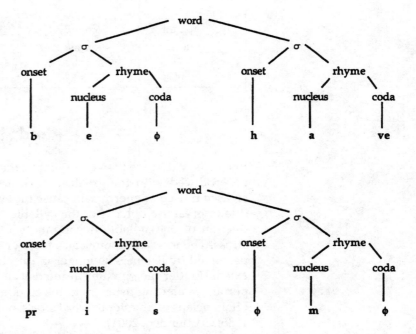

FIGURE 2.3   Syllable structure of the two-syllable words "behave" and "prism."

Words with Open Syllables		*Words with Closed Syllables*	
One-Syllable	*Two-Syllable*	*One-Syllable*	*Two-Syllable*
he	allow	corn	captive
bow	daily	suave	chalice
may	belie	wish	dentist
rye	zebra	charge	English
through	hobo	slammed	invest

EXERCISE 2.14

Examine the following two-syllable words. Indicate whether the *first* syllable is open (O) or closed (C) by filling in the blank with the appropriate letter.

Example: __O__ around   __C__ blistered

____ pliant   ____ comply   ____ coerced   ____ minutes
____ decree   ____ encase   ____ flatly   ____ preface

EXERCISE 2.15

Examine the same two-syllable words as those in the previous exercise. Indicate whether the *second* syllable is open (O) or closed (C) by filling in the blank with the appropriate letter.

Example: __C__ around   __C__ blistered

____ pliant   ____ comply   ____ coerced   ____ minutes
____ decree   ____ encase   ____ flatly   ____ preface

Word Stress

In words with more than one syllable, there will often be one syllable that will be produced with the greatest force or greatest muscular energy. The increased muscular energy will cause the syllable to stand apart from the others due to greater emphasis of the syllable. This increased emphasis in the production of one syllable is commonly referred to as **word stress** or **lexical stress**. The increase in muscular force or emphasis results in a syllable that is perceived by listeners as longer in duration, higher in pitch, and, to a lesser extent, louder (i.e., greater in intensity). The rise in pitch is particularly important in alerting listeners to the stressed syllable in a word (Lehiste, 1970). Phoneticians often refer to word stress, or lexical stress, as *word accent* (Calvert, 1986; Cruttenden, 2001).

Stress is not a trivial matter in learning and understanding spoken language. When we hear a word such as "confuse," we recognize it not only because of the particular phonemes that comprise it, but also because of the inherent stress pattern of the word. Try saying this word by changing the stress to the first syllable, that is, CONfuse. The word now sounds somewhat odd to you because the string of phonemes does not coincide with the new stress pattern. The unique combination of these individual phonemes and this particular stress pattern does not match any item stored in your mental dictionary. As language is developed, children (not just those learning English) must master not only the phonemes that make up individual words, but also their associated stress patterns. However, the stress patterns of different languages vary remarkably. One major reason why foreign speakers of English (or any second language) have difficulty with pronunciation is due to lack of knowledge of the stress patterns of the new language being learned. Second-language learners will often sound "foreign" when using their native language's stress patterns while speaking the new language.

In English, words that have more than one syllable will always have one particular syllable that will receive *primary stress* (i.e., the greatest emphasis). For example, the bisyllabic (two-syllable) word "SISter" has primary stress on the first syllable. The multisyllabic (more than two-syllable) word "courAgeous" has primary stress on the second syllable. Syllables in bisyllabic and multisyllabic words that do not receive primary stress may receive *secondary stress* or no stress, depending on the level of emphasis given to the individual syllable.

Word (lexical) stress is extremely important in learning the phonetic transcription of English because some of the IPA symbols indicate which syllable in a word receives primary stress. Although it is possible to learn how to mark levels of stress in multisyllabic words (i.e., primary vs. secondary stress), for now, we will focus primarily on indicating whether a syllable receives primary stress.

Some students will experience little difficulty in identifying the syllable with primary stress in bisyllabic and multisyllabic words. Unfortunately, for many this ability is extremely trying. Part of the reason for this difficulty is that although we know how to use stress correctly in *production of speech*, we are not accustomed to thinking about stress patterns in the *perception of speech*. As communicators, we simply are not used to listening to speech and identifying stressed syllables in words. Researchers have been successful in enumerating the rules that govern the location of primary stress in words (Chomsky & Halle, 1968; Cruttenden, 2001; Jones, 1967). However, the rules do have exceptions, and they are also difficult to remember. During transcription of speech, there is simply not enough time to think about the rules governing stress in words. For purposes of phonetic transcription, what is important is the ability to hear the location of primary stress in words, not the rules that govern how stress is assigned to syllables. Fortunately, the ability to identify (hear) the location of primary stress in words can be developed in time with much listening practice.

Examine the following bisyllabic words. Say them aloud. What do you notice about the stress patterns of these words? (**Hint**: They all have the *same* stress pattern.)

contain	aware	berserk	charade
inspect	reveal	suppose	detain

Hopefully, you have determined that the *second* syllable of each of these words receives primary stress. Say the words again, paying careful attention to the increased pitch and effort associated with the second syllable:

conTAIN	aWARE	berSERK	chaRADE
inSPECT	reVEAL	supPOSE	deTAIN

The IPA symbol used for indicating the primary stress of a word is a raised mark (ˈ) placed at the initiation of the stressed syllable. The words above would be marked in the following manner to indicate second-syllable stress:

conˈtain	aˈware	berˈserk	chaˈrade
inˈspect	reˈveal	supˈpose	deˈtain

Now, examine the following bisyllabic words. Each of these words contain *first* syllable primary stress:

ˈteacher	ˈcertain	ˈcareful	ˈpractice
ˈplural	ˈlarynx	ˈprimate	ˈcontact

Stress, in addition to its role in the proper pronunciation of words, plays a phonemic role in English as well. Word stress is capable of distinguishing between words that are spelled the same but vary in part of speech, or **word class** (i.e., whether a word is a noun, verb, adjective, adverb, etc.). For instance, the words "ˈcontract" (noun) and "conˈtract" (verb), although spelled the same, have different stress patterns. The noun form ˈ*contract* has stress placed on the first syllable, whereas the verb form *con*ˈ*tract* has word stress on the second syllable. Note that the change in the stress pattern not only changes the meaning of the word, but also changes the pronunciation of the word. Say these two words aloud. How do the two words differ in pronunciation? You probably noted that as stress changes, so does the pronunciation of the vowel in the first syllable. Other examples of two-syllable noun/verb pairs, differing in word stress, include:

Noun	*Verb*	*Noun*	*Verb*
ˈconflict	conˈflict	ˈpermit	perˈmit
ˈrecord	reˈcord	ˈsubject	subˈject
ˈdigest	diˈgest	ˈrebel	reˈbel
ˈconvert	conˈvert	ˈconduct	conˈduct

Note that in these word pairs, the noun form always receives first-syllable stress, and the verb form always receives second-syllable stress.

EXERCISE 2.16

Circle the words that can be spoken as both a *noun and a verb* by shifting the stress pattern between the first and second syllables.

propose	contest	protest	congress	research
project	consume	compress	reasoned	confines

Because identifying the primary stress in bisyllabic and multisyllabic words is a difficult chore, the following twelve word lists will provide you with some practice in listening for primary stress in words. These word lists (and accompanying exercises) are designed to make you focus on one particular stress pattern at a time. The lists begin with bisyllabic words and progress to multisyllabic words. As you examine each list, say the words aloud, focusing on the particular stress pattern being demonstrated. Listen to each list several times until you are comfortable with the stress pattern being demonstrated. If you experience any difficulty with Exercises 2.17, 2.18, and 2.19, review the word lists until you understand your errors.

List 1 - Bisyllabic words; first-syllable stress (words beginning with "e")

edict	easy	eager	Easter
Egypt	ether	either	even
Ethan	eagle	eater	ego

Note: Keep in mind that words beginning with the letter "e" do not always have first-syllable stress. Examine the words in List 2:

List 2 - Bisyllabic words; second-syllable stress (words beginning with "e")

eclipse	elapse	efface	effect
elate	elect	ellipse	elude
Elaine	emote	enough	erupt

List 3 - Bisyllabic words; first-syllable stress (words beginning with "o")

over	ocean	omen	owner
Oprah	onus	oboe	ogre
okra	open	ozone	odor

Note: Keep in mind that words beginning with the letter "o" do not always have first-syllable stress. Examine the words in List 4:

List 4 - Bisyllabic words; second-syllable stress (words beginning with "o")

overt	obey	oppress	olé
okay	oblique	obese	oblige

List 5 - Bisyllabic words; first-syllable stress (words beginning with "in")

invoice	instant	inbred	insect
inner	inches	ingrate	infant
income	index	infield	inlay

Note: Keep in mind that words beginning with the letters "in" do not always have first-syllable stress. Examine the words in List 6:

List 6 - Bisyllabic words; second-syllable stress (words beginning with "in")

inspire	instead	induce	inject
infect	inflict	indeed	inept
infer	inscribe	intrude	involve

List 7 - Bisyllabic words; second-syllable stress (words beginning with "a")

around	abuse	abort	amass	avoid	abode
away	aware	arise	alike	afloat	avenge
abrupt	adorn	accost	atone	aloof	aghast
alas	akin	avow	adapt	afraid	anoint

Note: There are many words in English (such as those in List 7) that begin with the letter "a." The vowel associated with the sound at the beginning of these words is called schwa—/ə/. This unstressed vowel constitutes its own syllable in all of the words in List 7.

List 8 - Bisyllabic words; first-syllable stress

engine	master	caring	lucky	staples	Harold
plastic	rowing	neither	happen	Dayton	careful
forest	whisper	quandary	listless	tantrum	nacho
siphon	solo	hidden	trophy	panda	Pittsburgh

Note: Most, but not all, two-syllable words in English have first-syllable primary stress. Examine List 9 for two-syllable words with second-syllable primary stress.

List 9 - Bisyllabic words; second-syllable stress

remove	control	serene	carafe	pertain	repulse
arranged	remain	caffeine	repute	suppose	untrue
perspire	beside	react	Brazil	invoke	humane
manure	discrete	compress	admire	assist	beguile

Note: The first syllable of many bisyllabic words with second-syllable stress (as those in List 9) are often bound morphemes (prefixes) such as re-, a-, pre-, in-, and dis-.

List 10 - Three-syllable words; first-syllable stress

realize	horrible	circulate	fidgety	element	hypnotize
hydrogen	insulin	character	mediate	critical	Michigan
premium	rivalry	sacrifice	tolerant	verbalize	readable
yesterday	xylophone	mystify	glorious	caraway	terrible

List 11 - Three-syllable words; second-syllable stress

Missouri	insipid	metallic	Ohio	betrayal	inscription
confusion	diploma	abortion	courageous	erosion	contagious
awareness	preparing	computer	neurotic	palatial	morphemic
repulsive	reminded	semantics	charisma	aroma	transistor

List 12 - Three-syllable words; third-syllable stress

interrupt	indiscreet	Illinois	prearrange	disrespect	contradict
minuet	intervene	buccaneer	decompose	interfere	masquerade
reprehend	obsolete	readjust	disinfect	reapply	connoisseur
reimburse	introduce	predispose	disenchant	represent	nondescript

Note: It is possible to pronounce some of words in List 12 with stress on the *first* syllable, depending on your own speaking habit and dialect. In addition, the location of stress in a multisyllabic word may change, depending on the message the speaker wishes to convey.

EXERCISE 2.17

Circle the words that have *second*-syllable stress.

decoy	mirage	pastel	puzzle	regret	platoon
stipend	thesis	undo	reason	falter	Maureen
timid	planted	derail	virtue	restricts	peon
transcend	parade	circus	suspend	movie	shoulder
lucid	cajole	devoid	cassette	provide	merchant

EXERCISE 2.18

Circle the three-syllable words that have *first*-syllable stress.

pondering	edited	consequent	misery	calendar	ebony
plentiful	asterisk	pharyngeal	persona	distinctive	example
surrounded	December	caribou	underling	Barbados	lasagna
terrified	hydrangea	telephoned	contended	perfected	India
musical	skeletal	courageous	umbrella	Philistine	perusal

EXERCISE 2.19

Circle the three-syllable words that have *second*-syllable stress.

stupendous	pliable	creative	carefully	elevate	magical
corporal	answering	spectacle	presumption	placenta	bananas
plantation	clarinet	murderer	predisposed	decorum	horribly
heroic	violin	integer	discover	clavicle	majestic
daffodil	subscription	expertise	immoral	muscular	Hawaii

Complete Assignment 2-2.

Review Exercises

A. How many phonemes are there in each of the following words? Circle the words that have the same number of phonemes as letters.

1. bread _____   5. plot _____   9. fat _____
2. coughs _____   6. stroke _____   10. tomb _____
3. throw _____   7. fluid _____   11. walked _____
4. news _____   8. spew _____   12. last _____

B. How many morphemes are there in the following words?

1. clueless _____   6. rewrite _____
2. tomato _____   7. winterized _____
3. pumpkin _____   8. edits _____
4. likable _____   9. thoughtlessness _____
5. cheddar _____   10. coexisting _____

C. Listed below are three columns of words. Decide if the words in columns 2 or 3 <u>end</u> in the same phoneme as the words in the first column. *Circle* the correct matches.

1. box   flack   puss
2. buzz   dogs   fits
3. flag   lounge   league
4. cooked   pant   nagged
5. throw   cow   beau
6. through   chow   flew
7. tomb   limb   bob
8. fleas   wheeze   mice
9. laugh   giraffe   bough
10. path   bathe   cloth

D. When the sounds in the words below are reversed, they make another word. What is the new word in each case, after reversing the sounds?

1. net _____   6. main _____
2. sell _____   7. pin _____
3. pots _____   8. ban _____
4. gnat _____   9. tack _____
5. need _____   10. tune _____

E. For the following set of items, circle the one that *begins* with a sound *different* from the other two.

1. church   chef   chop
2. see   cent   cut
3. think   this   these
4. knee   came   nut
5. phone   please   frost
6. song   sure   sheep
7. gnat   grim   groan

er4er444

8. cup   choir   chore
9. gerbil   goat   George
10. their   thanks   thing

F. Give a minimal pair for each of the following words by changing the underlined phoneme.

1. s<u>p</u>it _____   6. f<u>a</u>n _____
2. <u>h</u>and _____   7. <u>th</u>ink _____
3. <u>p</u>ink _____   8. h<u>a</u>d _____
4. <u>s</u>in _____   9. <u>t</u>ook _____
5. pai<u>l</u> _____   10. r<u>o</u>b _____

G. Circle the following pairs of words that are *minimal pairs*.

1. maybe, baby   6. bribe, tribe
2. plaid, prod   7. smart, dart
3. looks, lacks   8. dinner, runner
4. mail, snail   9. window, minnow
5. prance, prince   10. lumpy, bumpy

H. Indicate, for the underlined syllables, whether they are open (O) or closed (C).

1. mar<u>ble</u> _____   6. <u>awe</u>some _____
2. <u>pre</u>vious _____ 7. mis<u>take</u> _____
3. pa<u>tron</u> _____   8. luc<u>ky</u> _____
4. <u>tri</u>fle _____   9. pro<u>fit</u> _____
5. s<u>o</u>dium _____   10. <u>sys</u>tem _____

I. Examine the following words. Indicate whether the *first* syllable has an *onset* and/or a *coda* by placing an "X" in the appropriate column.

Examples:	Onset		Coda	
	Yes	No	Yes	No
social	X	___	___	X
picture	X	___	X	___
1. mentions	___	___	___	___
2. icon	___	___	___	___
3. camper	___	___	___	___
4. instinct	___	___	___	___
5. able	___	___	___	___
6. lotion	___	___	___	___
7. charming	___	___	___	___
8. asterisk	___	___	___	___
9. Japan	___	___	___	___
10. aloof	___	___	___	___

J. Indicate the primary stress for each of the following two-syllable words. Write "1" if the first syllable has primary stress or "2" if the second syllable has primary stress.

____ 1. loser	____ 6. provoke	____ 11. plastic
____ 2. unsure	____ 7. stagnant	____ 12. divorce
____ 3. anxious	____ 8. beside	____ 13. western
____ 4. disturb	____ 9. germane	____ 14. language
____ 5. Grecian	____ 10. gourmet	____ 15. defer

K. Indicate the primary stress for each of the following three-syllable items. Write "1", "2," or "3" to indicate the syllable with primary stress.

____ 1. provincial	____ 6. hypocrite	____ 11. picturesque
____ 2. sorceress	____ 7. indisposed	____ 12. relegate
____ 3. indigent	____ 8. uncertain	____ 13. foundation
____ 4. commander	____ 9. magenta	____ 14. contagious
____ 5. arabesque	____ 10. platypus	____ 15. constable

L. Indicate the primary stress for each of the following four-syllable words. Write "1," "2," "3," or "4" to indicate the syllable with primary stress.

____ 1. problematic	____ 6. correlation	____ 11. protozoan
____ 2. mercenary	____ 7. catamaran	____ 12. contradiction
____ 3. statistical	____ 8. continuant	____ 13. protoplasm
____ 4. ecosystem	____ 9. allegory	____ 14. Argentina
____ 5. gregarious	____ 10. carnivorous	____ 15. obstructionist

Study Questions

1. What is a phonetic alphabet?

2. What is the difference between a *digraph* and an *allograph?*

3. Discuss three ways in which English spelling principles deviate markedly from the ways words are pronounced.

4. Define the following terms:

    a. morpheme

    b. phoneme

    c. grapheme

5. Why are *allophones* not considered to be *phonemes?*

6. Contrast the terms *complementary distribution* and *free variation.*

7. What is the difference between *phonemic, allophonic,* and *impressionistic* transcription?

8. What is the purpose of the IPA?

9. Why is the term *syllable* difficult to define?

10. Define the following terms: *onset, rhyme, coda, nucleus.*

11. What is the difference between an *open* and a *closed* syllable?

12. What is a *distinctive feature?*

13. Why are the words "spread" and "bread" not *minimal pairs?*

Assignment 2-1   Name _____

1. Indicate the number of phonemes in the following words.

   a. ____ queen
   b. ____ Christine
   c. ____ thought
   d. ____ ripped

   e. ____ treats
   f. ____ rough
   g. ____ diskette
   h. ____ extra

   i. ____ window
   j. ____ Toledo
   k. ____ received
   l. ____ sprints

2. Indicate the number of morphemes in the following words.

   a. ____ lasting
   b. ____ wonders
   c. ____ ideas
   d. ____ misplaced

   e. ____ paper
   f. ____ speedy
   g. ____ monkeys
   h. ____ devalue

   i. ____ currently
   j. ____ unchanging
   k. ____ cantaloupe
   l. ____ reapplied

3. For the following set of items, circle the words that *begin* with a sound different from the other two.

   a. train   think   Thomas
   b. Janet   genie   gaunt
   c. them   Theo   that
   d. capture   chaos   chowder
   e. fathom   phone   push
   f. chasm   king   chastity
   g. knot   gnu   guru
   h. genre   judge   gym
   i. chance   chortle   chord
   j. sail   candy   centipede

4. For the following set of items, circle the words that *end* with a sound different from the other two.

   a. wreath   breathe   breath
   b. coop   coup   flew
   c. keys   gnats   wheeze
   d. catch   splash   mesh
   e. blue   flow   chew
   f. rapt   rad   caulked
   g. was   floss   causes
   h. tract   trapped   trailed
   i. wax   laws   wicks
   j. below   brow   crow

Assignment 2-2   Name _____

1. Give a minimal pair for each of the following words by changing the underlined phonemes.

   a. b<u>i</u>nd _____   f. w<u>i</u>n _____

   b. lea<u>n</u> _____   g. pa<u>th</u> _____

   c. r<u>e</u>d _____   h. job _____

   d. wi<u>sh</u> _____   i. <u>t</u>rash _____

   e. l<u>oo</u>k _____   j. f<u>oa</u>m _____

2. Circle the following pairs of words that are *not* minimal pairs.

   a. one, sun   f. respire, perspire

   b. clasp, grasp   g. large, charge

   c. learn, turn   h. feud, rude

   d. slice, nice   i. thrash, crash

   e. spite, spot   j. gerbil, journal

3. Indicate, for the underlined syllables, whether they are open (O) or closed (C).

   a. grue<u>some</u> _____   f. con<u>spire</u> _____

   b. la<u>zy</u> _____   g. set<u>tee</u> _____

   c. <u>pre</u>dict _____   h. <u>sev</u>eral _____

   d. con<u>fuse</u> _____   i. sui<u>ta</u>ble _____

   e. <u>suc</u>cess _____   j. <u>thy</u>roid _____

4. Indicate (with an "X") the words that have an onset in the *second* syllable.

   a. concern _____   f. preempt _____

   b. inaugurate _____   g. request _____

   c. gigantic _____   h. earring _____

   d. bulkhead _____   i. barley _____

   e. cocoa _____   j. coaxial _____

5. Examine the following words. Indicate whether the *first* syllable has an onset and/or a coda by placing an "X" in the appropriate column.

Examples:	Onset		Coda	
	Yes	No	Yes	No
social	X	___	___	X
picture	X	___	X	___
a. sandbag	___	___	___	___
b. deactivate	___	___	___	___
c. auspicious	___	___	___	___
d. enunciate	___	___	___	___
e. sycamore	___	___	___	___
f. toxic	___	___	___	___
g. reflective	___	___	___	___
h. overtly	___	___	___	___
i. encapsule	___	___	___	___
j. fusion	___	___	___	___

Assignment 2-2 (cont.)   Name _____

6. Indicate the primary stress for each of the following four- or five-syllable words. Write "1", "2", "3," or "4" to indicate the syllable with primary stress.

    ____ a. intestinal   ____ f. devaluated   ____ k. unaccompanied
    ____ b. demarcation   ____ g. maniacal   ____ l. orthodontist
    ____ c. statuary   ____ h. sociology   ____ m. trigonometric
    ____ d. monetary   ____ i. coriander   ____ n. confederation
    ____ e. superfluous   ____ j. elasticity   ____ o. begrudgingly

7. For each of the following, indicate whether the underlined letters represent the onset (O), the nucleus (N), or the coda (C). Write O, N, or C in the blank.

    a. overt _____   f. handsome _____
    b. revered _____   g. seance _____
    c. spirits _____   h. grasped _____
    d. why _____   i. confined _____
    e. ledger _____   j. stoic _____

8. On a separate piece of paper, draw tree diagrams of the syllable structure for the following words.

    a. own
    b. crust
    c. lonely
    d. undo

CHAPTER

3

Anatomy and Physiology of the
Speech Mechanism

To fully understand the production of English phonemes, it is essential to have a basic understanding of the role of the speech organs. When you hear the term "speech organs," what comes to mind? Most likely, you think of the tongue, and perhaps the teeth and lips. If you already have taken an introductory course in speech-language pathology and audiology, you also may be familiar with the role of the alveolar ridge and the hard and soft palates. Speech production is, however, quite a complex process involving many other anatomical structures. For instance, the lungs are important in generating the breath stream for speech. The larynx is important for generating voice. The resonating capability of the vocal tract gives a unique sound quality to each of the speech sounds. In this chapter we will explore the function of the various components of the speech mechanism and also discuss their role in respiration, phonation, and articulation. To understand these processes we will explore three major biological systems, namely the *respiratory, laryngeal,* and *supralaryngeal* systems, respectively.

The Respiratory System and Respiration

Generally, when we think of respiration, we think of breathing for vegetative, or for life, purposes. As a matter of fact, that *is* the primary role of the respiratory system. However, respiration is vital in the production of speech, because speech could not occur without a steady supply of air from the lungs. We tend to think primarily of the lungs when we think of respiration. The respiratory system involves not only the lungs, but also the trachea, the rib cage, the thorax, the abdomen, the diaphragm, and other major muscle groups. Examine Figure 3.1, which displays the airway involved in respiration.

The process of speech production begins with the lungs. When a person begins to speak, a preparatory breath is taken (usually unconsciously) in order to have enough air to create an utterance (i.e., a word, phrase, or sentence). This

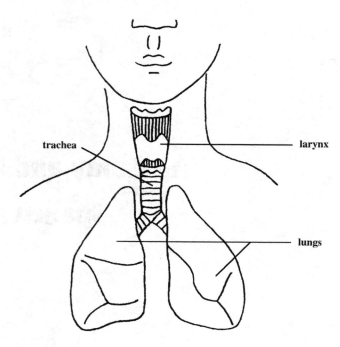

FIGURE 3.1   The anatomical relationship among the human larynx, trachea, and lungs.

preparatory breath uses more air volume than is needed when sleeping, or when sitting quietly reading a book, or watching a DVD. More air volume is necessary in order to speak. Try speaking without taking a preparatory breath—you will run out of air very quickly. You probably have tried to speak when you are "out of breath"—your speech is choppy and characterized by gasps for air. Therefore, good breath support is essential during speech production. Singers also need good breath support to sustain their notes while performing.

When sitting quietly, the period of time devoted to inhalation and exhalation is fairly equal. That is, inhalation and exhalation each comprise about 50 percent of one inhalation/exhalation cycle. When we breathe for speech, this fifty-fifty relationship drastically changes. For speech purposes, inhalation only takes up approximately 10 percent of the inhalation/exhalation cycle. The other 90 percent is devoted to exhalation (Borden, Harris, & Raphael, 1994). This is necessary to have enough breath support to sustain the airstream for speech.

During inhalation, the **thoracic cavity** (chest cavity) must expand in order to make room for the expansion of the lungs. This is accomplished, in part, by lowering the **diaphragm**. The diaphragm is a major muscle that separates the abdominal cavity from the thoracic cavity. The diaphragm contracts, thereby lowering, during inhalation. As the diaphragm lowers, the rib cage expands, enlarging the thoracic cavity and creating extra space for the inflating lungs. These actions are accomplished by several sets of muscles, most notably (but not limited to) the **external intercostal muscles**, located between the ribs. As the muscles of inhalation contract, the **sternum**, or breast bone, and the rib cage are also raised.

What causes the lungs to fill with air during inhalation? As the lungs expand, the air pressure in the lungs becomes less than the air pressure in the environment. This results in what is called a *negative pressure*, relative to atmospheric pressure, inside the lungs. That is, there is a drop in air pressure. To equalize the air pressure between the lungs and the environment, air rushes into the lungs.

During exhalation, the lungs deflate because they are composed of elastic tissue (not unlike letting the air out of a balloon). Simultaneously, the diaphragm begins to relax and rise, returning to its original position. Also, the rib cage becomes smaller as it lowers due to both the relaxation of the inhalation muscles and the contraction primarily of the **internal intercostal muscles** and the abdominal muscles. The internal intercostal muscles are located between the ribs, but are located *deep* to (beneath) the external intercostals. The end result is the expulsion of the airstream through the **trachea,** or windpipe. The trachea, which connects the lungs with the larynx, is a tube comprised of cartilaginous rings embedded in muscle tissue (see Figure 3.1).

The Laryngeal System and Phonation

The laryngeal system consists primarily of the **larynx,** or "voice box." The larynx is composed mainly of muscle and cartilages. It attaches inferiorly to (below) the trachea, and superiorly (above), by a broad curtain-like ligament, to a "floating" bone known as the **hyoid bone** (see Figures 3.2 and 3.3). This is the only bone in the human body that does not attach to another bone. The hyoid also has muscular attachments to the tongue and to the mandible.

Figure 3.2 displays the major structures of the larynx from the anterior and posterior viewpoints. Located in the larynx are the vocal cords, or **vocal folds**.

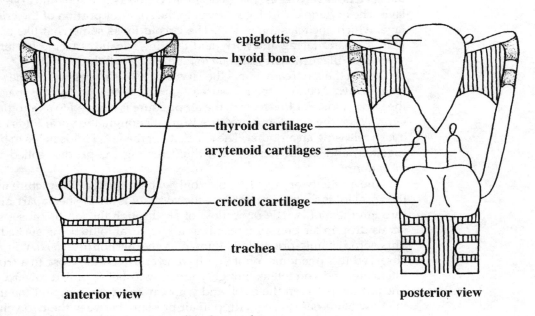

epiglottis
hyoid bone

thyroid cartilage

arytenoid cartilages

cricoid cartilage

trachea

anterior view   **posterior view**

FIGURE 3.2 Anterior and posterior views of the human larynx.

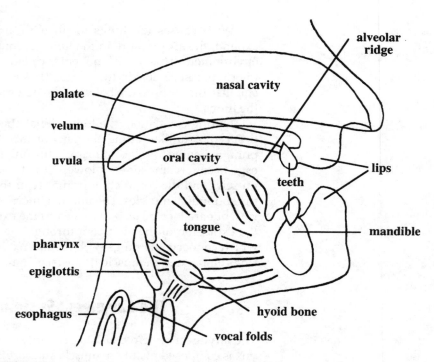

FIGURE 3.3   The vocal tract and related supralaryngeal structures.

The vocal folds are elastic folds of tissue, primarily composed of muscle. They attach *anteriorly* to (in the front of) the **thyroid cartilage**. The thyroid cartilage is more sharply angled in males than in females, explaining why males have more prominent thyroid cartilages. The vocal folds attach *posteriorly* to (in the back of) the **arytenoid cartilages**. Each vocal fold connects to a separate arytenoid cartilage. The arytenoid cartilages attach to the superior portion of the **cricoid cartilage**, which encircles the larynx. The cricoid looks somewhat like a class ring, with the band facing anteriorly and the ring's features facing posteriorly. The thyroid cartilage attaches *laterally* to (at the sides of) the cricoid.

When the airstream enters the larynx, it exerts a pressure on the vocal folds from below. Actually, the pressure is applied to the **glottis**, the space between the vocal folds. For this reason, the air pressure is referred to as **subglottal pressure**. When the subglottal pressure is great enough, the vocal folds are pushed apart, releasing an air burst. The elasticity of the vocal folds helps to bring them together, and the action repeats, thus creating the process called vocal fold vibration.

The elasticity of the vocal folds only explains half of the picture in bringing the vocal folds back together. Once the vocal folds are pushed apart, air is forced through the glottis. The rapid flow of air through the glottis causes a simultaneous drop in air pressure, resulting in the vocal folds being sucked together. This aerodynamic principle is known as the **Bernoulli effect**. You may have observed this phenomenon if you have ever driven too close to a truck on the interstate, and you felt as though your car was being pulled toward the truck. The airflow between the truck and your car has increased, and the increase in the flow of air has caused a drop in air pressure between the two vehicles. The

Bernoulli effect also explains how planes become airborne. Due to wing design, a pressure difference exists between the top and bottom of the wing as the plane picks up speed. As airflow increases across the wing (as the plane gains speed), the air pressure below the wing becomes greater than the pressure above the wing, causing the plane to lift off.

The vibration of the vocal folds in creation of a vocal sound is called **phonation**. You can feel the vocal folds vibrating if you place your fingertips on your "Adam's apple" (the notch in the thyroid cartilage in the front of your neck) while sustaining, or prolonging, the phoneme /z/ ("zzzzzzzzz"). You should be able to feel the vocal fold vibration. The phoneme /z/ is called a **voiced** sound due to vocal fold vibration during its production. Some other examples of voiced phonemes include all of the vowels and several of the consonants, for example, /b/, /r/, /m/, /v/, and /g/.

Now place your fingers on your larynx while sustaining the phoneme /s/ ("sssssssss"). The production of the phoneme /s/ does *not* involve phonation. Because the vocal folds do not vibrate, the phoneme /s/ is called a **voiceless** phoneme. It is important to keep in mind that not all speech sounds require participation of the vocal folds. Many sounds such as /s/ and /f/ are formed by forcing the airstream through a narrow constriction formed by the speech organs in the oral cavity, without participation of the vocal folds.

EXERCISE 3.1

Think of at least two other phonemes that are voiced and two others that are voiceless.

voiced _____   voiceless _____

During quiet breathing (when not speaking), the vocal folds remain apart, that is, in a state of **abduction**, to allow air to flow from the lungs through the glottis to the oral and nasal cavities. The vocal folds also remain apart during the production of voiceless sounds. However, when producing voiced phonemes, the vocal folds are in a state of **adduction**, that is, they are brought together. The vocal folds then alternate during phonation between periods of abduction and adduction.

During phonation, the vocal folds open and close at the rate of approximately 125 times per second in the male larynx, and approximately 215 times per second in the female larynx (Boone & McFarlane, 1994). This basic rate of vibration of the vocal folds is called the **fundamental frequency** of the voice. The fundamental frequency is responsible for the inherent voice pitch, or **habitual pitch,** of an individual. The pitch of the male voice is usually perceived to be lower than the pitch of the female voice due to the lower fundamental frequency. The pitch of the voice is largely dependent on the size of the individual larynx. Because the vocal fold tissue in the male larynx has greater mass than that of the female larynx, the male vocal folds vibrate more slowly. Hence, the male voice is perceived as being lower in pitch. Because children have smaller larynges than adults, their vocal pitch is the highest of all.

The fundamental frequency of the voice is not constant; voice pitch changes continually over time during speech production. When a word is given stress for emphasis (i.e., the *blue* car), the fundamental frequency rises. When someone asks a question, their voice pitch also rises, *doesn't it?* Singers change the fundamental frequency of their voices to sing a scale. Individuals who speak in a *monotone* ("one tone") rarely change the pitch of their voice. If you have ever had a professor who spoke in a monotone, you know how *monotonous* it was for the class. The pitch of the voice also conveys information regarding our moods, that is, whether we are happy, sad, excited, bored, or angry.

In addition to phonation, the larynx serves other important purposes. During a meal, the **epiglottis**, another cartilage of the larynx, diverts food away from the trachea and towards the esophagus to avoid food from "going down the wrong pipe" (see Figure 3.2). The larynx also is important in maintaining air pressure in the thoracic cavity during strenuous activities such as giving birth, lifting heavy weights, and elimination. During these activities, air is held in the lungs to provide extra muscular strength derived from the thorax. The vocal folds are held tightly together along their margins during these activities in order to stop the escape of air from the lungs. If you lift weights, you know the importance of good breath control to help you with your workout.

The Supralaryngeal System and Articulation

The supralaryngeal system is comprised of the **pharynx**, or throat, the oral cavity, the nasal cavity, and the articulators (see Figure 3.3). Collectively, these structures comprise what is known as the **vocal tract**. The length of the vocal tract from larynx to lips is about 17 cm (almost 7 inches) in the average adult male, and about 14 or 15 cm in the average adult female (Kent, 1997).

The pharynx directs airflow from the larynx to the oral and nasal cavities. It connects to the esophagus, which lies posteriorly to the larynx. The pharynx can be divided into three major sections. In ascending order from the larynx, they are (1) the *laryngopharynx*, the portion of the pharynx adjoining the larynx; (2) the *oropharynx*, adjacent to the posterior portion of the oral cavity; and (3) the *nasopharynx*, adjacent to the posterior portion of the nasal cavity. The **eustachian tubes**, important in equalizing changes in air pressure (when flying or diving in water), connect the nasopharynx with the middle ear systems on either side of the head.

The *nasal cavity* begins at the nostrils, or **nares**, and continues to the nasopharynx, posteriorly. Directly inferior to the nasal cavity (separated by the palate) is the oral cavity. The *oral cavity*, or mouth, begins at the lips and continues posteriorly to the oropharynx. The oral and nasal cavities join at the pharynx.

During phonation (vocal fold vibration), air bursts or pulses escape from the glottis when subglottal pressure becomes sufficient to push the folds apart. These pulses are modulated by the opening and closing of the vocal folds. The air bursts collide with a column of air residing in the vocal tract. This collision sends acoustic vibrations at the speed of sound through the vocal tract to the lips (Daniloff, Shuckers, & Feth, 1980).

During production of voiceless phonemes, the vocal folds do not modulate the air stream because the vocal folds are abducted. Instead, acoustic vibrations are created when air, streaming from the lungs, is impeded by a constriction formed by the speech organs in the oral cavity. As the flow of air is forced through the constriction, a turbulent airstream is generated. The turbulence generates acoustic vibrations, which then travel toward the lips along with the airstream.

As the airstream from the lungs (and the accompanying acoustic vibrations) is directed to the oral and nasal cavities, the vibrations are modified by the speech organs to produce the individual phonemes of a language. This process is called **articulation**. The term articulation means to "join together." Articulation of speech, therefore, involves the joining together of the speech organs for the production of phonemes.

The major articulators of the vocal tract are located in the oral cavity. It is these structures that are directly responsible for the production of speech sounds. A detailed description of these organs and their role in the production of speech follows. While reading the descriptions of the articulators in the next few paragraphs, you may find it helpful to refer to Figures 3.3 and 3.4.

The Lips

The purpose of the lips is to open and close in the production of several English speech sounds. The upper lip is supported by the **maxilla**, or upper jaw, and the lower lip is supported by the **mandible**, or lower jaw. In production of English sounds, the lower lip is more mobile because the mandible is quite active in the production of speech. The sounds associated with the lips are called **labial** sounds. When both lips are involved in the production of these sounds, they are also called **bilabial** phonemes. During production of speech, the lips may

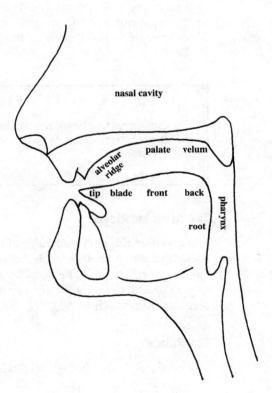

FIGURE 3.4 The landmarks of the tongue in relation to the other structures in the vocal tract.

become rounded, as in the word "who," or retracted (unrounded), as in the word "see."

Examples of labial (bilabial) sounds are the initial phonemes in the words "pear," "boy," "meet," and "witch." Notice that the formation of the phoneme /w/ is slightly different from the other three labial phonemes.

EXERCISE 3.2

Say the words "witch" and "pear," and pay attention to your lips in the formation of /w/ and /p/. What is the difference in the way the lips come together in the formation of these sounds?

The Teeth

The role of the teeth in the production of speech is more important than one might imagine. The top front teeth, the **central incisors**, and the lower lip are used in combination to produce the phonemes /f/ and /v/ as in the words "fat" and "vat." Phonemes that involve the articulation of the lower lip and the teeth are called **labiodental** (lips and teeth). The top and bottom central incisors (with the assistance of the tongue) are important in production of the initial phonemes in the words "think" and "that." Phonemes that are produced by the tongue and the teeth are called **dental** or **interdental**. In addition to being directly involved in the production of several phonemes, the teeth (most notably the *molars*) also help guide the tongue in production of other speech sounds, such as the initial sounds in "top," "sit," "ship," and "zebra."

EXERCISE 3.3

The phonemes that begin the words "think" and "that" both have a "th" sound, yet they are considered to be two separate phonemes. What is the difference in their production?

The Alveolar Ridge

The **alveolar ridge** (or *gum ridge* of the maxilla) is the bony ridge containing the sockets of the teeth. It is located directly posterior to the upper central incisors. Say the word "team." The tip of your tongue touches the anterior alveolar ridge as you produce the initial /t/ phoneme. Other phonemes produced using the alveolar ridge, such as /d/, /l/, /s/, and /z/, are called **alveolar**.

The Palate

The **hard palate** (or simply, palate) is the bony structure located just posterior to the alveolar ridge. You can feel the palate by sliding the tip of your tongue from the alveolar ridge towards the back of the mouth. The palate, often referred to as the roof of the mouth, separates the oral cavity from the nasal cavity. Individuals born with a *cleft palate* may have an incomplete closure of the hard palate that allows air to escape from the oral cavity directly into the nasal cavity. Sounds produced in conjunction with the palate (and tongue) are called **palatal**. Examples of palatal sounds include the sounds at the beginning of the words "ship" and "you."

The Velum

The **velum**, another name for the soft palate, is a muscular structure located directly posterior to the hard palate. (Some of you may be able to touch the soft palate with your tongue tip.) **Velar** sounds are those produced by articulation of the soft palate with the back of the tongue. Examples include the initial sounds in the words "kite" and "goat" and "ng" in the word "king."

The **uvula** is the rounded, tablike, fleshy structure located at the posterior tip of the velum. Although the uvula is not used in production of speech sounds in English, it is used in other languages, such as French and Arabic.

Because the velum is muscular, it is capable of movement. The velum acts as a switching mechanism that directs the flow of air coming from the lungs and larynx. When the velum is raised, it contacts the back wall of the pharynx, closing off the nasopharynx from the oropharynx. This process is called **velopharyngeal closure**. Closure of the velopharyngeal port prevents air from entering the nasal cavity. On the other hand, when the velum is lowered, air flows into both the oral and nasal cavities.

Phonemes produced with a raised (closed) velum are called oral phonemes; the airstream is directed solely into the oral cavity. Phonemes produced while the mouth is closed and the velum is lowered are called nasal phonemes because the breath stream flows into the nasal cavity as well. In English, there are only three nasal phonemes: /m/, /n/, and /ŋ/. The symbol /ŋ/ represents "ng" as in the words "sing" and "hunger." All of the other phonemes in English are oral.

The Glottis

The *glottis* is the place of production for the English phoneme /h/. This phoneme is considered a **glottal** sound because it is produced when the airstream from the lungs is forced through the opening between the vocal folds. Because the vocal folds do not vibrate during the production of /h/, it is considered to be voiceless.

The Tongue

The tongue is the major articulator in the production of speech. It is composed of muscle and is a quite active and mobile structure. The tongue is supported by the mandible and the hyoid bone through muscular attachments. The tongue also has muscular attachments to several other structures including the epiglottis, the palate, and the pharynx.

Sounds produced with the tongue are called **lingual** sounds. The tongue is the primary articulator for all of the English vowels. In addition, the tongue articulates with the lips, teeth, alveolar ridge, palate, and velum in production of the consonants. The **root** of the tongue arises from the anterior wall of the pharynx and is attached to the mandible (see Figure 3.4). As a result, tongue movement is very much related to movements of the lower jaw.

In addition to the root, the tongue has several other geographical landmarks (see Figure 3.4). These landmarks include the **tip** of the tongue (also known as the **apex**) and the **blade**, which lies immediately posterior to the tip. The **body** of the tongue is found just posterior to the blade. The body is comprised of two portions, the **front** and the **back**. The front of the tongue generally lies inferior to the hard palate, and the back lies inferior to the velum. The entire tongue body is sometimes referred to as the tongue **dorsum**. (The term *dorsum* is also used to refer specifically to just the back of the tongue.) The landmarks are useful in describing the portion of the tongue involved in production of the various English phonemes. For instance, the /t/ phoneme is produced by placing the apex or blade of the tongue against the alveolar ridge, and the phoneme /g/ is produced by articulation of the back of the tongue and the soft palate.

The Vocal Tract and Resonance

Every phoneme in a language has a unique sound quality associated with it due to a unique vocal tract shape and accompanying vibratory pattern, or **resonance**. Resonance deals with the vibratory properties of *any* vibrating body (including the vocal tract, a guitar, a harmonica, or a tuning fork). All objects have natural frequencies of vibration, or resonances. Consider blowing across the top of a pop bottle. When you blow across the opening, a particular tone is produced due to the inherent vibratory properties of the air mass in the bottle. Imagine adding some water to the bottle. Now what happens when you blow across the bottle? The tone that is produced will be higher in pitch because the mass of air is less than before.

During the process of articulation, the tongue and other articulators constantly change their positions to produce different sounds as acoustic vibrations from the larynx (or from a vocal tract constriction) flow through the vocal tract on their way to the lips. As the articulators move from one position to the next, the natural frequencies of vibration (or resonances) of the vocal tract change accordingly. These resonance changes are the direct result of modifications in the air mass in the vocal tract brought about by the ever-changing shape of the tongue, pharynx, lips, and jaw during production of speech. (This process is similar to changing the water level in the pop bottle.)

Now, consider how the resonance of the vocal tract differs between an oral and a nasal sound. During production of an oral sound, only the oral and pharyngeal cavities resonate. During production of a nasal sound, the oral cavity is closed, the velum is lowered, and the acoustic vibrations entering the nasal cavity undergo resonance there as well. The addition of the nasal cavity in production of nasal phonemes dramatically alters the resonance of the vocal tract. Hence, the sound quality varies markedly when comparing oral and nasal phonemes.

Alterations in the resonance of the vocal tract are what allow you to recognize differences among the individual English phonemes. As a child, you learned that a particular sound quality is associated with the /r/ phoneme (for example) and that a totally different sound quality is associated with the /s/ phoneme. It is your ability to recognize these differences that allow you to perceive speech.

Although the term *quality* has been used freely in this discussion of resonance, it has not yet been defined. **Quality** is the perceptual character of a sound based on its acoustic resonance patterns. **Timbre** is a synonym often used for sound quality.

The size, shape, and composition of any vibrating body help to determine its unique resonance characteristic (timbre). A middle "C" played on a piano has a different timbre than middle "C" on a clarinet even though both instruments produce the same note on the musical scale. The contrasting timbre allows you to recognize the difference in middle "C" played by these two instruments. Similarly, the vocal tract has a recognizable quality due to its own characteristic resonance and sounds nothing like the sounds produced from a pop bottle or a piano.

Review Exercises

A. Provide the name of the articulator referenced by each of the following adjectives.

velar _____   palatal _____

alveolar _____   glottal _____

lingual _____   dental _____

labial _____

B. Matching

Match each of the laryngeal cartilages at the right with its correct description.

____ 1. shaped like a signet ring   a. epiglottis

____ 2. forms the Adam's apple   b. cricoid

____ 3. situated atop the cricoid   c. thyroid

____ 4. prevents food from entering the larynx   d. arytenoids

C. Fill in the blank.

1. The basic rate of vocal fold vibration is called _____ .

2. The _____ is another name for the lower jaw.

3. The anatomical term anterior means _____ .

4. The anatomical term inferior means _____ .

5. The _____ is a major muscle that separates the chest cavity from the abdomen.

6. _____ pressure is the air pressure *below* the vocal folds.

7. Inherent voice pitch is also known as _____ pitch.

8. The _____ connect both middle ears with the nasopharynx.

9. The _____ is the portion of the tongue just posterior to the tip. The tip is also known as the _____ .

10. The tongue dorsum is composed of the _____ and the _____ .

Study Questions

1. Describe the process of inhalation and exhalation. Which anatomical structures are involved in these processes?

2. What is the Bernoulli effect? What is its importance in the production of speech?

3. Define the following terms:
   a. glottis
   b. abduction/adduction
   c. hyoid bone
   d. uvula

4. Which structures comprise the vocal tract?

5. What is the difference between a voiced and voiceless sound?

6. What is the pharynx, and what are its three major components?

7. What is the larynx, and what are its major cartilaginous components?

8. What is phonation? Which anatomical structures are involved in phonation?

9. What is articulation?

10. Identify and describe each of the geographical landmarks of the tongue.

11. What is resonance? Of what importance is resonance in the process of speech production?

12. What is the difference between an oral sound and a nasal sound?

13. What is timbre?

14. Why does an adult male have a different habitual pitch than an adult female?

Vowel Transcription

Beginning with this chapter, the focus will be on phonetic transcription. Chapter 4 will emphasize the vowel sounds, and Chapter 5 will introduce the consonants. In these two chapters, each phoneme of English will be identified in terms of the manner in which it is articulated. In addition, its phonetic symbol will be introduced in transcription practice.

As previously stated in Chapter 1, learning phonetics is much like learning a new language. In order for you to feel comfortable with the use of the IPA, ample opportunity will be given for practice. The importance of practice can not be emphasized enough in the study of phonetic transcription. Therefore, in addition to the printed exercises in this text, you will also have the opportunity to transcribe speech while listening to the instructor and other speakers, either in class or on the optional audio CDs.

What Is a Vowel?

Vowels are phonemes that are produced without any appreciable constriction or blockage of air flow in the vocal tract. As you know, English has many more vowel sounds than those represented by the five Roman alphabet letters, "a, e, i, o, and u." Table 4.1 lists all of the vowel phonemes in English along with the way in which they are classified.

The tongue is the primary articulator in the production of vowels. Because the tongue has muscular attachments to the mandible, changes in jaw position also are linked directly to vowel production. As the tongue changes position for production of the individual vowels, the size and shape of the pharynx also change correspondingly. The airstream passes through the oral cavity with virtually no obstruction by the tongue or other major articulators. If the tongue did create a constriction in the vocal tract, a consonant phoneme would be produced. How then are vowels produced if no obstruction occurs in the vocal tract? To answer this question, say the following words aloud. Pay particular attention to the position of your tongue as you produce the vowel (the middle element) in each word.

b<u>ea</u>d, b<u>i</u>d, b<u>ay</u>ed, b<u>e</u>d, b<u>a</u>d

Now say the words again and leave off the consonant phonemes /b/ and /d/ so that you are saying only the vowel. Once again, pay attention to the position of the tongue. What did you observe? Hopefully, you noted that as you said these words in order, the position of your tongue continually lowered. Specifically, it was the body of the tongue that lowered during the production of these vowels. Also, you may have noted that your jaw lowered at the same time.

Vowel phonemes are categorized in relation to the position of the body of the tongue in the mouth during their production. Specifically, vowels are characterized by height and advancement of the tongue body. **Tongue height** refers to how high (or low) in the oral cavity the tongue is when producing a particular vowel. **Tongue advancement** relates to how far forward (or backward) in the mouth the tongue is when producing a particular vowel. All of the vowels in English can be described by using these two dimensions of tongue position in the oral cavity.

To better understand the idea of tongue height and advancement, it is convenient to think of the oral cavity as the space schematically represented in Figure 4.1. This figure is called the **vowel quadrilateral** due to its characteristic shape. All of the vowels in English are plotted on this two-dimensional figure to represent tongue advancement and height. Examination of Figure 4.1 shows that tongue height can be divided into three dimensions: high, mid, and low. Tongue advancement also is divided into three dimensions: front, central, and back. It is these dimensions that will be discussed as each of the vowels are introduced in the following sections. Keep in mind that the vowel quadrilateral is only an approximation of tongue positions for the production of vowels.

A secondary characteristic of vowels involves lip rounding, that is, whether the lips are **rounded** or **retracted** (unrounded) in their production. For example, compare the vowel sounds in the following two words: "moon" and "mean." Notice that the first vowel is produced with the lips protruded or rounded,

TABLE 4.1 The Fourteen Vowels of English (Diphthongs Not Included)

Vowel Phoneme	Key Word	Tongue Height	Tongue Advancement	Tense/ Lax	Lip Rounding
/i/	*key*	high	front	tense	retracted
/ɪ/	*win*	high	front	lax	retracted
/e/	*reb<u>ate</u>*	high-mid	front	tense	retracted
/ɛ/	*red*	low-mid	front	lax	retracted
/æ/	*had*	low	front	lax	retracted
/u/	*moon*	high	back	tense	rounded
/ʊ/	*wood*	high	back	lax	rounded
/o/	*<u>o</u>kay*	high-mid	back	tense	rounded
/ɔ/	*law*	low-mid	back	tense	rounded
/ɑ/	*cod*	low	back	tense	retracted
/ə/	*<u>a</u>bout*	mid	central	lax	retracted
/ʌ/	*bud*	low-mid	back-central	lax	retracted
/ɚ/	*butt<u>er</u>*	mid	central	lax	rounded
/ɝ/	*bird*	mid	central	tense	rounded

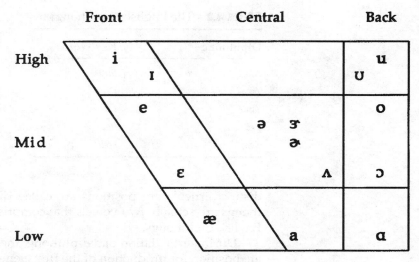

FIGURE 4.1 The vowel quadrilateral.

whereas the lips are retracted in association with the second vowel. In English, most vowels produced in the back of the mouth are rounded; the front vowels are all retracted. Other languages, such as German and French, have rounded front vowels (those produced in the front of the mouth). A summary of the rounded and retracted vowels of English follows:

Retracted: /i, ɪ, e, ɛ, æ, ɑ, ə, ʌ/
Rounded: /u, ʊ, o, ɔ, ɚ, ɝ/

Every vowel in English has a unique articulatory position based on the combination of tongue height, tongue advancement, and lip rounding.

PRELIMINARY EXERCISE 1—ROUNDED AND RETRACTED VOWELS

Using Table 4.1 as your guide, indicate whether the following one-syllable words have a rounded or an unrounded (retracted) vowel (vowel graphemes are in **bold letters**). Write either R (rounded) or U (unrounded/retracted) in the blanks.

____ 1. l**ea**n	____ 6. thr**ow**
____ 2. h**oo**k	____ 7. b**a**ck
____ 3. r**oa**d	____ 8. th**e**n
____ 4. m**i**nt	____ 9. w**ai**t
____ 5. ch**ew**	____ 10. sh**ou**ld

Because the oral structures (especially the tongue and pharynx) change during the production of each individual vowel, there is a corresponding change in the resonance of the vocal tract. These changes in resonance not only give each separate vowel a unique acoustic characteristic or quality, they also provide acoustic cues to listeners so that each vowel can be recognized individually.

Most English vowels are **monophthongs** ("one sound"), because they have one primary articulatory position in the vocal tract. Vowel sounds that have two

TABLE 4.2   The English Diphthongs

Diphthong	Key Word
/aɪ/	*buy*
/aʊ/	*cow*
/ɔɪ/	*toy*
/eɪ/	*hate*
/oʊ/	*coat*

distinct articulatory positions are called **diphthongs** ("two sounds"). Diphthongs are actually two vowels that comprise one phoneme. Table 4.2 lists the English diphthongs.

During articulation of a diphthong, the tongue is placed in the appropriate position for production of the first element. The tongue then moves to the second element in a continuous gliding motion. The first element of a diphthong is referred to as the **onglide** portion, and the second element is referred to as the **offglide**. The tongue rises in the oral cavity when moving from the onglide to the offglide for all of the English diphthongs. Therefore, the offglide is always produced at a higher position in the oral cavity than the onglide. Note that all English offglides consist of only two vowels, either /ɪ/ (a front vowel) or /ʊ/ (a back vowel).

The terms **tense** and **lax** also are used to classify vowels. Tense vowels are generally longer in duration and require more muscular effort than lax vowels. Below is a list of the English tense and lax vowels:

> Tense: /i, e, u, o, ɔ, ɑ, ɝ/
> Lax: /ɪ, ɛ, æ, ʊ, ə, ʌ, ɚ/

The best way to distinguish tense and lax vowels is to examine the way they are apportioned among English syllables when speaking. Tense vowels are capable of ending stressed open syllables. Examples of tense vowels can be found in the open syllables "he" /hi/ and "too" /tu/ and in the first syllable of the word "purchase" /ˈpɝtʃəs/. (Tense vowels also occur in closed syllables, as in the words "feet" /fit/ and "goose" /gus/.)

Conversely, lax vowels never end a stressed open syllable. Placing a lax vowel at the end of a one-syllable word, for instance, would result in the creation of a nonsense string. Say the word "him" without the final /m/, for example, /hɪ/. This is obviously not a real word. Examples of lax vowels can be found in the words "had" /hæd/ and "look" /lʊk/ (closed syllables) and in the first syllable of the word "aloud" /əlaʊd/ (an *unstressed* open syllable).

PRELIMINARY EXERCISE 2—TENSE AND LAX VOWELS

Using Table 4.1 as your guide, indicate whether the following one-syllable words have a tense or a lax vowel (vowel graphemes are in **bold letters**). Write either T (tense) or L (lax) in the blanks.

____ 1. s**ee**k	____ 3. s**i**nge	____ 5. h**o**t	____ 7. m**a**p
____ 2. p**u**sh	____ 4. h**ea**d	____ 6. h**oo**t	____ 8. cl**e**rk

Because all English vowels are oral sounds, the velum is generally raised to prevent air from being directed into the nasal cavity during their production. In some instances, vowels may become nasalized due to the phonemic environment of a word. In these cases, the velum would be lowered. For example, the vowel /i/ would be nasalized in articulation of the word "mean"—/mĩn/. (The tilde over the /ĩ/ indicates nasalization.) Because the /m/ and /n/ are both nasal consonants, the vowel would become nasalized due to the fact that the velum remains lowered throughout the production of the word. Say the word aloud and you will be able to observe the nasalization of the vowel. Nasalized vowels are typical of some dialects of English and, in some cases, also may be characteristic of a speech disorder.

The English Vowels

In the following sections, the vowels of English will be introduced using the following format:

1. **Pronunciation Guide** for the phonemes being discussed.
2. **Description** of each vowel on four dimensions: tongue height, tongue advancement, lip rounding, and tense/lax.
3. **Sample Words** containing the phoneme being discussed.
4. **Allographs** commonly used to represent the phoneme in spelling.
5. **Discussion** involving the production of the vowel, and some examples of dialectal variants.
6. **Practice Exercises.**

The Front Vowels

Pronunciation Guide

/i/	as in "keep"	/kip/
/ɪ/	as in "hit"	/hɪt/
/e/	as in "reb<u>a</u>te"	/ribet/
/eɪ/	as in "state"	/steɪt/
/ɛ/	as in "led"	/lɛd/
/æ/	as in "mat"	/mæt/

/i/

Description

Height:	high
Advancement:	front
Lip rounding:	retracted
Tense/lax:	tense

Sample Words

fleet	we	eke	t<u>ea</u>cher
<u>TV</u>	eaves	creek	cr<u>e</u>dence
<u>Ea</u>ster	yeast	reach	piece
seeks	<u>e</u>dict	r<u>ecei</u>pt	p<u>i</u>laf

Allographs

Grapheme	Example	Grapheme	Example
i	mosquito	ee	keel
e	she	ey	key
ei	seizure	ie	relieve
ea	reach	oe	amoeba

Discussion   The vowel /i/ is produced by raising the body of the tongue to a high front position in the oral cavity. During production of /i/ (as well as for the other front vowels), the tongue is raised in the vicinity of the hard palate (Figure 4.2). If you examine the vowel quadrilateral (Figure 4.1), you will see that the vowel /i/ is the highest and most fronted of all vowels. Because it represents an extreme point or corner of the vowel quadrilateral, it is referred to as one of the **point vowels**. The other point vowels in English include the front vowel /æ/ and the back vowels /u/ and /ɑ/. The lips are unrounded, or retracted, in production of /i/. In addition, /i/ is considered to be tense, because it is capable of ending a one-syllable word (open monosyllable), for example, "key" /ki/ and "pea" /pi/.

The mandible is raised during production of /i/, because the tongue is in a high position. In fact, the jaw is in a somewhat closed position. Also, the oropharynx enlarges during production of /i/ because the tongue body and root move superiorly and anteriorly away from the pharynx. As the tongue lowers in production of the front vowels (from /i/ to /æ/), the jaw lowers, and the size of the oropharynx decreases (as the tongue moves closer to the pharyngeal area). See Figure 4.3 for a comparison of the tongue, jaw, and pharyngeal positions for the two front vowels /i/ and /æ/.

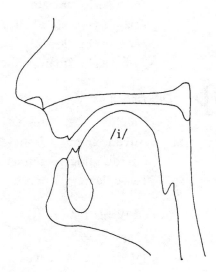

FIGURE 4.2   /i/ articulation.

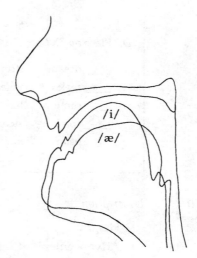

FIGURE 4.3 /i/ and /æ/ articulation.

Practice Exercises

EXERCISE 4.1—THE VOWEL /i/

A. Circle the words that contain the /i/ phoneme.

paper	train	Cleveland	seaside
please	picture	trip	trail
tribal	machine	labor	trees
settle	screen	Toledo	lip
nice	foreign	Levi	jeans

B. Circle the phonetic transcriptions that represent English words.

(*Note*: In this exercise and several others in this chapter, consonant IPA symbols are used. The IPA consonant symbols to be used are the same as their Roman alphabet counterparts. These consonant phoneme symbols include: /b, d, f, g, h, k, l, m, n p, r, s, t, v, w, z/.) For example: /iz/—"ease"; /din/—"dean"

/ist/	/flip/	/min/	/hid/
/iv/	/hig/	/lim/	/wins/
/rift/	/if/	/trit/	/lik/

C. In the blanks, write each of the words using English orthography (i.e., use the Roman alphabet to write the words).

/lip/ _____	/it/ _____	/brizd/ _____
/pip/ _____	/hip/ _____	/spik/ _____
/mit/ _____	/sip/ _____	/klin/ _____
/rid/ _____	/did/ _____	/krist/ _____

Continues

EXERCISE 4.1 (*cont.*)

D. Place an "X" next to the pairs of words that share the same vowel sound.

____	dream	drip	____	east	eaves
____	seek	wheel	____	chief	vein
____	same	land	____	base	lease
____	creek	steam	____	need	pain
____	bean	heed	____	creed	cream

/ɪ/

Description

Height:	high (lower than /i/)
Advancement:	front
Lip rounding:	retracted
Tense/lax:	lax

Sample Words

flit	wh<u>i</u>ttle	<u>i</u>nside	dr<u>ea</u>ry
b<u>u</u>siness	king	s<u>i</u>ster	steer
l<u>i</u>sten	p<u>i</u>stol	<u>i</u>ntend	prince
reall<u>y</u>	stink	choos<u>y</u>	k<u>i</u>tt<u>y</u>

Allographs

Grapheme	Example	Grapheme	Example
i	with, ring	e	England, pretty
y	gym	ea(r)	fear
ui	guilt	ee(r)	deer
u	business	i(r)	mirror
-y	baby	ei(r)	weird
ee	been	ie(r)	pierce
o	women	e(re)	here
ie	sieve		

Discussion   The body of the tongue is only slightly lower in production of /ɪ/ when compared to /i/ (Figure 4.4). This is why it is also classified as a high vowel. The jaw is in a fairly closed position during production of /ɪ/, and the lips are retracted. One distinction between /ɪ/ and /i/ is that /ɪ/ is lax. Placing /ɪ/ in the final position of a monosyllable would result in a nonsense string, that is, /bɪ/ or /wɪ/. The phoneme /ɪ/ does occur in closed syllables such as in "l<u>i</u>sten" and "<u>i</u>ndent."

The vowel /ɪ/ has some peculiarities in phonetic transcription. In unstressed syllables that end in "y," like "crazy," "gloomy," and "partly," it is debatable whether the phoneme /i/ or /ɪ/ should be used in the transcription of the final sound. In reality, this phoneme tends to be shorter in duration (when

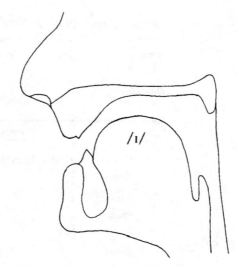

FIGURE 4.4   /ɪ/ articulation.

compared to the phoneme /i/). In this book, /ɪ/ will be used when transcribing the final "y" in unstressed syllables. Keep in mind that some individuals will use the phoneme /i/ in this context.

Another peculiarity with /ɪ/ involves words that contain the letter string "ing," such as in the words "running," "finger," and "thing." Their actual transcriptions are /rʌnɪŋ/, /fɪŋgɚ/, and /θɪŋ/. Notice the use of the phoneme /ɪ/. Again, you might be tempted to use /i/ in the transcription of these words. If you listen carefully, you will observe that the vowel in "ing" does not really sound like the high front vowel /i/, as in "key" /ki/ or "meet" /mit/. In the "ing" context, /ɪ/ becomes nasalized due to the lowered velum associated with the production of /ŋ/. The altered sound quality of the nasalized /ɪ/ causes it to sound different from the nonnasalized /ɪ/. Therefore, it is considered preferable to transcribe this vowel with the phoneme symbol /ɪ/ in words which contain "ing."

Last, /ɪ/ is often found preceding the consonant /r/ as in the words "hear" /hɪr/ and "ear" /ɪr/. In this case, /ɪ/ becomes an **r-colored vowel**. This means that the vowel partially assumes the quality of the consonant /r/ following it. Some phoneticians use the term **rhotic diphthong** when referring to the combination of the /ɪ/ + /r/ phonemes. The term *rhotic* simply means that the diphthong has r-coloring, or an "r" quality, associated with it.

The r-colored vowel, or rhotic diphthong, /ɪr/, also may be transcribed as /ɪɚ/ or /ɪ͡ɚ/. The connecting mark in the last example is used by some phoneticians and clinicians when transcribing a diphthong to signify the production of two sounds as one phoneme. This text will adopt the use of /ɪr/, as opposed to /ɪɚ/ or /ɪ͡ɚ/, when transcribing r-colored vowels. /ɪr/ is only one of several r-colored vowels found in English.

There are a few dialectal variants involving the phoneme /ɪ/. For instance, in the southeastern United States, some people pronounce the r-colored vowel /ɪr/ with /i/, as in "here" /hir/ or "ear" /ir/ (Hartman, 1985). /ɪ/ is also found to occur before /l/ in some southern pronunciations, as in "really" /rɪlɪ/ and "meal" /mɪl/. Both in African American Vernacular English and in southern American dialect, words such as "many," "pen," and "cents" might be pronounced as /mɪnɪ/, /pɪn/, and /sɪnts/, respectively.

Practice Exercises

EXERCISE 4.2–THE VOWEL /ɪ/

A. Contrast the vowels in the following pairs of words (minimal pairs) by saying them aloud.

/i/	/ɪ/		/i/	/ɪ/
reed	rid		keel	kill
heed	hid		deal	dill
deep	dip		ceased	cyst
seat	sit		bean	been
sleek	slick		feet	fit

B. Circle the words that contain the /ɪ/ phoneme.

peace	friend	enthrall	bitter
mythical	silver	woman	tryst
click	ingest	build	fear
thread	pink	bowling	tried
pride	clear	sporty	synchronize

C. Circle the phonetic transcriptions that represent English words.

/vɪl/	/sɪst/	/fɪld/	/wɪns/
/izɪ/	/klip/	/spid/	/hik/
/hɪr/	/ɪl/	/sɪg/	/pɪgɪ/

D. In the blanks, write each of the words using English orthography.

/stɪp/ _____		/pɪk/ _____	
/pliz/ _____		/kɪst/ _____	
/mɪt/ _____		/bik/ _____	
/dɪd/ _____		/pɪp/ _____	
/fɪr/ _____		/mɪstɪ/ _____	
/rilɪ/ _____		/ɪndid/ _____	

E. Place an "X" next to the pairs of words that share the same vowel sound.

____ feel	teach		____ win	king
____ lip	thread		____ mint	inch
____ been	drink		____ deed	flea
____ vent	list		____ dish	ill
____ tied	pig		____ kick	mill

Continues

F. Indicate with an "X" the words that contain the r-colored vowel /ɪr/.

1. ____ flirt	5. ____ smeared	9. ____ stirred	
2. ____ peerless	6. ____ worried	10. ____ stared	
3. ____ bird	7. ____ steered	11. ____ earring	
4. ____ shrill	8. ____ harder	12. ____ cursor	

/e, eɪ/

Description

Height:	high-mid
Advancement:	front
Lip rounding:	retracted
Tense/lax:	tense

Sample Words   The following set of words all take the allophone /e/ in their transcriptions because the syllables that contain the vowel do not receive primary stress.

ch<u>a</u>Otic	UNdul<u>ate</u>
GYr<u>ate</u>	l<u>ay</u>ETTE
PHOn<u>ate</u>	DEC<u>a</u>de
MANd<u>ate</u>	ROt<u>ate</u>

The following words all take the allophone /eɪ/because the syllables are either stressed or at the end of a word.

aW<u>AY</u>	(also ends the word)	conT<u>A</u>gious
touP<u>EE</u>	(also ends the word)	ST<u>A</u>Ted
cre<u>ATE</u>		B<u>A</u>by
T<u>A</u>ble		BR<u>AI</u>D

Allographs

Grapheme	Example	Grapheme	Example
ea	great	ei	veil
a..e	hate	ay	stray
au	gauge	ey	grey
ai	faint		

Discussion   The /e/ vowel is produced with the body of the tongue slightly higher than the exact middle of the mouth, therefore it is referred to as a *high-mid vowel* (see Figure 4.5). /e/ also is retracted. Like the vowel /i/, it is tense, and can be found in the word "bay." The stressed form of the vowel /e/ is actually a diphthong, written as /eɪ/. The use of this diphthong in speech (as opposed to the monophthong /e/) varies with syllable context as well as

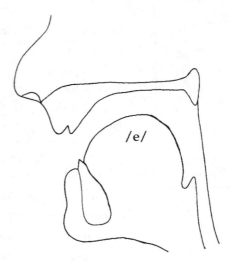

FIGURE 4.5   /e/ articulation.

regional pronunciation. Because /e/ and /eɪ/ represent the same sound, they are considered to be allophones. Substituting the articulatory production of /e/ for /eɪ/ or vice versa would not result in the creation of a different phoneme or of a minimal pair.

The diphthongal form of the vowel is longer in duration than the monophthongal /e/, because it is comprised of the onglide /e/ plus the offglide /ɪ/. In producing /eɪ/, the tongue and vocal tract assume the initial position for the /e/ vowel. The tongue then continues to glide to the high, front position for /ɪ/ (see Figure 4.16). The diphthongal form, /eɪ/, is usually produced in stressed syllables, and at the end of words (regardless of stress), because in these cases, the vowel tends to become lengthened or drawn out. The shorter monophthong /e/ generally occurs in unstressed syllables.

Some southern speakers in the United States use the diphthong /eɪ/ in words such as "fresh" /freɪʃ/ and "mesh" /meɪʃ/. In addition, /eɪ/ may be found in southern speech preceding the consonant /g/ as in "leg" /leɪg/ and "egg" /eɪg/.

Practice Exercises

EXERCISE 4.3 — THE VOWEL /e/ - /eɪ/

A. Contrast the vowels in the following minimal pairs.

/eɪ/	/ɪ/		/eɪ/	/i/
grade	grid		tame	team
tape	tip		grain	green
drape	drip		trait	treat
take	tick		sale	seal
late	lit		Grace	grease
tale	till		wade	weed
faze	fizz		raid	reed

Continues

B. Circle the words that contain the /eɪ/ phoneme.

trail	rage	wheel	palatial
vice	razor	manage	green
transit	machine	whale	potato
lazy	bread	football	temperate
dale	tackle	daily	bright

C. Circle the phonetic transcriptions that represent English words.

/freɪd/	/deɪs/	/dɪnt/	/deɪlɪ/
/kreɪt/	/biz/	/spid/	/deɪm/
/neɪp/	/trips/	/treɪ/	/fril/
/pɪln/	/blid/	/feɪlm/	/streɪp/

D. In the blanks, write each of the words using English orthography.

/bleɪz/ _____	/pleɪket/ _____
/pleɪd/ _____	/rimeɪn/ _____
/beɪn/ _____	/ɪnmet/ _____
/iveɪd/ _____	/ribet/ _____
/krɪmp/ _____	/steɪnd/ _____
/rikt/ _____	/deɪzi/ _____

E. Indicate whether the syllable that contains /eɪ/ is either open or closed by writing O or C in the blank.

____ crayon	____ unmade
____ prepay	____ stay
____ baking	____ tailor
____ masonry	____ betrayed

F. Place an "X" next to the pairs of words that share the same vowel sound.

____ braid	hid		____ state	rain
____ feed	hate		____ fist	flea
____ lane	aim		____ cringe	hid
____ fill	kissed		____ deal	will
____ treat	sling		____ wheel	meat

/ɛ/

Description

Height:	low-mid
Advancement:	front
Lip rounding:	retracted
Tense/lax:	lax

Sample Words

met	etch	bury	intend
steady	where	terror	tender
pretend	repent	heather	elephant
relish	stencil	marry	pleasures

Allographs

Grapheme	Example	Grapheme	Example
e	let	ai	said
ei	heifer	ai(r)	flair
ea	meant	ei(r)	their
a	many	ea(r)	bear
ie	friend	u(r)	bury
ue	guest	a(re)	bare
eo	Leonard	e(re)	where

Discussion   The /ɛ/ vowel is commonly referred to as "epsilon," an IPA symbol borrowed from the Greek alphabet. It is categorized as a low-mid, front vowel (see Figure 4.6). Examination of the vowel quadrilateral indicates the tongue body is located midway between the mid and low positions in the mouth for its production. Epsilon is a retracted and lax vowel. (Placing /ɛ/ at the end of a monosyllabic word creates a nonsense string, e.g., /tɛ/ or /wɛ/.) The vowel /ɛ/ often occurs before the consonant /r/ in words such as "hair" /hɛr/ and "fair" /fɛr/. /ɛr/ is another example of an r-colored vowel. This phoneme sequence is transcribed by some individuals as /ɛɚ/. In the northeastern and southeastern United States, the r-colored vowel /ɛr/ may be pronounced as /er/ as in /her/ and /fer/ (Hartman, 1985). Also, some speakers in the Great Lakes region pronounce words like "pillow" and "milk" as /pɛloʊ/ and /mɛlk/ (Hartman, 1985).

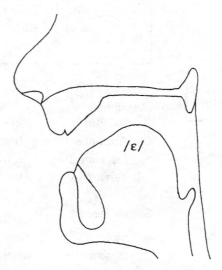

FIGURE 4.6   /ɛ/ articulation.

Practice Exercises

EXERCISE 4.4—THE VOWEL /ɛ/

A. Contrast the vowels in the following minimal pairs by saying them aloud.

/ɛ/	/ɪ/	/ɛ/	/eɪ/
red	rid	wed	wade
dead	did	tread	trade
head	hid	shed	shade
etch	itch	met	mate
bell	bill	bread	braid
bear	beer	every	Avery
fair	fear	bell	bale

B. Circle the words that contain the /ɛ/ phoneme.

pimple	trip	ensure	tryst
syrup	caring	women	contend
pencil	butter	build	pretzel
thing	thread	prepare	tried
jeep	pistol	unscented	remember

C. Circle the phonetic transcriptions that represent English words.

/mɛrɪ/	/hint/	/split/	/istɚ/
/slɛpt/	/fɛr/	/ɪrk/	/meɪd/
/sɪsɪ/	/kleɪ/	/wɛl/	/krip/

D. In the blanks, write each of the words using English orthography.

/reɪk/	_____	/stɛr/	_____
/fɪz/	_____	/treɪl/	_____
/smɛl/	_____	/pritɛnd/	_____
/sid/	_____	/hɛvɪ/	_____
/kreɪn/	_____	/friz/	_____
/breɪzd/	_____	/blɛst/	_____

E. Place an "X" next to the pairs of words that share the same vowel sound.

____	fill	fear	____	step	edge
____	made	cage	____	bread	breathe
____	wind	best	____	flit	red
____	trade	peel	____	sill	kit
____	rid	sing	____	care	meant

Continues

EXERCISE 4.4 *(cont.)*

F. Indicate whether the words below end with an open (O) or closed (C) syllable (write C or O in the blanks).

____	1. trail	____	6. spree
____	2. repay	____	7. arouse
____	3. strike	____	8. rough
____	4. plea	____	9. undo
____	5. late	____	10. chow

G. Indicate with an "X" the words that contain the r-colored vowel /ɛr/.

____	1. share	____	6. careful
____	2. early	____	7. sparrow
____	3. dearly	____	8. third
____	4. compare	____	9. corridor
____	5. fluoride	____	10. certain

/æ/

Description

Height:	low
Advancement:	front
Lip rounding:	retracted
Tense/lax:	lax

Sample Words

trash	jazz	smacked	language
thank	stand	asterisk	Capricorn
manage	batter	aster	blasphemy
Alabama	tamper	fantastic	trespass

Allographs

Grapheme	Example	Grapheme	Example
a	back	au	laugh
a(ng)	hang	ai	plaid
a(nk)	tank		

Discussion   The vowel /æ/, referred to as "ash," is the lowest of the five front vowels. (The vowel /a/, found in some eastern American dialects, is slightly lower). It is also one of the four point vowels. In reference to the front vowels, the mandible and tongue are in their lowest position for /æ/ (see Figure 4.7). The size of the oropharynx is small for /æ/ because the tongue body is in an inferior and posterior position (see Figure 4.3). Like all of the other front vowels, /æ/ is retracted. Also, /æ/ is lax; no monosyllables end with this sound. The one peculiarity of "ash" is its use in words in which it precedes the nasal

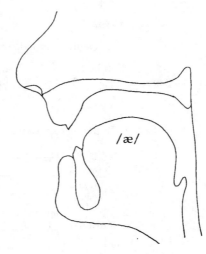

FIGURE 4.7   /æ/ articulation

/ŋ/, as in "rank" (/ræŋk/) and "bang" (/bæŋ/). You might be tempted to use the vowel /eɪ/ in these words. Keep in mind that it is the vowel /æ/ in this context; its perception is affected by nasalization due to the /ŋ/ that follows.

In the eastern and southern United States, speakers will use the vowel /æ/ in words such as "marry," "Harry," and "carry," that is, /mærɪ/, /hærɪ/, and /kærɪ/.

Practice Exercises

EXERCISE 4.5 – THE VOWEL /æ/

A. Contrast the vowels in the following pairs of words by saying them aloud.

/ɛ/	/æ/	/eɪ/	/æ/
led	lad	bade	bad
tend	tanned	haze	has
den	Dan	shale	shall
Ben	ban	mate	mat
bed	bad	lane	language
Kent	can't	bane	bank
spend	spanned	Dane	dank

B. Circle the words that contain the /æ/ phoneme.

straddle	practice	lapse	revamp
pale	panther	repast	straight
Lester	pacific	pacify	farmer
baseball	hanged	chances	cards
jazz	pistol	tamed	bombastic

Continues

EXERCISE 4.5 (*cont.*)

C. Circle the phonetic transcriptions that represent English words.

/klæd/	/prɪd/	/strɪv/	/wæd/
/slæpt/	/bɪrd/	/bæz/	/trækt/
/wɛb/	/steɪp/	/sprɪg/	/læzɪ/

D. In the blanks, write each of the words using English orthography.

/klæn/	_____	/spɪr/	_____
/sprɪnt/	_____	/hɛrɪ/	_____
/rɛk/	_____	/pækt/	_____
/teɪstɪ/	_____	/dræg/	_____
/præns/	_____	/bɛrɪ/	_____
/læft/	_____	/tinz/	_____

E. Place an "X" next to the pairs of words that share the same vowel sound.

____	badge	rage	____	hair	bend
____	seed	shade	____	lick	beer
____	cab	blonde	____	beak	bless
____	tray	whale	____	trap	bake
____	crank	shag	____	lapse	crag

Complete Assignment 4-1.

The Back Vowels

Pronunciation Guide

/u/	as in "toot"	/tut/
/ʊ/	as in "look"	/lʊk/
/o/	as in "<u>o</u>bese"	/obis/
/oʊ/	as in "vote"	/voʊt/
/ɔ/	as in "dawn"	/dɔn/
/ɑ/	as in "not"	/nɑt/

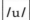

Description

Height:	high
Advancement:	back
Lip rounding:	rounded
Tense/lax:	tense

Sample Words

chew	ewe	unc<u>ou</u>th	strewn
f<u>u</u>tile	truth	spew	loot
Tr<u>u</u>man	cr<u>u</u>el	c<u>u</u>cumber	t<u>u</u>lip
clue	st<u>u</u>pid	t<u>u</u>na	s<u>u</u>per

Allographs

Grapheme	Example	Grapheme	Example
u	Pluto	wo	two
ue	true	oe	shoe
u..e	tune	o	to
ui	suit	ew	stew
ou	through	ieu	lieu
oo	moon	eu	maneuver
o..e	move	ioux	Sioux

Discussion   If you compare the placement of /u/ with the placement of /i/ in the vowel quadrilateral, you will see that these two vowels are mirror images of one another, that is, they are the two highest vowels in English. Actually, all of the back vowels are approximate mirror images of their front vowel counterparts in terms of height. Because of the extremely high back tongue body position, /u/ is considered to be another point, or corner, vowel in English (see Figure 4.8). /u/ is a rounded vowel. As previously stated, although all of the front vowels are produced with lip retraction, most of the English back vowels are rounded. The vowel /u/ is a tense vowel; it is found at the end of the one-syllable words "through," "you," and "true."

In raising the tongue to such a high position for /u/, the tongue root is forced to be somewhat advanced, widening the pharynx (see Figure 4.9). As the tongue lowers in production of the back vowels from /u/ to /ɑ/, the pharynx narrows accordingly, due to the retreating movement of the tongue root, posteriorly. Figure 4.9 displays the different tongue, jaw, lip, and pharyngeal positions for /u/ and /ɑ/.

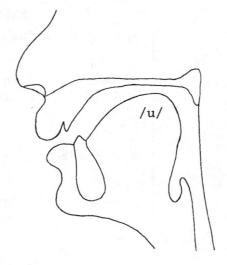

FIGURE 4.8   /u/ articulation.

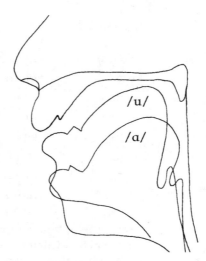

FIGURE 4.9   /u/ and /ɑ/ articulation.

There is one peculiarity associated with the phoneme /u/ and its transcription. Notice that in words like "you," "few," and "music," /u/ is actually preceded by the consonant phoneme /j/ (/ju/, /fju/ and /mjuzɪk/). (The /j/ phoneme is the palatal "y" sound.) Without the /j/ phoneme, these words would sound like "oo," "foo," and "moosic." Some phonetics texts do treat the phoneme sequence /ju/ as a diphthong. In this text, however, we will treat /j/ + /u/ as separate phonemes. As you examine the allographs of /u/ above, you will see several varied spellings for this phoneme.

Practice Exercises

EXERCISE 4.6–THE VOWEL /u/

A. Circle the words that contain the /u/ phoneme.

ghoul	oboe	crew	plural
butter	stuck	Lucifer	must
should	luck	lusty	shook
fuchsia	look	molding	stupor
loosely	glue	blouse	choose

B. Circle the phonetic transcriptions that represent English words.

/ust/	/krud/	/prus/	/tul/
/suv/	/tug/	/pus/	/wund/
/pul/	/rup/	/lus/	/slug/

Continues

C. In the blanks, write each of the words using English orthography.

/spun/ _____   /sup/ _____
/tun/ _____   /lud/ _____
/rut/ _____   /stru/ _____
/mud/ _____   /flu/ _____
/klu/ _____   /grum/ _____
/ruf/ _____   /snut/ _____

D. Indicate with an "X" the pairs of words that share the same vowel phoneme.

_____ 1. could   showed   _____ 6. brood   hood
_____ 2. suit   loon   _____ 7. stood   could
_____ 3. lute   book   _____ 8. hoops   poor
_____ 4. crew   scoot   _____ 9. feud   moose
_____ 5. push   foot   _____ 10. muse   cook

E. Indicate with an "X" the words that have the phoneme sequence /j/ + /u/, as in "you."

_____ 1. oozing   _____ 6. fuming
_____ 2. cute   _____ 7. Pluto
_____ 3. huge   _____ 8. useful
_____ 4. ruined   _____ 9. viewing
_____ 5. sloop   _____ 10. spooky

/ʊ/

Description

Height: high (lower than /u/)
Advancement: back
Lip rounding: rounded
Tense/lax: lax

Sample Words

could   sugar   pushed   bull
should   would   cushion   lure*
obscure*   unsure*   took   hood
wolf   full   stood   put

*/ʊ/ in these words may be pronounced differently, depending on a speaker's dialect.

Allographs

Grapheme	Example	Grapheme	Example
u	push	oo	book
ou	could	o	wolf
u(r)	secure		

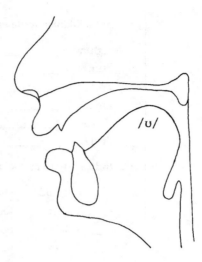

FIGURE 4.10   /ʊ/ articulation.

Discussion   The vowel /ʊ/ is produced with the tongue body only slightly lower in the oral cavity than for /u/ (see Figure 4.10). Therefore, it also is termed high. Like /u/, the vowel /ʊ/ is rounded; unlike /u/, it is lax. You will never see open syllables ending with this phoneme, as in /bʊ/ or /tʊ/. This vowel, in combination with the consonant /r/, forms the r-colored vowel /ʊr/ (or /ʊɚ/). The combination of /ʊ/ + /r/ may be used in the pronunciation of the words "tour" /tʊr/ and "lure" /lʊr/ by some individuals. Others may pronounce these words as if they rhymed with "core," that is, /tɔr/ and /lɔr/ (see the vowel /ɔ/ below). Notice that there are many fewer allographs associated with /ʊ/ than for the vowel /u/.

When the allograph "oo" is followed by /l/ (as in pool, cool, fool, and tool), the resulting pronunciation may be either /ʊ/ or /u/, depending on a speaker's dialect (especially in the South). Examine the following possible pronunciations of these words:

pool	/pʊl/	or	/pul/
cool	/kʊl/	or	/kul/
fool	/fʊl/	or	/ful/
tool	/tʊl/	or	/tul/

Some eastern speakers use the vowel /ʊ/ in words such as "room" /rʊm/ and "broom" /brʊm/.

Practice Exercises

EXERCISE 4.7—THE VOWEL /ʊ/

A. Contrast the vowels in the following words.

/u/	/ʊ/	/u/	/ʊ/
who'd	hood	food	foot
cooed	could	shoed	should
Luke	look	stewed	stood

Continues

B. Circle the words that contain the /ʊ/ phoneme.

hole	wooden	snooze	stunned
shut	punched	luscious	spook
hood	couldn't	pulled	shook
flushed	mistook	beauty	person
rudely	cooker	brood	stood

C. Circle the phonetic transcriptions that represent English words.

/buk/	/stʊ/	/rul/	/sul/
/lʊv/	/lum/	/rʊk/	/frut/
/trups/	/stʊr/	/buts/	/slʊg/

D. In the blanks, write each of the words using English orthography.

/pʊs/	_____	/tʊr/	_____
/tru/	_____	/hʊk/	_____
/stʊd/	_____	/lum/	_____
/dum/	_____	/fluk/	_____
/gru/	_____	/prun/	_____
/gʊd/	_____	/krʊk/	_____

E. Place an "X" next to the pairs of words that share the same vowel sound.

____	1. loot	foot		____	6. what	look
____	2. tune	mute		____	7. nook	stood
____	3. coupe	soon		____	8. rust	rook
____	4. flood	cute		____	9. goof	cruise
____	5. would	soot		____	10. mutt	look

/o/, /oʊ/

Description

Height:	high-mid
Advancement:	back
Lip rounding:	rounded
Tense/lax:	tense

Sample Words   The following words all take the allophone /o/ in their transcription because the syllables that contain the vowel are not stressed.

boDAcious	RIboflavin
CroAtian	floTILla
broCADE	proHIBit
ptoMAINE	roTAtion

The following words all take the allophone /ou/ because the syllables are either stressed (including monosyllables), or are at the end of a word.

cone	flow
bowl	whole
PR<u>O</u>bate	t<u>oa</u>d
ST<u>O</u>ic	SL<u>OW</u>er
BL<u>OA</u>Ted	reM<u>O</u>TE
beL<u>OW</u> (also end of word)	BELL<u>ow</u> (also end of word)

Be sure to compare and contrast the words "below" and bellow." The second syllable in "below" is stressed and the second syllable in "bellow" is not. However, both words are transcribed with /ou/ because this sound ends both words. In either case, the final phoneme is correspondingly lengthened.

Allographs

Grapheme	Example	Grapheme	Example
o	open	oe	foe
o..e	rose	oh	oh
oa	road	ou	soul
ow	bowl	eau	beau
ew	sew	au	cafe <u>au</u> lait

Discussion   The body of the tongue is in the high-middle portion of the oral cavity during production of /o/ (see Figure 4.11). In many ways this phoneme is similar to the front allophones /e/ and /eɪ/. That is, the stressed form of the vowel is written as the diphthong /ou/ and the unstressed form is written as the monophthong /o/. Therefore, /ou/ and /o/ should be considered allophones of the same phoneme. The production of the diphthong begins with the tongue in position for the onglide /o/, in the mid-back portion of the mouth. The tongue then glides to a higher position for production of the offglide /ʊ/ (see Figure 4.16). Similar to /eɪ/, the diphthong /ou/ is used when transcribing words that end with this sound.

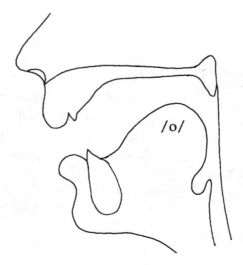

FIGURE 4.11   /o/ articulation.

Practice Exercises

EXERCISE 4.8 — THE VOWEL /o/ - /oʊ/

A. Contrast the vowels in the following minimal pairs.

/oʊ/	/u/	/oʊ/	/ʊ/
grow	grew	coke	cook
slope	sloop	broke	brook
cope	coop	code	could
lobe	lube	hoed	hood
grope	group	showed	should
stowed	stewed	croak	crook

B. Circle the words that contain the /oʊ/ phoneme.

mope	aloof	root	toll
noose	slowed	pond	push
soda	lost	loaded	lasso
nosy	book	sugar	remote
dole	spoke	doily	wholly

C. Circle the phonetic transcriptions that represent English words.

/toʊ/	/boʊn/	/stup/	/prʊb/
/bʊt/	/floʊd/	/boʊd/	/krud/
/stub/	/stud/	/flʊk/	/woʊnt/

D. In the blanks, write each of the words using English orthography.

/moʊld/ _____   /tupeɪ/ _____

/kupt/ _____   /bruzd/ _____

/boʊnɪ/ _____   /bændeɪd/ _____

/ivoʊk/ _____   /kʊkɪ/ _____

/stoʊd/ _____   /koʊɛd/ _____

/doʊpɪ/ _____   /rizum/ _____

E. Indicate whether you should use /o/ or /oʊ/ when transcribing the following words.

____ Romania   ____ snowman

____ corroded   ____ location

____ stolen   ____ jello

____ magnolia   ____ coagulate

/ɔ/

Description

Height:	low-mid
Advancement:	back
Lip rounding:	rounded
Tense/lax:	tense

Sample Words

prawn	thought	vault	wrong
awl	ought	autumn	haul
all	sought	off	gone
cord	frog	hoard	soar

Note: Some speakers may use the phoneme /ɑ/ in the production of some of these words.

Allographs

Grapheme	Example	Grapheme	Example
ou	wrought	o	log
au	laud	a	call
aw	lawn	oa	broad

Discussion   The /ɔ/ vowel is often referred to as "open o." This rounded vowel is produced with the tongue slightly lower in the oral cavity than /o/, in the low-mid position (see Figure 4.12). In addition, it is a tense vowel, and it is found in some individuals' pronunciations of the words "saw," "haul," "caught," and "awl." This vowel is difficult for many students to recognize since it is not produced by all speakers of American English; its use varies considerably with regional dialect. This vowel is prevalent among speakers in the eastern and southern United States. In the Midwest, the western United States, and New England, the production of this phoneme is more variable. Some speakers from these regions use this vowel; others do not.

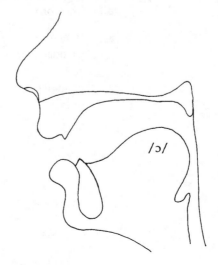

FIGURE 4.12   /ɔ/ articulation.

Speakers who do not use /ɔ/ often replace it with /ɑ/ (to be discussed in the next section).

One use of this vowel is more common in American English. In words like "corn," "bored," and "foreign," it is the r-colored vowel /ɔr/ (or /ɔɚ/) that is used in their transcriptions—that is, /kɔrn/, /bɔrd/, and /fɔrən/. Also, some individuals will pronounce the words "lure" and "tour" as /lɔr/ and /tɔr/, respectively. Some individuals will use /ɔr/ in the production of the word "sure," that is, /ʃɔr/.

Practice Exercises

EXERCISE 4.9—THE VOWEL /ɔ/

A. Circle the phonetic transcriptions that represent possible pronunciations of English words.

/bɔt/	/drʊm/	/stɔn/	/brɔn/
/koʊt/	/grɔn/	/tɔk/	/pʊl/
/lʊps/	/fɔrt/	/flum/	/ɔrn/

B. In the blanks, write each of the words using English orthography.

/spɔrt/	_____	/sprɔl/	_____
/kʊd/	_____	/stʊd/	_____
/proʊb/	_____	/frɔt/	_____
/pruv/	_____	/kɔrps/	_____
/stɔrd/	_____	/hʊkt/	_____
/ɔfʊl/	_____	/doʊnet/	_____

C. Indicate with an X the words that contain the r-colored vowel /ɔr/.

1. ____ farm   4. ____ storm   7. ____ lured
2. ____ third   5. ____ worm   8. ____ worth
3. ____ horrid   6. ____ thorn   9. ____ spar

/ɑ/

Description

Height:	low
Advancement:	back
Lip rounding:	retracted
Tense/lax:	tense

Sample Words

r<u>o</u>tten	<u>o</u>strich	p<u>o</u>sse	cause
f<u>a</u>ther	ap<u>a</u>rt	l<u>a</u>tte	watch
bond	stop	car	pr<u>o</u>blem
plod	bronze	Hans	smart

Note: Some speakers may use the phoneme /ɔ/ in production of some of these sample words.

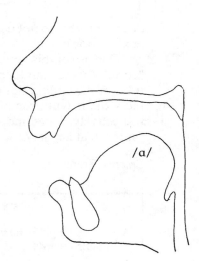

FIGURE 4.13   /ɑ/ articulation.

Allographs

Grapheme	Example	Grapheme	Example
a	shawl	ea(r)	heart
o	rob	e(r)	sergeant
a(r)	mart		

Discussion   /ɑ/ is a point vowel due to the tongue's extremely low, back articulatory position in the oral cavity during its production (see Figure 4.13). It is the only retracted back vowel in English. /ɑ/ is also tense. Due to dialectal variation in pronunciation, some individuals use this vowel instead of /ɔ/, especially in pronunciation of words such as "saw," "haul," "caught," and "awl." The /ɑ/ vowel is most commonly used in combination with /r/ to form the r-colored vowel /ɑr/ (or /ɑɚ/) as in the words "bark" /bɑrk/ and "art" /ɑrt/.

   This vowel is used by some speakers in the South and East in words like "florist" and "horrid," that is /flɑrɪst/ and /hɑrɪd/. Some eastern U.S. speakers use this vowel in words like "dance" /dɑns/ and "pass" /pɑs/.

Practice Exercises

EXERCISE 4.10–THE VOWEL /ɑ/

A. Contrast the vowels in the following words.

/oʊ/	/ɑ/ (or) /ɔ/ (depending on dialect)
boat	bought
bowl	ball
coat	caught
load	laud
sewed	sawed
loan	lawn

Continues

B. Circle the phonetic transcriptions that represent possible pronunciations of English words.

/wɑnd/	/tɔb/	/hɑrm/	/blɑb/
/koʊd/	/sɔt/	/blɑd/	/ɑrmɪ/
/frɔd/	/pʊnt/	/ɑd/	/kɑd/

C. In the blanks, write each of the words using English orthography.

/frɑst/	_____	/zɑr/	_____
/lʊkt/	_____	/prund/	_____
/bɔrd/	_____	/blɔnd/	_____
/kroʊm/	_____	/ɑnsɛt/	_____
/wɑnt/	_____	/krɔdæd/	_____
/stɑrvd/	_____	/ɑrdvɑrk/	_____

D. Indicate with an "X" the words that contain the r-colored vowel /ɑr/.

1. ____ war	5. ____ starred	9. ____ poorly
2. ____ cleared	6. ____ dirt	10. ____ smarter
3. ____ quartz	7. ____ orchard	11. ____ carbon
4. ____ flare	8. ____ March	12. ____ spore

Complete Assignment 4-2.

The Central Vowels

Pronunciation Guide

/ə/	as in "<u>a</u>lone"	/<u>ə</u>loʊn/	(unstressed)
/ʌ/	as in "b<u>u</u>t"	/bʌt/	(stressed)
/ɚ/	as in "p<u>er</u>haps"	/p<u>ɚ</u>hæps/	(unstressed)
/ɝ/	as in "h<u>ear</u>d"	/hɝd/	(stressed)

/ə/

Description

Height:	mid
Advancement:	central
Lip rounding:	retracted
Tense/lax:	lax

Sample Words

<u>a</u>stound	par<u>a</u>d<u>e</u>d	plantat<u>io</u>n	c<u>o</u>mmand
re<u>a</u>rrange	tang<u>e</u>nt	sp<u>u</u>moni	rel<u>e</u>v<u>a</u>nt
roast<u>e</u>d	s<u>a</u>lami	mount<u>ai</u>n	car<u>ou</u>sel
rans<u>o</u>m	ketch<u>u</u>p	tun<u>a</u>	<u>u</u>ndone

Note: /ə/ occurs in unstressed syllables in all of these words.

Allographs

Grapheme	Example	Grapheme	Example
u	<u>u</u>ntrue	ou	jeal<u>ou</u>s
o	c<u>o</u>logne	i	merr<u>i</u>ly
a	m<u>a</u>chine	oi	porp<u>oi</u>se
ai	vill<u>ai</u>n	e	happ<u>e</u>n
ia	parl<u>ia</u>ment	eo	surg<u>eo</u>n
io	nat<u>io</u>n		

Discussion   /ə/ is commonly known as "schwa." Schwa is produced with the tongue body in the most central portion of the mouth cavity. The entire vocal tract is in its most neutral configuration during production of /ə/. It is difficult to discuss this vowel without discussing another vowel concurrently, namely /ʌ/, referred to as *turned v*. These vowels are used to represent allophones of the same sound, even though most phoneticians and clinicians treat them as two separate vowel phonemes. (There *is* actually a slight difference in their place of production in the oral cavity.) The basic distinction between these vowels is that */ə/ occurs only in unstressed syllables* and */ʌ/ occurs only in stressed syllables*. The distribution of these vowels is similar to /e/ and /eɪ/ and /o/ and /oʊ/ in reference to their occurrence in stressed and unstressed syllables:

Stressed	**Unstressed**
eɪ	e
oʊ	o
ʌ	ə

The schwa vowel is retracted because the lips do not protrude in its production. It is also a lax vowel.

Practice Exercises

EXERCISE 4.11–THE VOWEL /ə/

A. Circle the words that contain the /ə/ phoneme.

rowing	decision	control	untamed	laundry
lasagna	injure	glamor	opera	petunia
wooded	poorly	motion	puppy	cockroach
Laverne	ruled	holding	fuchsia	lotion

B. Circle the phonetic transcriptions that represent English words.

/sətɪn/	/zəbrɑ/	/əbeɪt/	/əluf/
/drɑmə/	/ləpʊr/	/bəlun/	/rədæn/
/səpoʊz/	/rəpik/	/brəzɪl/	/əndu/

Continues

C. In the blanks, write each of the words using English orthography.

/pinət/	_____	/kənteɪn/	_____
/əkrɔs/	_____	/lɛmən/	_____
/vəlɔr/	_____	/bətɑn/	_____
/səpɔrt/	_____	/əwɔrd/	_____
/kɔfɪn/	_____	/eɪprəl/	_____
/plətun/	_____	/kəsɛt/	_____

/ʌ/

Description

Height:	low-mid
Advancement:	back-central
Lip rounding:	retracted
Tense/lax:	lax

Sample Words

r<u>u</u>b	b<u>u</u>tton	M<u>o</u>nday	m<u>u</u>stard
tr<u>ou</u>ble	l<u>u</u>ncheon	l<u>u</u>ckily	scr<u>u</u>mptious
fl<u>oo</u>d	und<u>o</u>ne	r<u>u</u>shing	p<u>u</u>blic
ab<u>u</u>ndance	st<u>u</u>mble	red<u>u</u>ndant	w<u>o</u>nderful

Note: /ʌ/ occurs in only the stressed syllables of these words.

Allographs

Grapheme	Example	Grapheme	Example
u	crumb	oe	does
o	done	ou	double
oo	flood		

Discussion   /ʌ/ is the stressed version of schwa (see above). As such, it is found in monosyllabic words and stressed syllables. /ʌ/ is produced slightly lower and farther back in the oral cavity than /ə/ (see Figure 4.14). Like /ə/, /ʌ/ is retracted and lax. Although /ʌ/ can occur in one-syllable words, it does not usually occur in open syllables in English. One exception might be in the production of the word "the," which usually does not receive stress in conversational English.

Students often confuse /ʌ/ with the vowel /ʊ/. Compare the minimal pairs in Exercise 4.12A below that contrast these two phonemes.

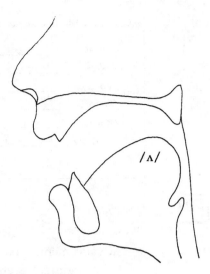

FIGURE 4.14   /ʌ/ articulation.

Practice Exercises

EXERCISE 4.12—THE VOWEL /ʌ/

A. Contrast the vowel /ʌ/ in the following minimal pairs.

/ʌ/	/ʊ/	/ʌ/	/u/	/ʌ/	/ɑ, ɔ/
cud	could	rub	rube	hut	hot
shuck	shook	done	dune	mum	mom
tuck	took	bust	boost	hug	hog
buck	book	dumb	doom	bust	bossed
stud	stood	rum	room	rub	rob
putt	put	spun	spoon	gun	gone
luck	look	glum	gloom	rubbed	robbed

B. Circle the words that contain the /ʌ/ phoneme.

awful	blunder	laundry	Hoover
custard	laborious	Sunday	lawyer
pushy	cushion	hundred	trumpet
cologne	abundant	plural	shouldn't
charades	mundane	wander	conducive

Continues

C. Examine the English words in the first column and the transcriptions in the second column. Place an "X" next to the transcription if it is wrong.

Examples:

| book | /bʊk/ | ____ |
| subbed | /sʊbd/ | X |

1.	hooked	/hʌkt/	____
2.	bond	/bʊnd/	____
3.	bluff	/blʌf/	____
4.	hood	/hud/	____
5.	cluck	/klʌk/	____
6.	rookie	/rʌkɪ/	____
7.	mistook	/mɪstʊk/	____
8.	lucky	/lʌkɪ/	____
9.	rubbing	/rʊbɪŋ/	____
10.	crooked	/krɔkəd/	____

D. Circle the phonetic transcriptions that represent English words.

/klʊstɪ/	/əpʊft/	/dʊkɪ/	/sʌntæn/
/rizən/	/krɑmd/	/pʊlɪ/	/vɪstʌ/
/mʌstɪ/	/əndʌn/	/plʌmət/	/plæzə/

E. In the blanks, write each of the words using English orthography.

/pɛrəs/	_____	/robʌst/	_____
/hʌnɪ/	_____	/sʌdən/	_____
/əlɑt/	_____	/kəbus/	_____
/kənvɪns/	_____	/tʌndrə/	_____
/gɑrdəd/	_____	/kəlæps/	_____
/flʌbd/	_____	/bəfun/	_____

F. Indicate whether /ʌ/ or /ə/ should be used in transcribing the following words by circling the appropriate symbol.

lumber	/ʌ/	/ə/		suspend	/ʌ/	/ə/
abort	/ʌ/	/ə/		suppose	/ʌ/	/ə/
shaken	/ʌ/	/ə/		induct	/ʌ/	/ə/
contain	/ʌ/	/ə/		serpent	/ʌ/	/ə/
thunder	/ʌ/	/ə/		rusty	/ʌ/	/ə/

G. Indicate with an "X" the following pairs of words that share the same vowel phoneme.

____	1.	nuts	could		____	6.	crook	fund
____	2.	foot	stoop		____	7.	blood	crust
____	3.	done	rubbed		____	8.	runs	floods
____	4.	crumb	rust		____	9.	loom	food
____	5.	cook	should		____	10.	rush	look

/ɚ/

Description

Height:	mid
Advancement:	central
Lip rounding:	rounded
Tense/lax:	lax

Sample Words

pertain	luxury	cursor*	percussion
surround	treasure	flirtatious	mattered
runner	under	countered	Herbert*
ergonomic	ferocious	Saturday	harbor

*Note: /ɚ/ occurs only in the unstressed syllables in the sample words above. (The words "Herbert" and "cursor" have stress on the first syllable and would use the phoneme /ɝ/—for example, /hɝbɚt/ and /kɝsɚ/.)

Allographs

Grapheme	Example	Grapheme	Example
or	labor	er	winner
ar	lunar	ir	flirtatious
ur	urbane	yr	martyr

Discussion   /ɚ/ is referred to as "schwar" because the phonetic symbol visually resembles schwa, but in addition, reflects the auditory quality known as **rhotacization**, or r-coloring, of the phoneme. The term rhotacization simply means that /ɚ/ has an "r" quality (or "r" sound) associated with it. /ɚ/ is not easily defined by referring only to the four categories used previously to describe the other English vowels—that is, height, advancement, lip rounding, and tense/lax. Production of schwar involves additional tongue movement and is formed either by: (1) raising the tongue tip, and curling it posteriorly toward the alveolar ridge or (2) lowering the tongue tip while bunching the tongue body in the region of the palate (Ladefoged, 2001; MacKay, 1987). In either case, the associated "r" quality is due to a constriction in the pharynx brought about by retraction of the portion of the tongue below the epiglottis (Ladefoged, 2001).

Like schwa, /ɚ/ is produced only in unstressed syllables. Therefore, it is lax. One distinguishing feature of schwar is that it is produced with lip rounding. The degree of lip rounding varies from speaker to speaker. (Some phoneticians argue that this vowel is retracted.) The tense version of this vowel, /ɝ/, is found only in stressed syllables (see the next section). We now can add these two phonemes to the table of stressed and unstressed vowel allophones:

Stressed	*Unstressed*
eɪ	e
oʊ	o
ʌ	ə
ɝ	ɚ

Note: Words such as "ring" and "raisin" begin with the phoneme /r/, *not* with the phoneme /ɚ/.

Practice Exercises

EXERCISE 4.13 — THE VOWEL /ɚ/

A. Contrast the underlined sounds in the words below.

/ɚ/	/r/	/r/-colored vowels
slumb<u>er</u>	<u>dr</u>ess	quee<u>r</u>
p<u>er</u>use	<u>r</u>ibbon	me<u>re</u>
ov<u>er</u>	<u>cr</u>eam	sna<u>re</u>
stup<u>or</u>	<u>thr</u>ead	chai<u>r</u>
walk<u>er</u>	<u>fr</u>ost	sto<u>red</u>
must<u>ard</u>	a<u>r</u>ound	floo<u>r</u>

B. Circle the words that contain the /ɚ/ phoneme.

clover	rebel	barley	dearly
fearless	endear	perjure	fester
carbon	torment	harbor	electric
tremor	written	poorly	breezy
laundered	perhaps	torpedo	surprise

C. Circle the phonetic transcriptions that represent English words.

/kɑnvɚt/	/pɚteɪn/	/pɚsɛnt/	/lɛpɚd/
/rɑbɚ/	/tɚoud/	/drimɚ/	/fɚɚst/
/sɚvɛs/	/ɚɛdɪ/	/ʌnfɛr/	/hɪndɚ/

D. In the blanks, write each of the words using English orthography.

/drɛsɚ/ _____		/kɚntɔrt/ _____
/kæmrɚ/ _____		/pɚɑnɚ/ _____
/rʌbɚ/ _____		/pɚu/ _____
/mɑrbəl/ _____		/sɪmɚ/ _____
/tɚeɪn/ _____		/kɛrosin/ _____
/flʌstɚd/ _____		/ɚweɪtɚd/ _____

/ɝ/

Description

Height:	mid
Advancement:	central
Lip rounding:	rounded
Tense/lax:	tense

Sample Words

<u>c</u>urse	thi<u>r</u>d	Thu<u>r</u>sday	mu<u>r</u>der*
det<u>er</u>	<u>s</u>u<u>r</u>geon	w<u>orr</u>y	reve<u>r</u>se
rehea<u>r</u>se	pu<u>r</u>ple	thi<u>r</u>sty	nu<u>r</u>sery
f<u>ur</u>nace	s<u>er</u>vice	pe<u>r</u>colate	ave<u>r</u>sion

Note: The word "murder" would be transcribed as /mɝdɚ/.

Allographs

Grapheme	Example	Grapheme	Example
or	word	ir	shirt
ear	learn	ur	curt
er	perk	yr	Myrtle

Discussion   The stressed schwar, /ɝ/, is the partner of /ɚ/. This vowel is produced in a manner similar to /ɚ/ with the lips rounded, although the degree of rounding varies among speakers (see Figure 4.15). (Like schwa, this vowel is considered retracted by some phoneticians.) Stressed schwar is the only central vowel that is considered to be tense. It is found at the end of the one-syllable words "her," "stir," and "fur," and for some speakers "sure." Keep in mind that /ɝ/ occurs in only the stressed syllables of the sample words provided above.

Stressed schwar is often confused with the rhotic diphthongs, previously introduced in this chapter. Especially confusing are /ɝ/ versus /ɪr/ and /ɛr/. Examine the following word combinations, paying close attention to the distinction between /ɝ/ and the rhotic diphthongs. Each of the words in the left column contain a different rhotic diphthong. All of the words in the right column contain /ɝ/. Say each word pair (i.e., fear-fur; hair-her, etc.) listening to the differences between the rhotic diphthongs and schwar. Also, be sure to look at Exercise 4.14A.

		/ɝ/			/ɝ/
/ɪr/	fear	— fur	/ɪr/	beer	— burr
/ɛr/	hair	— her	/ɛr/	spare	— spur
/ɑr/	star	— stir	/ɑr/	shark	— shirk
/ɔr/	court	— curt	/ɔr/	ward	— word
/ʊr/	tour	— tur(n)	/ʊr/	lure	— lear(n)

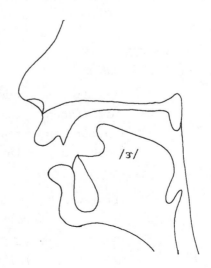

FIGURE 4.15   /ɝ/ articulation.

Practice Exercises

EXERCISE 4.14—THE VOWEL /ɝ/

A. Contrast the vowel /ɝ/ with the rhotic diphthongs in the following minimal contrasts.

/ɝ/	/ɑr/	/ɔr/	/ɪr/	/ɛr/
stir	star	store	steer	stare
purr	par	pore	peer	pair
fur	far	for	fear	fair
burr	bar	bore	beer	bare
myrrh	mar	more	mere	mare

B. Circle the words that contain the /ɝ/ phoneme.

forward	muster	warship	steered	morale
disturbed	pretend	wordy	distort	persistent
terrible	turban	January	conserve	choir
conversion	arid	stirrup	barren	fearless

C. Circle the phonetic transcriptions that represent English words.

/kʌstəd/	/lɝdɪ/	/kərɪr/	/vɝsəz/
/pɝsən/	/hɝdəd/	/fɝmɚ/	/dɝsənt/
/plædɝ/	/fɔrən/	/ɝbɔrt/	/kɝsɚ/

D. In the blanks, write each of the words using English orthography.

/smɝkt/	_____	/kənvɝt/	_____
/ovɝt/	_____	/wɪspɚ/	_____
/kɛrət/	_____	/bɝbən/	_____
/sʌbɚb/	_____	/skwɝəl/	_____
/supɝb/	_____	/səhɛrə/	_____

E. Indicate whether /ɝ/ or /ɚ/ should be used in transcribing the following words by circling the appropriate symbol.

erasure	/ɝ/	/ɚ/	ermine	/ɝ/	/ɚ/
surprise	/ɝ/	/ɚ/	color	/ɝ/	/ɚ/
furnace	/ɝ/	/ɚ/	infer	/ɝ/	/ɚ/
curtail	/ɝ/	/ɚ/	terror	/ɝ/	/ɚ/
immerse	/ɝ/	/ɚ/	duster	/ɝ/	/ɚ/

Continues

EXERCISE 4.14 (*cont.*)

F. Indicate with an "X" the pairs of words that share the same vowel phoneme.

_____ 1. herd   cheered   _____ 6. hair   queer

_____ 2. cord   word   _____ 7. birch   lurk

_____ 3. lured   stored   _____ 8. hoard   lord

_____ 4. ark   smart   _____ 9. pear   heard

_____ 5. fears   cheer   _____ 10. term   peered

G. For the following, indicate whether the word contains a rhotic diphthong or the stressed schwar (in any syllable) by placing the correct symbol in the blank.

Examples:

/ɪr/   cheer   /ɝ/   stir

_____ 1. mirth   _____ 11. appearance

_____ 2. flared   _____ 12. Carol

_____ 3. cirrus   _____ 13. furtive

_____ 4. serenade   _____ 14. larynx

_____ 5. Merlin   _____ 15. experience

_____ 6. cherub   _____ 16. disturbing

_____ 7. portion   _____ 17. clearance

_____ 8. farming   _____ 18. nervous

_____ 9. sparrow   _____ 19. furious

_____ 10. nervous   _____ 20. clairvoyant

Complete Assignment 4-3.

More on Diphthongs

The diphthongs /eɪ/ and /oʊ/ were discussed earlier in conjunction with the /e/ and /o/ vowels, respectively. In English, there are three additional diphthong phonemes that do not exist in a monophthongal form. These three diphthongs are /aɪ/ as in "kite," /aʊ/ as in "loud," and /ɔɪ/ as in "void."

There is considerable variation in the symbols use to transcribe these three diphthongs. This is due to the fact that the exact articulation of these phonemes varies by dialect and by phonetic context. Similar to /eɪ/ and /oʊ/, these diphthongs should be thought of as having two distinctive articulations. That is, there is a gliding of the tongue from the first articulatory position (the onglide) to the second position (the offglide); the exact starting and ending position varies from speaker to speaker. The one commonality among all of the diphthongs (including /eɪ/ and /oʊ/) is the fact that the tongue always glides from a lower to a higher position in the oral cavity (see Figure 4.16). The symbols cho-

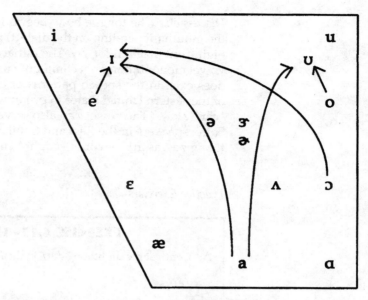

FIGURE 4.16 Onglide and offglide positions for the diphthongs /eɪ/, /oʊ/, /aɪ/, /ɔɪ/, and /aʊ/ (in reference to the traditional vowel quadrilateral).

sen for this text to represent the three diphthongs are the ones most often adopted by most phonetics texts. They also represent a fairly close approximation of the actual articulation of these sounds.

Pronunciation Guide

/aɪ/	as in "buy"	/baɪ/
/aʊ/	as in "bough"	/baʊ/
/ɔɪ/	as in "boy"	/bɔɪ/

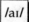

Description

Sample Words

lye	ice
fiber	light
thyme	tie
buy	feisty

Allographs

Grapheme	Example	Grapheme	Example
i..e	write	uy	buy
i	sigh	ie	tried
ai	aisle	ei	height
ae	maestro	ey	eye
y	my	ay	aye

Discussion   The tongue body begins in the low central or low back portion of the mouth (depending on the dialect) in the production of /a/ and glides to the high front position for /ɪ/. The initial phoneme in this diphthong represents a vowel monophthong not commonly used by all speakers in the United States. It does exist in the speech patterns of individuals from Boston and other areas of the eastern United States in pronunciation of words such as "park" /pak/ or "car" /ka/. (The vowel /a/ also serves as the onglide in the diphthong /aʊ/.) Some speakers in the East and South produce this diphthong as the monophthong /a/ as in the words "might" /mat/ and "ice" /as/.

Practice Exercises

EXERCISE 4.15—THE DIPHTHONG /aɪ/

A. Contrast the diphthong /aɪ/ in the following minimal pairs.

/aɪ/	/ɪ/	/eɪ/
kite	kit	Kate
height	hit	hate
sight	sit	sate
wind (verb)	wind (noun)	waned
lime	limb	lame
style	still	stale
tyke	tick	take

B. Circle the words that contain the /aɪ/ phoneme.

power	spacious	machine	replaced
slice	delicious	formica	traded
contrite	spider	maybe	piped
lever	Cairo	cider	supplied
rivalry	razor	piano	spigot

C. Circle the phonetic transcriptions that represent English words.

/fraɪdeɪ/	/braɪmɚ/	/taɪfraɪn/	/rəvaɪz/
/məbaɪ/	/naɪlɔn/	/prədaɪt/	/traɪdɛnt/
/traɪd/	/laɪɚ/	/haɪəst/	/straɪpt/

D. In the blanks, write each of the words using English orthography.

/səpraɪz/	_____	/klaɪmæks/	_____
/kəlaɪd/	_____	/preɪlin/	_____
/treɪlɚ/	_____	/baɪsɛps/	_____
/praɪmet/	_____	/waɪəd/	_____
/vaɪrəs/	_____	/taɪred/	_____
/deɪlaɪt/	_____	/daɪmənd/	_____

/ɔɪ/

Description

Sample Words

toy	join	ah<u>oy</u>	flamb<u>oy</u>ant
expl<u>oi</u>t	b<u>oi</u>sterous	f<u>oi</u>ble	c<u>oi</u>ned

Allographs

Grapheme	**Example**
oy	soy
oi	foil

Discussion The tongue body begins in the low-mid back position of the mouth (for /ɔ/) and glides to a high front position (for /ɪ/). When initiating this diphthong, the lips are rounded. As the tongue glides upward in the oral cavity towards the offglide portion, the lips become retracted. In the East and South, some speakers will produce this diphthong as the monophthong /ɔ/, as in "oil" /ɔl/ and "soil" /sɔl/.

Practice Exercises

EXERCISE 4.16—THE DIPHTHONG /ɔɪ/

A. Contrast the diphthong /ɔɪ/ in the following minimal pairs.

/ɔɪ/	/aɪ/	/eɪ/
Boyd	bide	bade
soy	sigh	say
coil	Kyle	kale
hoist	heist	haste
loin	line	lane
boys	buys	bays
poise	pies	pays

B. Circle the words that contain the /ɔɪ/ phoneme.

repay	hoisted	voiceless	reward
loiter	crowded	fiery	tiled
straight	feisty	coy	cloying
crime	broiler	stoic	destroy
goiter	razor	avoid	supplied

C. Circle the phonetic transcriptions that represent English words.

/kwaɪət/	/sprɔɪdɪn/	/dɔɪəz/	/plɔɪdənt/
/mɝdɚ/	/blaɪndlɪ/	/ənstraɪt/	/taɪpsɛt/
/pɔɪzən/	/vɔɪdəd/	/rikɔɪld/	/taɪwɑn/

Continues

EXERCISE 4.16 (*cont.*)

D. In the blanks, write each of the words using English orthography.

/ɔɪlɪ/ _____   /ændrɔɪd/ _____

/maɪstroʊ/ _____   /laɪvlɪ/ _____

/taɪfɔɪd/ _____   /ɪnvɔɪs/ _____

/pɑrbɔɪl/ _____   /ɔɪstɚ/ _____

/haɪndsaɪt/ _____   /haɪɔɪd/ _____

/baɪaʊt/ _____   /deɪlaɪt/ _____

/aʊ/

Description

Sample Words

loud	s<u>our</u>
clown	tr<u>ou</u>sers
ar<u>ou</u>nd	p<u>ow</u>der
fl<u>ow</u>er	r<u>ou</u>sed

Allographs

Grapheme	Example
ou	house
ow	cow

Discussion   The tongue begins in the low back position of the mouth for the onglide /a/ and glides upward to the high back position for the production of the offglide /ʊ/. When initiating this diphthong, the lips are retracted. As the glide progresses towards the second component, the lips become rounded.

Practice Exercises

EXERCISE 4.17—THE DIPHTHONG /aʊ/

A. Contrast the diphthong /aʊ/ in the following minimal pairs.

/aʊ/	/oʊ/	/aɪ/	/ɔɪ/
bough	bow	buy	boy
sow	sew	sigh	soy
cowl	coal	Kyle	coil
row (fight)	row	rye	Roy
towel	toll	tile	toil
fowls	foals	files	foils

Continues

EXERCISE 4.17 (*cont.*)

B. Circle the words that contain the /aʊ/ phoneme.

toilet	dowdy	frown	bounty
mousy	allowed	loaded	probate
beauty	explode	soils	proud
astound	toil	chowder	crowbar
hello	toad	chastise	scrolled

C. Circle the phonetic transcriptions that represent English words.

/taɪəd/	/laʊzɪ/	/aɪvrɪ/	/hoʊmbɔɪ/
/rɪbaʊ/	/blaʊkɚ/	/rɔɪdɪ/	/kaʊtaʊ/
/waʊntɪd/	/roʊgbɪ/	/pauzɚ/	/aʊəlɪ/

D. In the blanks, write each of the words using English orthography.

/bɔɪfrɛnd/ _____   /roʊboʊt/ _____

/klɑndaɪk/ _____   /pɪspaɪp/ _____

/daʊntaʊn/ _____   /sɚaʊnd/ _____

/sloʊɚ/ _____   /doʊnʌt/ _____

/faʊndəd/ _____   /klaɪənt/ _____

/vaɪzɚ/ _____   /braʊzɚ/ _____

Complete Assignment 4-4.

Review Exercises

A. Describe each of the following vowels by providing their tongue height, tongue advancement, lip rounding, and tense/lax characteristics.

	Height	Advancement	Rounded	Tense/Lax
i	high	front	no	tense
ʊ				
ɝ				
ə				
o				
u				
ɛ				
ɚ				
ʌ				
e				
ɪ				
ɑ				
ɔ				
æ				

B. For the following items, fill in the blank with the appropriate vowels from the description given. Then write the word in English orthography.

Example:

/m i̲ t/	high, front, tense vowel	_____meat_____

1. /b__d/	low, front	_____
2. /s__n/	low-mid, back-central	_____
3. /sl__pt/	low-mid, front	_____
4. /s__p/	high, back, tense	_____
5. /k__rd/	low-mid, back	_____
6. /f__t/	high, back, lax	_____
7. /f__z/	high, front, lax	_____
8. /p__rk/	low, back	_____
9. /w__d/	mid-central, tense	_____
10. /kr__z/	high-mid, back	_____

C. For each of the the following two-syllable words, indicate whether each vowel is tense (T) or lax (L).

   Example:

        lasso   <u>L</u>   <u>T</u>

   1. Sunday   ____   ____   6. concern   ____   ____
   2. bashful   ____   ____   7. regroup   ____   ____
   3. laundry   ____   ____   8. obese   ____   ____
   4. confused   ____   ____   9. layette   ____   ____
   5. fender   ____   ____   10. abrupt   ____   ____

D. For the following two-syllable words, indicate whether each vowel is rounded (R) or unrounded (U).

   Example:

        lasso   <u>U</u>   <u>R</u>

   1. foolish   ____   ____   6. Pluto   ____   ____
   2. curfew   ____   ____   7. person   ____   ____
   3. decade   ____   ____   8. pursuit   ____   ____
   4. collate   ____   ____   9. rugby   ____   ____
   5. football   ____   ____   10. lower   ____   ____

E. Transcription Practice—Front Vowels

   Use the correct IPA symbol(s) (i, ɪ, e, eɪ, ɛ, æ) for each of the front vowels in the following words.

   ____ 1. straight   ____ ____ 11. empty
   ____ 2. bees   ____ ____ 12. rabies
   ____ 3. bread   ____ ____ 13. instead
   ____ 4. can   ____ ____ 14. stampede
   ____ 5. filled   ____ ____ 15. vacate
   ____ 6. bring   ____ ____ 16. pleasing
   ____ 7. lapse   ____ ____ 17. transit
   ____ 8. sang   ____ ____ 18. beer can
   ____ 9. fair   ____ ____ 19. implant
   ____ 10. mean   ____ ____ 20. barely

F. Transcription Practice—Back Vowels

   Use the correct IPA symbol(s) (u, ʊ, o, oʊ, ɔ, ɑ) for each of the back vowels in the following words.

   ____ 1. moat   ____ ____ 11. awful
   ____ 2. push   ____ ____ 12. Clorox
   ____ 3. laud   ____ ____ 13. loco
   ____ 4. locks   ____ ____ 14. oboe
   ____ 5. crude   ____ ____ 15. taco
   ____ 6. chose   ____ ____ 16. monarch
   ____ 7. raw   ____ ____ 17. popcorn
   ____ 8. lure   ____ ____ 18. truthful
   ____ 9. sword   ____ ____ 19. costume
   ____ 10. card   ____ ____ 20. crouton

G. Transcription Practice—Central Vowels

Use the correct IPA symbol(s) (ə, ʌ, ɚ, ɝ) for each of the central vowels in the following words.

___ ___	1. certain	___ ___ 11. purpose
___ ___	2. rusted	___ ___ 12. sudden
___ ___	3. perturb	___ ___ 13. luster
___ ___	4. assert	___ ___ 14. purchase
___ ___	5. upper	___ ___ 15. sherbet
___ ___	6. merger	___ ___ 16. mother
___ ___	7. clutter	___ ___ 17. converge
___ ___	8. verbal	___ ___ 18. herder
___ ___	9. traverse	___ ___ 19. worded
___ ___	10. learner	___ ___ 20. mustard

H. Diphthong Practice

Some of the following words have the wrong diphthong/vowel symbol in their transcriptions. If there is an error, write the correct symbol in the blank.

1. word	/wɝd/	_____	16. maestro	/maɪstroʊ/	_____
2. lard	/lɔrd/	_____	17. flour	/floʊɚ/	_____
3. carp	/kɝp/	_____	18. pouring	/pɔrɪŋ/	_____
4. war	/wɑr/	_____	19. liar	/laɪɚ/	_____
5. mere	/mɪr/	_____	20. appear	/əpɛr/	_____
6. wide	/weɪd/	_____	21. tighter	/taɪtɝ/	_____
7. curd	/kʊrd/	_____	22. parrot	/pɝət/	_____
8. stay	/steɪ/	_____	23. corner	/kɔrnɚ/	_____
9. pray	/praɪ/	_____	24. oyster	/ɔɪstɛr/	_____
10. crow	/kraʊ/	_____	25. squarely	/skwɛrlɪ/	_____
11. coin	/kɔɪn/	_____	26. silence	/sɪləns/	_____
12. pride	/praɪd/	_____	27. smarter	/smɔrtɚ/	_____
13. firm	/fɪrm/	_____	28. avoid	/əvaɪd/	_____
14. tour	/tʊr/	_____	29. prowess	/prowəs/	_____
15. fair	/fɛr/	_____	30. license	/leɪsəns/	_____

I. Using /ɝ/ and the rhotic diphthongs listed below, create as many meaningful English words as possible for each of the following items.

/ɪr, ʊr, ɔr, ɑr, ɛr, ɝ/

Example:

b _____   beer, boor, bore, bar, bear, burr _____

1. p _____   _____
2. r _____   _____
3. d _____ t   _____
4. w_____ d   _____
5. k _____ d   _____

J. Using the vowels listed below, create as many meaningful English words as possible for each of the following items.

/i, ɪ, eɪ, ɛ, æ, u, ʊ, oʊ, ɔ, ɑ, ɝ, ʌ/

Example:

    _____ z   ease, is, as, ooze, owes, awes, Oz

1.   _____ d
2.   _____ n
3. l _____ st
4. sk _____ n
5. st _____ d
6. b _____ rd
7. t _____ nt
8. s _____ t
9. r _____ t
10. r _____ bd
11. sp _____ t
12. w _____ d

K. Write each of the following transcribed words in English orthography.

1. /kʌstəmz/ _____
2. /əbaʊnd/ _____
3. /twɔrd/ _____
4. /slɛndɚ/ _____
5. /kɛrfri/ _____
6. /veɪkənt/ _____
7. /bʌntəd/ _____
8. /klaʊdɪ/ _____
9. /steɪplɚ/ _____
10. /kəntɔrt/ _____
11. /saɪrənz/ _____
12. /klɔɪstəd/ _____
13. /ohaɪoʊ/ _____
14. /reɪdɪoʊ/ _____
15. /kɚoʊsɪv/ _____
16. /plətɑnək/ _____
17. /rɛzənet/ _____
18. /daɪgrɛs/ _____
19. /saɪfənd/ _____
20. /ɑrkənsɔ/ _____
21. /wʌndɚful/ _____
22. /kæləndɚ/ _____

23. /rimɔrsfʊl/ _____

24. /stupɛndəs/ _____

25. /læksətɪv/ _____

26. /sɪnsɪrlɪ/ _____

27. /kɑləndɚ/ _____

28. /rezənɛts/ _____

29. /bɛrəton/ _____

30. /disɛmbɚ/ _____

31. /mɛksɪkoʊ/ _____

32. /kwægmaɪɚ/ _____

33. /ɔrdəlɪ/ _____

34. /hɝbəsaɪd/ _____

35. /rəpʌlsɪv/ _____

36. /kɛrəktɚ/ _____

37. /sæsəfræs/ _____

38. /zaɪləfon/ _____

39. /kwɑrtɚbæk/ _____

40. /ɛmbɛrəst/ _____

L. Transcription Practice—Front, Back, and Central Vowels

Use the correct IPA symbol(s) for each of the vowels in the following words.

____ ____	1. epic	____ ____	21. inkling
____ ____	2. faster	____ ____	22. Fairbanks
____ ____	3. wonder	____ ____	23. car pool
____ ____	4. octet	____ ____	24. machine
____ ____	5. woolen	____ ____	25. Athens
____ ____	6. depot	____ ____	26. autumn
____ ____	7. soldier	____ ____	27. rebus
____ ____	8. itchy	____ ____	28. torment
____ ____	9. worship	____ ____	29. utter
____ ____	10. palace	____ ____	30. bushel
____ ____	11. barely	____ ____	31. corner
____ ____	12. nation	____ ____	32. quandary
____ ____	13. genius	____ ____	33. aster
____ ____	14. cupboard	____ ____	34. phone booth
____ ____	15. cartoon	____ ____	35. turban
____ ____	16. nasty	____ ____	36. key case
____ ____	17. fearless	____ ____	37. boarder
____ ____	18. number	____ ____	38. blaring
____ ____	19. sanction	____ ____	39. strangle
____ ____	20. ocean	____ ____	40. awesome

M. Transcribe the vowels in the following words.

___ ___	1. broiler	___ ___ 16. gender
___ ___	2. mousetrap	___ ___ 17. China
___ ___	3. boardwalk	___ ___ 18. jaundiced
___ ___	4. closure	___ ___ 19. turquoise
___ ___	5. nylons	___ ___ 20. invoice
___ ___	6. steroid	___ ___ 21. financed
___ ___	7. starstruck	___ ___ 22. merchant
___ ___	8. regime	___ ___ 23. proclaim
___ ___	9. bashful	___ ___ 24. probate
___ ___	10. perjure	___ ___ 25. July
___ ___	11. spearmint	___ ___ 26. martian
___ ___	12. lightbulb	___ ___ 27. future
___ ___	13. destroy	___ ___ 28. prospect
___ ___	14. banquet	___ ___ 29. product
___ ___	15. eyesore	___ ___ 30. tofu

Study Questions

1. What is the vowel quadrilateral and what is its importance in the study of phonetics?

2. Which vowels in English are tense? Which ones are lax? How does your understanding of syllables help in understanding the use of tense and lax vowels in English?

3. How are vowels produced in the vocal tract?

4. Which vowels in English are rounded? Which ones are retracted?

5. What is a point vowel? List the English point vowels.

6. Why isn't the final sound in the word "lucky" transcribed with /i/?

7. Define the terms onglide and offglide.

8. Which vowels in English are affected by syllable stress?

9. What is the difference between a monophthong and a diphthong?

10. What is the relationship between tongue movement and pharyngeal shape during vowel production?

Assignment 4-1
Front Vowels

Name _____

Transcribe the front vowels in the following words.

_____ 1. cramp	_____ _____ 21. bandaid
_____ 2. stared	_____ _____ 22. headband
_____ 3. each	_____ _____ 23. keychain
_____ 4. spleen	_____ _____ 24. cheery
_____ 5. skim	_____ _____ 25. barely
_____ 6. bless	_____ _____ 26. pin head
_____ 7. mist	_____ _____ 27. revamp
_____ 8. trapped	_____ _____ 28. cherry
_____ 9. fears	_____ _____ 29. invest
_____ 10. axe	_____ _____ 30. chin strap
_____ _____ 11. impasse	_____ _____ 31. welfare
_____ _____ 12. hearsay	_____ _____ 32. immense
_____ _____ 13. eclipse	_____ _____ 33. farewell
_____ _____ 14. cheesecake	_____ _____ 34. baby
_____ _____ 15. skinflint	_____ _____ 35. filly
_____ _____ 16. banish	_____ _____ 36. bareback
_____ _____ 17. Sinbad	_____ _____ 37. staircase
_____ _____ 18. herring	_____ _____ 38. bereft
_____ _____ 19. reindeer	_____ _____ 39. playpen
_____ _____ 20. kinship	_____ _____ 40. eggplant

Assignment 4-2
Front and Back Vowels

Name

Transcribe the front and back vowels in the following words.

____ 1. feud	____ ____ 21. arrow
____ 2. bull	____ ____ 22. borax
____ 3. spore	____ ____ 23. faux pas
____ 4. rocks	____ ____ 24. forceps
____ 5. strew	____ ____ 25. footstool
____ 6. rook	____ ____ 26. boorish
____ 7. lost	____ ____ 27. Fargo
____ 8. bog	____ ____ 28. ballroom
____ 9. oats	____ ____ 29. romance
____ 10. crone	____ ____ 30. offshoot
____ ____ 11. carpool	____ ____ 31. meatballs
____ ____ 12. wrongful	____ ____ 32. jaw bone
____ ____ 13. pseudo	____ ____ 33. awning
____ ____ 14. oxbow	____ ____ 34. inkblot
____ ____ 15. doorknob	____ ____ 35. romaine
____ ____ 16. careful	____ ____ 36. armhole
____ ____ 17. bookshelf	____ ____ 37. hardware
____ ____ 18. bootleg	____ ____ 38. previewed
____ ____ 19. bamboo	____ ____ 39. artful
____ ____ 20. barnyard	____ ____ 40. airborne

Assignment 4-3
Front, Back, and Central Vowels

Name _____

Transcribe the front, back, and central vowels in the following words.

____ ____ 1. bedbug

____ ____ 2. revered

____ ____ 3. yogurt

____ ____ 4. yuppie

____ ____ 5. virtue

____ ____ 6. uproar

____ ____ 7. tortoise

____ ____ 8. performed

____ ____ 9. tether

____ ____ 10. terror

____ ____ 11. suburb

____ ____ 12. soldier

____ ____ 13. quasar

____ ____ 14. circus

____ ____ 15. gumdrop

____ ____ 16. ogre

____ ____ 17. gorgeous

____ ____ 18. mirthful

____ ____ 19. luggage

____ ____ 20. frontier

____ ____ 21. placard

____ ____ 22. opposed

____ ____ 23. hurrah

____ ____ 24. ferment

____ ____ 25. drunkard

____ ____ 26. govern

____ ____ 27. pewter

____ ____ 28. bonus

____ ____ 29. arrest

____ ____ 30. pungent

____ ____ 31. Thursday

____ ____ 32. parcel

____ ____ 33. goulash

____ ____ 34. cupcake

____ ____ 35. gleeful

____ ____ 36. morale

____ ____ 37. golfer

____ ____ 38. footage

____ ____ 39. exhaust

____ ____ 40. drama

____ ____ 41. conceit

____ ____ 42. teardrop

____ ____ 43. slogan

____ ____ 44. secrete

____ ____ 45. proclaim

____ ____ 46. dormant

____ ____ 47. bunker

____ ____ 48. acute

____ ____ 49. hundred

____ ____ 50. cedar

Assignment 4-4
Vowel/Diphthong Review

Name _____

Transcribe all of the vowels and diphthongs in the following words.

____ ____	1. corker	____ ____ 26. bauxite
____ ____	2. irate	____ ____ 27. crackdown
____ ____	3. absurd	____ ____ 28. perturb
____ ____	4. bagpipe	____ ____ 29. highbrow
____ ____	5. Boise	____ ____ 30. playwear
____ ____	6. clubhouse	____ ____ 31. poem
____ ____	7. bullfrog	____ ____ 32. ion
____ ____	8. conjoin	____ ____ 33. proclaim
____ ____	9. commute	____ ____ 34. beehive
____ ____	10. grotto	____ ____ 35. procure
____ ____	11. errand	____ ____ 36. import
____ ____	12. fervor	____ ____ 37. punster
____ ____	13. birthright	____ ____ 38. carbide
____ ____	14. jousting	____ ____ 39. toystore
____ ____	15. deltoid	____ ____ 40. outlaw
____ ____	16. discount	____ ____ 41. unfair
____ ____	17. honor	____ ____ 42. employed
____ ____	18. inform	____ ____ 43. icebox
____ ____	19. mastoid	____ ____ 44. x-ray
____ ____	20. oblique	____ ____ 45. furtive
____ ____	21. outbreak	____ ____ 46. eyesore
____ ____	22. goiter	____ ____ 47. blowtorch
____ ____	23. bloodshot	____ ____ 48. ozone
____ ____	24. parsnip	____ ____ 49. suburb
____ ____	25. downward	____ ____ 50. voiceless

CHAPTER

5

Consonant Transcription

What Is a Consonant?

Although this seems like a simple question, unfortunately the answer is not so simple. The term **consonant** can be defined in several ways. It is possible to define consonants in terms of the letters used to represent them or by the way they are formed by the articulators. Consonants also can be defined in terms of their particular role in the structure of syllables, or by their acoustic and physical properties. To best answer the question *"What is a consonant?"* we need to consider all of these issues.

We already know that there are many more consonant letters in the Roman alphabet than vowels. Likewise, there are more consonant than vowel phonemes. In the last chapter, we learned that there are 14 vowel phonemes in English plus the 3 phonemic diphthongs. In this chapter, 24 consonant phonemes will be introduced. As you are aware, the IPA symbols for the consonants are well represented by the letters of the Roman alphabet. There are only a few new symbols to learn in order to transcribe English consonants. In this respect, consonant transcription is easier to learn than vowel transcription. In addition to the 24 consonant phonemes, some of the more common allophonic variations of some of the consonants will be discussed.

Vowels versus Consonants

In terms of production, vowels and consonants vary considerably. Unlike vowels, consonants are not produced solely by changes in tongue and lip positioning. Consonants are produced by vocal tract constrictions that modify the breath stream coming from the larynx. Consonant production generally involves the coming together of two articulators to modify the flow of air as it passes through the oral and/or nasal cavities. The tongue, the primary articulator in production of consonants, often makes contact with other articulators to form most of the English consonants. In addition, there are several consonants that do not utilize the tongue in their production, for example, /h/, /b/, and /f/.

Another way in which vowels and consonants vary is in relation to where the sound generator (or sound source) is located during their production. The sound source for all of the vowels is at the level of the vocal folds. That is, for vowel production, the breath stream coming from the larynx is voiced (with the vocal folds vibrating). As you recall, changes in lip and tongue position cause alterations in the resonant frequencies of the vocal tract, giving each vowel its characteristic quality. Similar to the vowels, the **resonant consonants**, or simply *resonants*, are produced with resonance occurring throughout the entire vocal tract. The resonant consonants include the nasals, the liquids, and the glides, all of which are voiced. Refer to Table 5.1 for a classification of all the English consonants.

The sound source for several consonants, however, is not in the larynx. For some consonants, the sound source is the noise (or turbulence) created at the point of constriction in the oral cavity, formed by the articulators, as air flows through the supralaryngeal system. Consonants produced in this manner are called **nonresonant consonants**, or **obstruents** (because the airflow is obstructed during their articulation). Obstruents include the stop, fricative, and affricate consonants. In the production of obstruents, resonance does not occur throughout the entire vocal tract, as it does for the vowels and the resonant consonants. Instead, resonance occurs primarily in the portion of the vocal tract anterior to the constriction formed by the articulators. For voiceless obstruent sounds, such as /s, f, t, and k/, the sound source is solely at the point of constriction in the vocal tract. However, for voiced obstruents, such as /z, v, d, and g/, the vibrating vocal folds do provide a second sound source, creating a modulation of the breath stream coming from the lungs.

In addition to the degree of vocal tract constriction involved in their production, vowels and consonants differ markedly in terms of their physical and acoustic characteristics. With respect to duration (the time its takes to articulate them), vowels are generally longer than consonants in any particular syllable. Because vowels are longer than consonants, they comprise the largest part of any individual syllable. The actual length of any vowel or consonant phoneme varies in relation to the following: (1) whether the phoneme occurs in a stressed syllable; (2) the phonemic context (the other vowels and consonants that sur-

TABLE 5.1   The Classification of English Consonant Phonemes

	Bilabial		Labiodental		Interdental		Alveolar		Palatal		Velar		Glottal
	vl	v	vl	v	vl	v	vl	v	vl	v	vl	v	vl
Nonresonants													
Stops (Plosives)	p	b					t	d			k	g	ʔ
Fricatives			f	v	θ	ð	s	z	ʃ	ʒ			h
Affricates									tʃ	ʤ			
Resonants													
Nasals		m						n				ŋ	
Approximants													
Glides		w								j		w	
Liquids								l		r			

vl = voiceless v = voiced

round a particular phoneme in a word); and (3) the importance of the meaning of a word in an utterance that contains the phoneme.

In relation to intensity, vowels are greater in intensity than consonants. That is, vowels are perceived as being louder. This is mainly because of the greater acoustic energy associated with the resonance of the vocal tract during their production, when compared to consonants.

Consonants and vowels also differ in terms of their frequency specifications. During vowel production, each specific articulatory shape results in a unique resonant frequency pattern throughout the vocal tract. Resonant frequencies of the vocal tract are called **formants**. Each vowel has a distinct formant pattern, comprised of several resonant frequencies, which distinguishes it from the other vowels, perceptually. The resonances of the vocal tract associated with vowel production contain primarily low-frequency energy (although higher than the fundamental frequency of the voice). The frequency array, or energy pattern, associated with a particular phoneme is called its **spectrum**. Therefore, vowels are considered to have low frequency spectra and are perceived as being low in spectral pitch. The resonant consonants (nasals, glides, and liquids) also are characterized as having low-frequency spectra and, therefore, are perceived as low-pitched phonemes. The obstruents (especially the fricatives) have spectra higher in frequency than the vowels and resonant consonants and are perceived as having higher spectral pitch. This is due to the high frequency noise (turbulence) generally associated with obstruent production.

Whereas vowels can stand alone and create a meaningful utterance, for example, "oh," "a," and "I," consonants do not have the ability to stand alone. Consonants are generally found at the beginning and/or the end of syllables. As such, they are often classified as to their position in relation to the vowel in each syllable. Consonants that occur before a vowel in any syllable are referred to as **prevocalic** and those that occur after a vowel are referred to as **postvocalic**. Consonants located between two vowels are termed **intervocalic**. See Table 5.2 for some examples of prevocalic, postvocalic, and intervocalic consonants.

As you learned in Chapter 2, vowels generally serve as the center or nucleus of a syllable. Vowels are considered to be the nucleus of a syllable because they are of greater intensity than consonants and, therefore, are the prominent aspect of a syllable. Because vowels can form the nucleus of a syllable, they are said to be **syllabic**. We will see later that in some instances a few consonants may become syllabic in some phonetic contexts. Consequently, they have the special ability to become the nucleus of a syllable as well.

TABLE 5.2 Examples of Prevocalic, Postvocalic, and Intervocalic Consonants—Consonant Graphemes Are Underlined

Prevocalic	Postvocalic	Intervocalic
tee	eat	easy
hoe	ouch	anew
cow	Oz	okay
see	ail	away
ray	eyes	utter

PRELIMINARY EXERCISE 1—PREVOCALIC, INTERVOCALIC, AND POSTVOCALIC CONSONANTS

Match the appropriate term to each of the words below to indicate whether the <u>underlined</u> consonant is in the prevocalic, intervocalic, or postvocalic position.

a. prevocalic   b. intervocalic   c. postvocalic

____ 1. <u>s</u>eem   ____ 6. oi<u>l</u>y
____ 2. tra<u>d</u>e   ____ 7. hot<u>d</u>og
____ 3. a<u>w</u>ay   ____ 8. ha<u>s</u>ten
____ 4. <u>c</u>ruise   ____ 9. o<u>p</u>en
____ 5. oa<u>f</u>   ____ 10. foo<u>t</u>ball

Manner, Place, and Voicing

One last way in which consonants and vowels differ is the way in which consonant articulation is classified. Vowels are usually classified in terms of lip and tongue position. Consonants, on the other hand, are classified according to three different phonemic dimensions: *manner of production, place of articulation, and voicing.*

Manner of production refers to *the way in which the airstream is modified* as it passes through the vocal tract. For instance, stops are produced when the articulators completely impede the airstream passing through the vocal tract. Fricatives, on the other hand, are produced by forcing air through a narrow channel formed by the articulators in the oral cavity. Stop and fricative consonants belong to separate manners of production. In addition to stops and fricatives, the other English manners of production include affricates, nasals, glides, and liquids. Examine Table 5.1 in order to see the distribution of the English consonants among the various manners of production.

PRELIMINARY EXERCISE 2—MANNER OF PRODUCTION

Referring to Table 5.1, match each of the following consonants to their manner of production.

____ 1. /r/   a. stop
____ 2. /d/   b. fricative
____ 3. /w/   c. affricate
____ 4. /f/   d. nasal
____ 5. /n/   e. glide
____ 6. /tʃ/   f. liquid

To define **place of articulation** we must answer the question, *Where* in the vocal tract is the constriction located during the production of a particular consonant? In other words, to determine place of articulation, we need to know which speech organs are active in production of that consonant. From Chapter 3, you should be familiar with the various adjectives that refer to specific articulators located in the vocal tract. It is these adjectives that are used to refer to place of articulation. For example, if both lips are used to produce a phoneme, the place of production is bilabial. Likewise, if a phoneme is created by placing the tongue against the alveolar ridge, the place of articulation is considered to be lingua-alveolar or simply alveolar. (It is redundant to say lingua-alveolar because it is understood that the primary articulator is the tongue.) Table 5.3 reviews the various places of articulation most common to spoken English.

The last dimension used in classifying consonants is **voicing**. Voicing refers to whether the vocal folds are vibrating during the production of a particular consonant. Several phonemes in English share the same manner of production and place of articulation, yet differ only in the voicing dimension (/s/ and /z/, for example). Phonemes that differ only in voicing are called **cognates**. Other examples of voiceless/voiced cognates include /k/ and /g/, /f/ and /v/, and /p/ and /b/. Keep in mind that word pairs differing only in the voicing dimension of one phoneme also are minimal pairs. For example, the word pairs "bit"/"pit" and "tuck"/"duck" are minimal pairs because they differ only in the voicing of the initial phoneme.

PRELIMINARY EXERCISE 3—
VOICED/VOICELESS COGNATES

Place an "X" by each word pair having initial consonants that are voiced/voiceless cognates. You may need to refer to Table 5.1 for assistance.

____ 1. me, we		____ 6. shoot, suit
____ 2. seal, zeal		____ 7. flame, blame
____ 3. plan, clan		____ 8. dram, tram
____ 4. lice, rice		____ 9. yes, chess
____ 5. grain, crane		____ 10. vender, fender

TABLE 5.3   Most Common Places of Articulation in English

Place of Articulation	Articulators Involved
bilabial	upper and lower lips
labiodental	lower lip and upper central incisors
dental	tongue apex or blade and teeth
alveolar	tongue apex or blade and alveolar ridge
palatal	blade of tongue and hard palate
velar	back of tongue and velum
glottal	vocal folds
lingual	tongue

The English Consonants

In the following sections, the consonants of English will be introduced using the following format:

1. **Pronunciation Guide** for each consonant within each manner class, along with a detailed explanation of each manner.
2. **Description** of each consonant on three dimensions: voicing, place of articulation, and manner. Voiced/voiceless cognates will be introduced together.
3. **Sample Words** and **Minimal Pairs** containing the phoneme(s) being discussed.
4. **Allographs** commonly used to represent the phoneme in spelling.
5. **Discussion** involving the production of each consonant.
6. **Practice Exercises** for the entire manner class—exercises will *not* be given for each separate phoneme, as with the vowels.

The Stop Consonants (Plosives)

Pronunciation Guide

/p/	as in "pan"	/pæn/	/b/	as in "ban"	/bæn/
/t/	as in "tune"	/tun/	/d/	as in "dune"	/dun/
/k/	as in "could"	/kʊd/	/g/	as in "good"	/gʊd/

/ɾ/ as in "better" /bɛɾɚ/
/ʔ/ as in "kitten" /kɪʔn̩/

Stop consonants (sometimes referred to as plosives) are produced by *completely* obstructing the airstream once it enters the oral cavity. This is why stops are considered to be part of the class of consonants labeled as obstruents. The obstruction in the vocal tract is more occluding for this manner of articulation than for any of the others. Stop production is marked not only by a closure in the oral cavity, but also by a closure of the velopharyngeal port. That is, the velum is raised to prevent the breath stream from entering the nasal cavity. The English stop consonants are produced by forming a closure in the oral cavity at one of three places of articulation: bilabial (both lips coming together), alveolar (the tip or blade of the tongue contacting the alveolar ridge), or velar (the back of the tongue contacting the velum).

During the period of closure, **intraoral pressure** (air pressure within the oral cavity) increases due to the fact that the impeded airstream cannot escape the oral cavity. Once the constriction is released, the intraoral air pressure is relieved, resulting in the expulsion of an audible noise burst from the oral cavity (hence the name *plosive*). The burst of air is referred to as noise, since the airflow becomes turbulent when the stop is released. The articulatory process in stop consonant production is very rapid. In fact, of all the phonemes in English, stops are among the shortest in duration. Although it is possible to prolong the production of a vowel (iiiiiiiiii), it is not possible to prolong the production of a stop consonant. Once the airstream has been released by the articulators, the production of the phoneme is complete.

One last thing to consider on the production of plosives is their sound source. Stops may have one or two sound sources, depending on whether they are voiced or not. In English there are three voiceless stops (/p,t,k/) and three voiced stops (/b,d,g/). The primary sound source for voiceless stop consonants is considered to be at the point of constriction in the vocal tract, formed by the articulators. More specifically, the source of sound is the turbulent airflow generated when the intraoral pressure is released. For this reason, the sound source for voiceless stops is considered to be a noise source.

For voiced stops, the vocal folds do vibrate in conjunction with the release of the stop in the oral cavity. Therefore, voiced stops have two separate sound sources: (1) the noise source produced at the constriction in the vocal tract and (2) the vocal tone produced by the vibrating vocal folds.

Each stop consonant has a characteristic vocal tract shape due to the position of the articulators that form the stop constriction. Therefore, there is a separate, characteristic vocal tract resonance for the labial, alveolar, and velar places of production. Vocal fold vibration causes modifications in the vocal tract resonance during production of the voiced stops. The differences in the resonance of the larynx, pharynx, and oral cavity during production of the various stop consonants provide listeners the auditory cues necessary to distinguish their place of articulation.

/p/, /b/

Description

/p/	voiceless, bilabial stop
/b/	voiced, bilabial stop

Sample Words

/p/	/b/
played	breeze
appear	rube
spite	stubborn
leapt	rubbed
ripped	club
stripe	abrade

Minimal Pairs

/p/	/b/	/p/	/b/
pet	bet	ape	Abe
punt	bunt	rip	rib
patch	batch	rope	robe
prim	brim	lap	lab
packed	backed	staple	stable
plead	bleed	ample	amble

Allographs

	/p/		/b/
Grapheme	**Example**	**Grapheme**	**Example**
p	pig	b	bear
pp	apple	bb	blubber

Discussion   The airstream is impeded as both lips are brought together during production of the stops /p/ and /b/. Therefore, these two phonemes are classified as bilabial (see Figure 5.1). The jaws are in an almost closed position so that the lips can come together. The velopharyngeal port remains closed so that air does not flow into the nasal cavity. Upon release, the burst of air for /p/ is more powerful than for /b/, because the amount of intraoral pressure is greater for voiceless phonemes. During production of /p/ or /b/, the tongue's position is determined by the following vowel.

The use of the /p/ and /b/ phonemes in transcription is fairly straightforward (see the sample words above).

/t/, /d/

Description

/t/   voiceless, alveolar stop

/d/   voiced, alveolar stop

Sample Words

/t/	/d/
taste	dunce
stick	address
attack	pedestal
sate	door
tempest	edict
walk<u>ed</u>	mail<u>ed</u>

/ɾ/ (allophone of /t/ and /d/)

whi<u>tt</u>le	ba<u>tt</u>le
To<u>t</u>o	cu<u>t</u>ie
co<u>dd</u>le	la<u>dd</u>er/la<u>tt</u>er

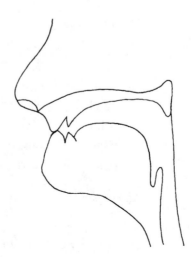

FIGURE 5.1   Bilabial articulation.

Minimal Pairs

/t/	/d/	/t/	/d/
talk	dock	pat	pad
to	do	trot	trod
touch	Dutch	state	stayed (staid)
troll	droll	straight	strayed
taffy	daffy	trait	trade
tram	dram	post	posed

Allographs

	/t/		/d/
Grapheme	*Example*	*Grapheme*	*Example*
t	toe	d	doe
ed	look<u>ed</u>	ed	wad<u>ed</u>

Discussion To produce the alveolar stops /t/ and /d/, the apex, or blade, of the tongue makes contact with the alveolar ridge, impeding oral airflow (see Figure 5.2). The sides of the tongue are placed against the upper molars so that air does not escape from the sides of the tongue. In essence, a small airtight cavity is formed by the tongue and teeth so that an increase in intraoral pressure may occur.

The air burst associated with the release of the voiceless /t/ is greater than for the voiced /d/, due to greater intraoral pressure for the voiceless cognate. In certain phonetic contexts, the velopharyngeal port may open during release of /t/ or /d/, allowing release of air through the nasal cavity instead of through

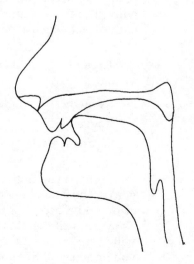

FIGURE 5.2 Alveolar articulation.

the oral cavity. In the words "mutton" and "sudden," for instance, the tongue remains in contact with the alveolar ridge during the release of the consonant; the stop is released through the nasal cavity instead of through the oral cavity. This maneuver is accomplished by lowering the velum. The release of air through the nasal cavity is called **nasal plosion** for obvious reasons.

There is an allophone of /t/ and /d/ that is often used in casual speech in words like "latter"/"ladder" and "Plato"/"play dough." Say these word pairs aloud to yourself, and you will not see a difference in their production. For example, the pronunciation of the word "latter" is not truly a /t/, as in the pronunciation /lætɚ/, nor is it truly a /d/, as in /lædɚ/—the pronunciation is somewhere between the two. In this context, the **tap** /ɾ/ is the allophone used to represent the combination of /t/ and /d/ as in /læɾɚ/ or /pleɪɾoʊ/. Tap articulation involves a very rapid movement of the tongue tip against the alveolar ridge creating a very brief stop consonant. The motion associated with a tapped stop consonant is more rapid than the "traditional" stop articulation of /t/ or /d/. The tap generally occurs in words with an intervocalic "t" or "d" digraph, in which the first syllable receives stress. Some examples include:

better	stutter	matted	battle
madder	huddle	coddle	riddle

The tap also is used in transcription when an intervocalic /t/ closes a stressed syllable. Examine the following words by saying them aloud:

fa̲t̲ed	flir̲t̲ed	sta̲t̲ic	da̲t̲a

Notice that the /t/ becomes partially voiced, due to the voiced environment provided by the vowels preceding and following the consonant. Using the tap would be appropriate when transcribing these words.

One last comment regarding /t/ and /d/ is their use in transcribing the morpheme "-ed," used to represent the past tense ending in words. Notice that the words "bagged" /bægd/ and "reaped" /ript/ each end with a different phoneme. In the first case, "ed" is represented by /d/ and in the second case with /t/. Now, examine the following words, and see if you can determine a pattern as to the use of /t/ and /d/ in representing the morpheme "-ed."

Example	*Final Phoneme*	*Example*	*Final Phoneme*
crowed	/d/	taped	/t/
teamed	/d/	hiked	/t/
hogged	/d/	lacked	/t/
carded (carted)	/d/	docked	/t/

Perhaps you noticed that if the phoneme preceding the "-ed" morpheme is voiced, the final phoneme also will be voiced, that is, /d/. Notice that a final /d/ also will be used if a tap precedes "-ed," as in the words "carded"/"carted." Conversely, if the phoneme preceding "-ed" is voiceless, then the voiceless /t/ will represent the morpheme "ed." Reexamine the words above to make sure you understand this concept.

/k/, /g/

Description

/k/   voiceless, velar stop

/g/   voiced, velar stop

Sample Words

/k/	/g/
cotton	gold
wreck	rugged
clique	Ghandi
queue	lager
squirts	aggressive

Minimal Pairs

/k/	/g/	/k/	/g/
crow	grow	luck	lug
cane	gain	back	bag
cut	gut	broke	brogue
cram	gram	shack	shag
kill	gill	pluck	plug
kale	gale	lacked	lagged

Allographs

/k/		/g/	
Grapheme	*Example*	*Grapheme*	*Example*
k	like	g	gone
ck	rock	gg	leggings
c	cat	gh	ghost
cc	occult	gu	guard
ch	chord		
cq	acquit		
cu	biscuit		
q	liquor		

Discussion   The constriction in the oral cavity for production of /k/ and /g/ is considered to be velar because the stop is formed between the back of the tongue and the anterior portion of the velum (see Figure 5.3). As you would expect, there is greater intraoral pressure for the voiceless /k/ than for the voiced /g/. The release for both /k/ and /g/ is through the oral cavity. It is interesting to note the many allographs of the phoneme /k/. Of all the stop consonants, /k/ has the most variant spellings.

In some phonetic contexts, the back of the tongue may move slightly forward to articulate with the posterior portion of the palate during production of /k/ or /g/. To demonstrate, let us compare the production of the phoneme /k/

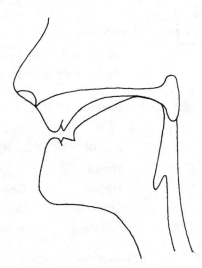

FIGURE 5.3   Velar articulation.

in two different phonetic contexts, that is, in the words "coop" and "keep." To produce the /k/ in /kup/, the back of the tongue would be close to the anterior portion of the velum because, in this context, it is followed by the back vowel /u/. To produce the /k/ in "keep," the tongue would be pulled forward, closer to the posterior portion of the palate, because /k/ is followed by the front vowel /i/. In anticipation of the forward place of articulation for /i/, the /k/ is produced more forward than normal.

The different articulatory gestures common for the production of /k/ help to demonstrate the process of coarticulation during speech production. Keep in mind that a phoneme's identity can be constantly altered by the other phonemes that precede or follow it.

/ ʔ /

Description

/ʔ/   voiceless, glottal stop

Sample Words

/ʔ/ (with the syllabic /n̩/)

Canton	fountain	bitten
written	fatten	rotten

The **glottal stop** /ʔ/ appears quite often in American English as an allophone of /t/. This stop is most readily noted in British English in the phrase, "Li'l bi' of tea" (Little bit of tea). The vocal folds are the articulators that both impede and release the flow of air in the production of this speech sound. Because the vocal folds do not vibrate during the production of the glottal stop, it is considered to be voiceless.

In American English, the glottal stop is found in some speakers' productions of words such as "kitten," "mountain," and "Dayton," where /t/ or /nt/

is followed by the /n/ phoneme. In saying these words, the /t/ is not released through the oral cavity. Instead, the release occurs at the level of the vocal folds. The reason for this is the tongue tip stays in place for both the /t/ and the following /n/ phonemes because they share the same (alveolar) place of articulation. Phonemes that share the same place of articulation are said to be **homorganic**. The transcription of the words "kitten," "mountain," and "Dayton" would be /kɪʔn̩/, /maʊnʔn̩/, and /deɪʔn̩/, respectively. The glottal stop also occurs between vowels in words such as "Hawaii" (/həwaɪʔɪ/). In connected speech, the glottal stop often occurs between vowels in adjacent words, as in "pay Amos" (/peɪʔeɪməs/).

Notice the use of the symbol /n̩/ in the transcription of the words /kɪʔn̩/, /maʊnʔn̩/ and /deɪʔn̩/. The /n̩/ represents an entire syllable, that is, both the consonant and the vowel, because there is no fully articulated vowel in these words. In this context, /n̩/ has become a syllabic consonant. (Remember that vowels are considered to be syllabic because they are the nucleus of a syllable.) The syllabic marking indicates that /n̩/ has become the nucleus of the syllable and therefore also represents the vowel in the syllable.

Syllabic consonants (or simply syllabics) result most often when adjacent homorganic consonants occur in either the same word or in separate words in connected speech. Syllabics also can be found in certain productions of "cat 'n dogs" /kæʔn̩dɑgz/ and "sittin'" /sɪʔn̩/ (note the use of the glottal stop here). We will return to the topic of syllabics in the sections focusing on nasals and liquids later in the chapter.

Practice Exercises

EXERCISE 5.1—THE STOP CONSONANTS

A. Place an "X" by the words with a stop consonant in their transcriptions.

____ 1. wish	____ 6. runs	____ 11. church	____ 16. think
____ 2. spring	____ 7. whisper	____ 12. tomb	____ 17. rummage
____ 3. loom	____ 8. question	____ 13. logical	____ 18. realm
____ 4. brush	____ 9. system	____ 14. jeans	____ 19. guess
____ 5. window	____ 10. phase	____ 15. Stephen	____ 20. fox

B. For each item, select the word(s) that have the specified criterion *in their transcriptions.* (There may be more than one correct response for each question.)

man   about   perky   could   plaque   green

Example:

Contains a bilabial sound   man, about, perky, plaque

1. Contains a high front vowel   _____
2. Contains a voiceless alveolar stop   _____
3. Contains no stops   _____
4. Contains a velar stop   _____
5. Contains a central vowel   _____
6. Ends with a voiceless sound   _____

Continues

EXERCISE 5.1 *(cont.)*

7. Begins with a voiced sound _____

8. Contains a back vowel and a voiced stop _____

9. Begins with a voiceless sound _____

10. Contains a front vowel and a voiceless stop _____

C. Indicate which of the following words have either a tap (T) or a glottal stop (G) in their transcriptions. Indicate which it would be by writing T or G in the blank.

____ 1. table   ____ 6. uncle   ____ 11. pushin'   ____ 16. talkin'

____ 2. better   ____ 7. written   ____ 12. splatter   ____ 17. bitten

____ 3. errand   ____ 8. beaten   ____ 13. rotted   ____ 18. wedded

____ 4. listen   ____ 9. walked   ____ 14. sweatin'   ____ 19. rotten

____ 5. quittin'   ____ 10. Lincoln   ____ 15. bottle   ____ 20. fodder

D. The words below all end with the "-ed" morpheme. Indicate in the blank whether the final phoneme should be transcribed as /t/ or /d/.

____ 1. wished   ____ 6. danced   ____ 11. sailed   ____ 16. crabbed

____ 2. loaded   ____ 7. wrapped   ____ 12. leased   ____ 17. placed

____ 3. endorsed   ____ 8. hanged   ____ 13. reached   ____ 18. meshed

____ 4. dangered   ____ 9. hoped   ____ 14. toted   ____ 19. burned

____ 5. robbed   ____ 10. traded   ____ 15. wrecked   ____ 20. carved

E. Circle the real English words given below.

1. /kipət/   5. /pɝkt/   9. /pɝpət/   13. /tʊkɪ/

2. /təkɪd/   6. /pækət/   10. /pɪkɪ/   14. /gækət/

3. /ədɛbt/   7. /tɛpɪd/   11. /ətæk/   15. /dɛrbɪ/

4. /paʊɾɚ/   8. /taɪɾɚ/   12. /tɔrkot/   16. /pipʔd/

F. In the blanks, write each of the words using English orthography.

1. /pɑɾɚ/ _____   7. /gʌpɪ/ _____

2. /pʌkəd/ _____   8. /pækɪŋ/ _____

3. /pəteɪɾou/ _____   9. /daɪpəd/ _____

4. /dɑktɚ/ _____   10. /peɪpəbɔɪ/ _____

5. /tɑrgət/ _____   11. /dækɚɪ/ _____

6. /pʌpət/ _____   12. /daɪətəd/ _____

G. For each item below, correct any vowel, diphthong, or stop consonant transcription errors by marking out the incorrect IPA symbol and placing the correct symbol above it. If no error is present, indicate by circling "no error."

Examples:

a. cap   /kæp/   (no error)

b. tick   /tɪk/   no error

1. direct   /dɚɛkt/   no error

2. tighter   /taɪɾɚ/   no error

Continues

3.	petted	/pɛɾed/	no error
4.	corker	/kɔrkɚ/	no error
5.	Carter	/cɑrɾɚ/	no error
6.	partake	/pɔrteɪk/	no error
7.	repeat	/repit/	no error
8.	poet	/poʊət/	no error
9.	oboe	/oʊboʊ/	no error
10.	paper	/pɑpɚ/	no error

H. Word Analysis

Read the phonetic descriptions of the following words. Then write the appropriate IPA symbols and the English orthography on the two lines.

Example:

voiceless alveolar stop + low front lax
vowel + voiced velar stop

/tæg/
tag

1. voiceless velar stop + high front lax
   vowel + voiced alveolar stop

   _____
   _____

2. high front tense vowel + voiced velar
   stop + mid-central lax rounded vowel

   _____
   _____

3. voiceless alveolar stop + low-mid front
   vowel + voiceless bilabial stop + high
   front lax vowel + voiced alveolar stop

   _____
   _____

4. mid-central unrounded lax vowel +
   voiced bilabial stop + low-mid back-
   central unrounded lax vowel +
   voiceless alveolar stop

   _____
   _____

5. voiced alveolar stop + low back tense
   vowel + voiceless velar stop + voiceless alveolar stop

   _____
   _____

6. voiced velar stop + low-mid back tense
   vowel + voiced alveolar stop + high
   front lax vowel

   _____
   _____

I. Written Transcription Practice

Transcribe the following words. Remember to enclose your transcriptions with virgules.

1.	cape _____		11.	peat _____
2.	pared _____		12.	taupe _____
3.	dog _____		13.	took _____
4.	tied _____		14.	putt _____
5.	kept _____		15.	coat _____
6.	debt _____		16.	apart _____
7.	bake _____		17.	guarded _____
8.	pour _____		18.	boater _____
9.	bored _____		19.	Bobby _____
10.	pork _____		20.	barter _____

Continues

EXERCISE 5.1 *(cont.)*

21. bigger   _____
22. beaker   _____
23. tuba   _____
24. cabby   _____
25. peered   _____
26. backed   _____
27. perky   _____
28. geared   _____
29. dagger   _____
30. giddy   _____

31. carpet   _____
32. doctor   _____
33. ticket   _____
34. decked   _____
35. tired   _____
36. bigger   _____
37. debate   _____
38. torrid   _____
39. parrot   _____
40. dirty   _____

Complete Assignment 5-1.

The Nasal Consonants

Pronunciation Guide

/m/   as in "man"   /mæn/
/n/   as in "new"   /nu/
/ŋ/   as in "ring"   /rɪŋ/

The three **nasal** consonants /m, n, and ŋ/are produced in a manner similar to the stop consonants. That is, the airstream is completely obstructed in the oral cavity during their production. Also, the obstruction occurs at the same three places of articulation as the stops, that is, bilabial, alveolar, and velar (see Figures 5.1, 5.2, and 5.3). However, this is where the similarity ends. Nasal consonants are produced with the velum lowered so that the airstream and acoustic vibrations continually flow into the nasal cavity. The obstruction at the lips, alveolar ridge, or velum is not released during the production of the nasal consonants as it is for stops. Therefore, there is no release of the intraoral pressure from the oral cavity. The articulators simply block the flow of air out of the oral cavity so that air may continually flow through the nostrils. For this reason, the nasal consonants are not considered to be obstruents. If you sustain the production of /m/, and place your index finger under your nose (as if you were trying to stifle a sneeze), you can feel a lightly escaping airstream.

Another difference between stop and nasal consonants is the fact that all nasal consonants are voiced; they have no voiceless counterparts in English. Like vowels, the sound source for nasals is the vibration of the vocal folds. Nasal consonants are classified as *nasal resonants* because resonance occurs throughout the vocal tract during their production.

Because airflow is directed through the nasal port during nasal consonant production, resonance occurs in the nasal cavity as well as in the oral cavity and pharynx. The oral cavity can be considered a sidebranch of the vocal tract. The size of the oral sidebranch decreases with the location of the constriction in the vocal tract from /m/ (bilabial) to /n/ (alveolar) to /ŋ/ (velar) (from anterior to posterior). Because the size of the oral cavity varies during production of the nasals, so does the resonance of the vocal tract during nasal consonant production. Due to the additional resonance provided by the nasal cavity, the nasal consonants have a sound quality quite different from the other phonemes in English.

Recall that in some instances, nasal phonemes may become syllabic. In the word "written" /rɪʔn̩/, the syllabic /n̩/ marks both the consonant and the vowel in the second syllable.

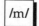

Description

/m/   voiced, bilabial nasal

Sample Words

/m/

mark	cramp
slam	dimpled
mend	alarming
maybe	amounted
drama	stomach
grump	mother

Minimal Pairs

/m/	/p/	/b/
mark	park	bark
roamed	roped	robed
messed	pest	best
crams	craps	crabs
sum	sup	sub
slam	slap	slab

Allographs

Grapheme	**Example**
m	cram
mm	hammer

Discussion   During production of /m/, the velum is lowered so that the airstream enters the nasal cavity. The lips are brought together in order to halt the airstream coming from the larynx (similar to the constriction for the phoneme /b/). Because /m/ is voiced, the vocal folds vibrate during its production. The oral resonating cavity for /m/ is the largest of the three nasals; it includes the entire oral cavity, extending from the lips to the oropharynx. The tongue is poised in position for the vowel following production of /m/. Figure 5.4 shows the articulation of the bilabial nasal /m/. Compare this figure with the articulation of a bilabial stop, as shown in Figure 5.1. Note the differing position of the velum in these two figures: It is lowered in Figure 5.4, and it is raised in Figure 5.1.

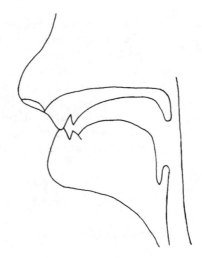

FIGURE 5.4   Bilabial nasal articulation.

In some instances, /m/ may become syllabic in conversational speech, depending on the phonetic environment. For example, the word "happen" becomes /hæpm̩/, and the phrase "wrap them up" becomes "wrap 'em up" /ræpm̩əp/.

/n/

Description

/n/   voiced, alveolar nasal

Sample Words

/n/

note	runner
nail	Andover
Nile	nervous
loaned	answered
tunes	astound
snowball	mannerism

Minimal Pairs

/n/	/m/	/n/	/m/
nail	mail (male)	nine	mine
note	mote (moat)	Nate	mate
loan	loam	cunning	coming
grin	grim	warned	warmed
noon	moon	sunning	summing
roan	roam	dinner	dimmer

Allographs

Grapheme	Example
n	nice
nn	dinner

Discussion   The phoneme /n/ is produced in a manner similar to /m/, except for its place of articulation. For /n/, the tongue tip (or blade) contacts the alveolar ridge in order to impede the flow of air coming from the larynx. Because the place of articulation is posterior to that for /m/, the oral cavity is slightly smaller, causing a different resonance to be created in the vocal tract.

Transcription of this sound is fairly straightforward. When /n/ occurs at the end of a word, and the preceding consonant is also alveolar (homorganic), such as /d, t, s, or l/, the /n/ often becomes the nucleus of the syllable (syllabic). Some examples are given below with the homorganic consonant allograph underlined.

"ri**dd**en"	/rɪdn̩/	"go**tt**en"	/gɑʔn̩/
"rea**s**on"	/rizn̩/	"cho**s**en"	/tʃouzn̩/
"le**ss**on"	/lɛsn̩/	"ea**t**en"	/iʔn̩/
"fa**ll**en"	/fɑln̩/		

Note that for the word "ridden," the stop /d/ may be released through the nasal cavity as the velum is lowered in production of /n/ (nasal plosion).

Examine the following words. Although the preceding consonant (underlined) is not homorganic, many individuals still use the syllabic /n̩/ in transcription because the vowel between the consonants is almost nonexistent.

"ri**bb**on"	/rɪbn̩/
"ha**pp**en"	/hæpn̩/ (or /hæpm̩/)
"wi**sh**in'"	/wɪʃn̩/
"co**ff**in"	/kɔfn̩/ or /kɑfn̩/
"le**g**ion"	/liʤn̩/

One last word about the use, or actually nonuse, of /n/. Keep in mind that in words containing the letter string "ing," the phoneme /ŋ/ is used, not /n/ (see the section on /ŋ/ below).

/ŋ/

Description

/ŋ/   voiced, velar nasal

Sample Words

/ŋ/

ring	clank	stinky
wrangler	ankle	lingo
being	dangle	wrinkle
finger	larynx	wrangler

Allographs

Grapheme	Example
ng	sing
nk	link

Discussion   /ŋ/ is produced similarly to the other two nasal consonants in terms of voicing and velar opening. However, for /ŋ/, the point of constricted airflow in the oral cavity is the most posterior, between the back of the tongue and the anterior portion of the velum (or sometimes the posterior portion of the hard palate, in a manner similar to /k/ and /g/). The oral resonating cavity for /ŋ/ is the shortest of all (when compared to /m/ and /n/) given that the constriction in the vocal tract is adjacent to the pharynx.

/ŋ/ never begins a word in English; it is found only in the middle or at the end of a word. In relation to transcription, /ŋ/ poses some interesting dilemmas for beginning transcribers. Note the use of /ŋ/ with the following letter strings:

Letter String	Sample Word	Transcription
"ink"	kink	/kɪŋk/
"ank"	lanky	/læŋkɪ/
"ynx"	lynx	/lɪŋks/
"inx"	sphinx	/sfɪŋks/

It would not be possible to say these words using /n/ instead of /ŋ/ (try it for yourself).

In some words, such as "English" and "finger," /ŋ/ is always followed by the voiced, velar stop /g/ in its pronunciation. However, there are other words in English, such as "longing" and "stinger," in which the production of /g/ is variable. Contrast the following two sets of words:

Word	Transcription	Word	Transcription
linger	/lɪŋgɚ/	hanger	/hæŋgɚ/ or /hæŋɚ/
ingot	/ɪŋgət/	singer	/sɪŋgɚ/ or /sɪŋɚ/
anger	/æŋgɚ/	clanging	/klæŋgɪŋ/ or /klæŋɪŋ/

Note that all of the words in the first set always have /g/ in their transcriptions, whereas the words in the second set may pronounced with or without the /g/, depending on individual speaker differences and/or dialect.

Practice Exercises

EXERCISE 5.2—THE NASAL CONSONANTS

A. Place an "X" by the words with a nasal phoneme in their transcription.

____ 1. ring   ____ 3. pet   ____ 5. tomb   ____ 7. crease

____ 2. bomb   ____ 4. stop   ____ 6. jasmine   ____ 8. inside

Continues

____ 9. trait   ____ 12. spanking   ____ 15. lung   ____ 18. monkey

____ 10. loaner   ____ 13. possible   ____ 16. ripen   ____ 19. lure

____ 11. moan   ____ 14. trench   ____ 17. unfair   ____ 20. failure

B. Indicate with an "X" the words that have /ŋ/ in their transcription.

____ 1. angle   ____ 8. singe   ____ 15. banging

____ 2. angel   ____ 9. ginger   ____ 16. manx

____ 3. brink   ____ 10. danger   ____ 17. ingest

____ 4. mango   ____ 11. blinker   ____ 18. singer

____ 5. Angie   ____ 12. hanger   ____ 19. hunger

____ 6. single   ____ 13. ringing   ____ 20. jangle

____ 7. conjure   ____ 14. mingle   ____ 21. congeal

C. Circle the words in B above that could have /ŋ/ followed by /g/ in their transcriptions. (Some words may be pronounced differently due to speaker dialect.)

D. Place an "X" next to the words that have /g/ in their transcriptions.

____ 1. hinge   ____ 7. ring   ____ 13. tango

____ 2. bangle   ____ 8. drank   ____ 14. flange

____ 3. wings   ____ 9. onyx   ____ 15. engine

____ 4. single   ____ 10. tingle   ____ 16. English

____ 5. wrong   ____ 11. bungee   ____ 17. tongue

____ 6. mangle   ____ 12. kangaroo   ____ 18. dangerous

E. Place an "X" next to the words that have /n/ in their transcriptions.

____ 1. pharynx   ____ 7. engine   ____ 13. ginger

____ 2. England   ____ 8. flank   ____ 14. blanket

____ 3. bungee   ____ 9. tingle   ____ 15. tongue

____ 4. length   ____ 10. lunge   ____ 16. danger

____ 5. lungs   ____ 11. strength   ____ 17. vengeance

____ 6. jungle   ____ 12. tango   ____ 18. ranges

F. For each item, select the word(s) that have the specified criterion *in their transcriptions*. (There may be more than one correct response for each question.)

good   mutton   curving   bank

napped   taken   carton   code

1. Contains an initial labial sound   _____

2. Contains a voiced initial sound   _____

3. Ends with a stop   _____

4. Contains a central vowel   _____

Continues

EXERCISE 5.2 (*cont.*)

5. Ends with a voiceless sound   _____

6. Contains a velar nasal   _____

7. Contains a syllabic consonant   _____

8. Contains no nasals   _____

9. Contains a low front vowel and
   a labial consonant   _____

10. Contains a velar consonant and a back vowel   _____

G. Circle the words that represent real English words.

1. /kæmp/   4. /pint/   7. /kræŋkɪ/   10. /bʌmpɪ/

2. /neɪm/   5. /tɪŋgə/   8. /kɔrn/   11. /pɪntoʊ/

3. /mɛlɪ/   6. /nɪŋgɪd/   9. /dænk/   12. /pɑrmɔɪ/

H. In the blanks, write each of the words using English orthography.

1. /næb/ _____   7. /kændɪ/   _____

2. /kɑnd/ _____   8. /əpɔɪnt/ _____

3. /əmæs/ _____   9. /kʊkɪŋ/   _____

4. /æŋgə/ _____   10. /tumɚ/   _____

5. /mɔrnɪŋ/_____   11. /taɪ ʔn̩/ _____

6. /bɛndɪŋ/_____   12. /maɪndəd/ _____

I. For each item below, correct any vowel, diphthong, nasal, or stop consonant transcription errors by marking out the incorrect IPA symbol and placing the correct symbol above it. If no error is present, so indicate by circling "no error."

1. camper   /kæmpɚ/   no error

2. adorn   /ədɔrn/   no error

3. duffer   /dəfɝ/   no error

4. bunting   /bʌntɪŋ/   no error

5. bingo   /bɪŋoʊ/   no error

6. pecking   /pɛckɪŋ/   no error

7. Dayton   /deɪʔən/   no error

8. batter   /bædɚ/   no error

9. baking   /bɑkɪŋ/   no error

10. doorknob   /dɔrknɑb/   no error

J. Word Analysis

Read the phonetic descriptions of the following words. Then write the appropriate IPA symbols and the English orthography on the two lines.

1. voiceless velar stop + low front   _____
   vowel + alveolar nasal + voiced   _____
   alveolar stop

Continues

2. voiced bilabial nasal + low-mid, _____
   back-central vowel + alveolar nasal _____
   + high front lax vowel

3. mid-central lax unrounded vowel _____
   + voiceless alveolar stop + high-mid _____
   front vowel + alveolar nasal

4. voiceless velar stop + low back _____
   vowel + velar nasal + voiced velar _____
   stop + high-mid back vowel

5. voiced bilabial stop + mid-central _____
   tense rounded vowel + voiceless _____
   bilabial stop + voiceless alveolar stop

K. Transcription Practice

Transcribe the following words, using the IPA.

1. mink   _____   22. tankard   _____
2. pert   _____   23. peanut   _____
3. tan   _____   24. dandy   _____
4. king   _____   25. partake   _____
5. done   _____   26. Monday   _____
6. knead   _____   27. nomad   _____
7. bang   _____   28. bongo   _____
8. gnome   _____   29. madam   _____
9. monk   _____   30. gander   _____
10. coin   _____   31. omit   _____
11. earn   _____   32. negate   _____
12. newt   _____   33. tunic   _____
13. town   _____   34. donkey   _____
14. mood   _____   35. command   _____
15. knight _____   36. mirror   _____
16. dumb   _____   37. countin' _____
17. could _____   38. daring   _____
18. torn   _____   39. empire   _____
19. tongue _____   40. coward   _____
20. gone   _____
21. under _____

Complete Assignment 5-2.

The Fricative Consonants

Pronunciation Guide

/f/	as in "form"	/fɔrm/	/v/	as in "van"	/væn/
/θ/	as in "thick"	/θɪk/	/ð/	as in "them"	/ðɛm/
/s/	as in "sip"	/sɪp/	/z/	as in "zoo"	/zu/
/ʃ/	as in "shell"	/ʃɛl/	/ʒ/	as in "rouge"	/ruʒ/
/h/	as in "ham"	/hæm/			

Fricatives are produced by forcing the breath stream (whether voiced or voiceless) through a narrow channel, or constriction, in the vocal tract. The articulators do not close completely during fricative production as they do in stop consonant production. They simply converge to form a slit to create the channel necessary for production of each fricative phoneme. There are five different places of articulation (points of constriction) in the vocal tract used for production of the nine English fricatives. These include the linguadental, labiodental, alveolar, palatal, and glottal places of articulation. Fricatives have voiced/voiceless cognate phonemes at each place of articulation. The only exception is the glottal fricative /h/, which is usually voiceless. Unlike stops and nasals, there are no bilabial or velar fricatives in English. However, these phonemes do exist in other languages. For instance, bilabial fricatives occur in Spanish and in Ewe, a West African language. Velar fricatives exist in German and Hebrew. Interestingly, bilabial and velar fricatives are sometimes produced by English-speaking children with phonological disorders.

Because the airstream from the lungs is being forced through a narrow channel, a turbulent, frictional noise is generated at the point of constriction. Fricatives, like stops, are considered to be obstruents, because their production involves an obstruction of the airstream in the vocal tract.

Voiceless fricatives, like voiceless stop consonants, are produced without the benefit of the vibrating vocal folds as the sound source. Therefore, the breath stream from the lungs must be forceful enough to create an audible turbulence at the point of constriction in the vocal tract. Like voiced stops, voiced fricatives have a second sound source—the vibrating vocal folds.

The alveolar and palatal fricatives /s, z, ʃ, ʒ/ are perceived as being louder than the other fricatives and are referred to collectively as **sibilants**.

/f/, /v/

Description

/f/	voiceless, labiodental fricative
/v/	voiced, labiodental fricative

Sample Words

/f/	/v/
free	veal
foam	love
phobia	calves
coffer	vane
rough	over
turf	vase

Minimal Pairs

/f/	/v/
fail	veil
fend	vend
fan	van
leaf	leave
first	versed
proof	prove

Allographs

	/f/		/v/
Grapheme	*Example*	*Grapheme*	*Example*
f	fix	v	vote
ff	muffin	f	of
gh	rough	ph	Stephen
ph	phone		

Discussion   The point of constriction for /f/ and /v/ is formed by bringing the lower lip close to the edges of the upper central incisors (see Figure 5.5). The lower jaw must be raised near the upper jaw to accomplish this maneuver. The breath stream is forced through the narrow constriction formed by the lower lip and upper teeth.

The labiodental fricatives are quite easy to transcribe. The only allographs associated with /f/ that may cause trouble at first are "ph" and "gh." /v/ is generally written with the letter "v" except in the rare case of "f" and "ph" (see allographs above for examples).

/θ/, /ð/

Description

/θ/	voiceless, interdental fricative
/ð/	voiced, interdental fricative

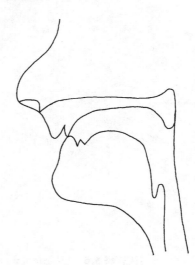

FIGURE 5.5   Labiodental articulation.

Sample Words

/θ/	/ð/	/θ/	/ð/
thermal	though	bath	bathe
thought	lathe	breath	breathe
froth	feather	thigh	thy
with	wither	ether	either

Note: "Either" and "ether" are minimal pairs, as are "thigh" and "thy."

Allographs

/θ/   /ð/

Grapheme	*Example*	*Grapheme*	*Example*
th	thistle	th	although

Discussion The interdental fricatives are named "theta" /θ/ (voiceless) and "eth" /ð/ (voiced). These phonemes are produced by forcing the breath stream through a constriction formed by the apex (or blade) of the tongue and the lower edge of the upper central incisors. The tongue is placed between the teeth for this articulation, hence the label *interdental*. Simultaneously, the sides of the tongue contact the upper molars to help direct the voiced or voiceless breath stream towards the constriction (see Figure 5.6).

A second way in which these phonemes may be produced is by forming a constriction between the apex of the tongue and the posterior portion of the upper central incisors. This particular articulation of these phonemes would be termed appropriately *dental*, as opposed to interdental.

/θ/ and /ð/ are both represented, in spelling, by the digraph "th." This is initially confusing to students new to the transcription of these sounds. If you listen carefully, the voicing difference should become readily apparent. The letter combination "th" is the only spelling representation of these two phonemes.

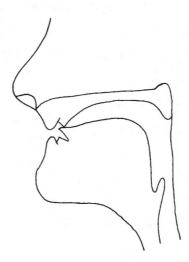

FIGURE 5.6   Interdental articulation.

/s/, /z/	*Description*

/s/   voiceless, alveolar fricative

/z/   voiced, alveolar fricative

Sample Words

/s/	/z/
sew	zenith
centaur	azalea
assert	fuzzy
lesson	xylophone
cease	pays
awesome	Aztec

Minimal Pairs

/s/	/z/		/s/	/z/
seal	zeal		brace	braise
lacy	lazy		spice	spies
sip	zip		seek	Zeke
close	close		sue	zoo
loose	lose		noose	news
race	raise		purse	purrs

Allographs

	/s/		/z/	
Grapheme	*Example*	*Grapheme*	*Example*
s	sink	z	zone
ss	press	zz	fizz
sc	science	s	was
c	ice	ss	scissors
		x	Xanadu

Discussion   The constriction for the alveolar fricatives is formed in one of two ways, depending on the individual speaker. The first involves the articulation of either the tongue apex or blade and the alveolar ridge. The tongue is raised so that it only approximates the ridge; the tongue does not make direct contact. At the same time, the tongue forms a tapering groove along its central or midline portion as the back of the tongue contacts the upper molars.

The second method for producing the alveolar fricatives is by placing the tip of the tongue behind the lower central incisors while the front of the tongue is raised to approximate the alveolar ridge. The tongue is still grooved along its central portion, and the sides of the tongue make contact with the upper molars. For both articulations, the channel formed by the tongue and teeth helps to direct the airstream anteriorly through the closely held upper and lower teeth.

In terms of transcription, the biggest problem for students is learning the correct use of /s/ and /z/ to represent the plural "s" morpheme in words. Examine the word pairs below. Is the final phoneme transcribed as /s/ or /z/?

taps	seats	walks	chicks
tabs	seeds	runs	hogs

Whenever the final consonant of a word is voiceless, its plural marker will be transcribed as the voiceless phoneme /s/. The words "taps," "seats," "walks," and "chicks" all have a voiceless phoneme immediately preceding the plural morpheme /s/. The remaining words, which all have a voiced phoneme prior the plural marker, are transcribed with /z/. Whenever the plural form of a word is "es" as in "babies" or "ladies," the plural phoneme is also represented by /z/, because it follows a (voiced) vowel. (The singular form of these words "baby" and "lady" ends with the vowel /ɪ/.) This rule should seem familiar to you because similar practice is involved in using the phonemes /t/ and /d/ to indicate the "-ed" morpheme.

The phoneme /z/ is used by some speakers in pronunciation of words that are normally transcribed with an /s/. Examples include:

resource → /rizɔrs/   greasy → /grizɪ/   absurd → /æbzɝd/

/ʃ/, /ʒ/

Description

/ʃ/ voiceless, palatal fricative
/ʒ/ voiced, palatal fricative

Sample Words

/ʃ/	/ʒ/
shook	fusion
sure	casual
mansion	profusion
machine	measure
cashier	regime
pressure	television
national	seizure
omniscient	erosion

Allographs

/ʃ/		/ʒ/	
Grapheme	*Example*	*Grapheme*	*Example*
sh	shape	z	azure
ss	pressure	g	garage
sci	conscience	s	measure
ce	ocean	si	vision
ch	machine	zi	brazier

/ʃ/ (cont.)

Grapheme	Example
ci	social
s	sugar
si	pension

Discussion   These two fricatives are created when the breath stream is forced through a constriction formed in a manner quite similar to the alveolar fricatives. The tongue has a groove along its central portion (although it is broader) and the sides of the tongue contact the upper molars. The airstream is directed anteriorly toward the front teeth. The more open constriction for /ʒ/ and /ʃ/ is formed by the closely held tongue blade and the hard palate. This articulation is posterior to the constriction formed for the alveolar fricatives /s/ and /z/. Therefore, /ʃ/ and /ʒ/ are considered by many phoneticians to have a **postalveolar** or **palatoalveolar** articulation (see Figure 5.7). Unlike /s/ and /z/, the lips are rounded in production of /ʃ/ and /ʒ/.

The transcription of the phonemes /ʃ/ and /ʒ/ is a bit tricky at first. Students will often confuse them with the two affricates /tʃ/ as in "cheap" and /dʒ/ as in "jam." Compare the following words:

"sheep" /ʃip/	—	"cheap" /tʃip/
"shoe" /ʃu/	—	"chew" /tʃu/
"leisure" /lɛʒɚ/	—	"ledger" /lɛdʒɚ/

Hopefully, you hear the difference in the pronunciation of these words. An explanation of the affricate manner of production will follow this section.

/h/

Description

/h/   voiceless, glottal fricative

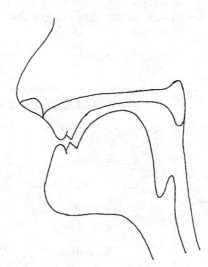

FIGURE 5.7   Palatal articulation.

Sample Words

/h/

hook	whose
helium	behave
hairy	ahead
Harold	unhook

Allographs

/h/

Grapheme	**Example**
h	hit
wh	who

Discussion   The fricative /h/ is created when the breath stream is forced through a constriction formed by the abducted vocal folds (the glottis). Because the vocal folds are not vibrating during production of this phoneme, it is considered to be voiceless. /h/ is the only fricative without a voiced cognate. In some phonetic contexts, however, it may take on a voiced quality. For instance, in the word "ahead" /əhɛd/, a vowel precedes and follows the /h/ causing it to become voiced, because the vowels are both voiced. When /h/ precedes the high vowels /i, ɪ, u, and ʊ/, the friction noise is created entirely, or nearly so, at the constriction formed by the tongue and palate, not at the glottis. Say the words "he" /hɪ/ and "who" /hu/ and you will see that this is so.

During the production of /h/, the articulators will take on the shape of whichever vowel follows. For example, compare the shape and position of your lips for the words "hoop" and "heap." You will immediately notice that your lips are rounded—even before you produce the /h/ phoneme—in the word "hoop." Similarly, your lips are retracted before the production of /h/ in "heap." The transcription of /h/ should pose few problems for students, because the only allographs of /h/ are "h" and "wh."

Practice Exercises

EXERCISE 5.3—THE FRICATIVE CONSONANTS

A. Place an "X" by the words with a fricative phoneme in their transcription.

____ 1. push	____ 6. brazen	____ 11. Montana	____ 16. hombre
____ 2. thesis	____ 7. cares	____ 12. pleasure	____ 17. leaks
____ 3. loom	____ 8. burlap	____ 13. leather	____ 18. worthy
____ 4. happy	____ 9. croissant	____ 14. marrow	____ 19. crouton
____ 5. caution	____ 10. vender	____ 15. other	____ 20. rajah

Continues

B. Indicate which of the following words have /ʃ/ or /ʒ/ in their transcription. Write the correct phoneme next to the word. (Hint: Watch out for /tʃ/ and /ʤ/!)

____ 1. mishap	____ 8. badge	____ 15. Sean
____ 2. usually	____ 9. lesion	____ 16. passion
____ 3. decision	____ 10. lotion	____ 17. ricochet
____ 4. cheese	____ 11. corsage	____ 18. college
____ 5. largest	____ 12. changed	____ 19. allusion
____ 6. reason	____ 13. friction	____ 20. inject
____ 7. election	____ 14. juice	____ 21. Persia

C. For the following words, indicate whether the "th" sound is voiced (/ð/) or voiceless (/θ/) by placing the correct IPA symbol in the blank.

____ 1. smoothly	____ 7. wrath	____ 13. thimble
____ 2. method	____ 8. writhe	____ 14. booth
____ 3. other	____ 9. lathe	____ 15. oath
____ 4. those	____ 10. thought	____ 16. scathing
____ 5. moth	____ 11. clothes	____ 17. another
____ 6. gather	____ 12. weather	____ 18. anything

D. For each item, create real words (or proper names) by placing one of the nine fricatives in the blank. Write your answers in the blank at the right of each item. More than one answer is possible for each item.

$$/f, v, θ, ð, s, z, ʃ, ʒ, h/$$

Example: /____u/   /s/, /z/, /ʃ/, /h/ _____

(The words created are "sue," "zoo," "shoe," and "who.")

1. /mu__/   _____
2. /wɪ__/   _____
3. /ʌ__ɚ/   _____
4. /lɛ__ɚ/   _____
5. /__ɛrɪ/   _____
6. /ru__/   _____
7. /__aɪ/   _____
8. /__ɪr/   _____

E. For each item, select the word(s) that have the specified criterion in their transcriptions.

them   beige   hug   wreath   tape   cash   soon   vend

1. Begins with a voiceless fricative   _____
2. Begins with a voiced obstruent   _____
3. Ends with a voiceless obstruent

Continues

EXERCISE 5.3 (*cont.*)

4. Contains a front vowel
   and a voiceless fricative   _____

5. Contains an alveolar sound   _____

6. Contains all voiced phonemes   _____

7. Contains a stop and a fricative   _____

8. Contains a nasal and a fricative   _____

9. Contains a fricative and a central vowel   _____

10. Contains no fricatives   _____

F. Indicate whether the following words should be transcribed with a final /s/
   or a final /z/.

____ 1. babes	____ 7. bananas	____ 13. dramas
____ 2. chafes	____ 8. drinks	____ 14. croaks
____ 3. cars	____ 9. passes	____ 15. meats
____ 4. books	____ 10. throws	____ 16. affairs
____ 5. carpets	____ 11. loaves	____ 17. loafs
____ 6. pushes	____ 12. roasts	____ 18. birds

G. Circle the words that represent real English words.

1. /ʃʊk/	5. /vɛrɪ/	9. /pɝs/	13. /feɪvɚ/
2. /ʒɪŋ/	6. /ðaɪ/	10. /ʃɑrk/	14. /kreɪzd/
3. /zɔrt/	7. /θru/	11. /ɪrðu/	15. /bɪʒɚ/
4. /θɝd/	8. /vɔɪnz/	12. /ʃæku/	16. /hoʊðɚ/

H. In the blanks, write each of the words using English orthography.

1. /eɪʒən/ _____	9. /sɝvəst/ _____
2. /vɔrtɛks/ _____	10. /ʌðɚz/ _____
3. /vɑrnɪʃ/ _____	11. /froʊzn̩/ _____
4. /bɑðɚ/ _____	12. /ʃɪvɚd/ _____
5. /spɛrd/ _____	13. /fæʔn̩/ _____
6. /θæŋks/ _____	14. /hɔrɚ/ _____
7. /hɪrseɪ/ _____	15. /gəziboʊ/ _____
8. /ɝbən/ _____	16. /bɝθdeɪz/ _____

I. For each item below, correct any vowel or consonant transcription errors by
   marking out the incorrect IPA symbol and placing the correct symbol above
   it. If no error is present, so indicate by circling "no error."

1. bijou	/biʃu/	no error
2. neither	/niθɚ/	no error
3. verify	/vɛrifaɪ/	no error

Continues

4.	hosed	/hosd/	no error
5.	Hoosier	/huʒɚ/	no error
6.	amnesia	/æmniʒə/	no error
7.	assure	/əʃʊr/	no error
8.	favored	/fevɚd/	no error
9.	shining	/ʃhaɪnɪŋ/	no error
10.	earthy	/ɛrθɪ/	no error

J. Transcription Practice

Transcribe the following words using the IPA.

1. Garth	_____	21. thunder	_____
2. fence	_____	22. heather	_____
3. sure	_____	23. satin	_____
4. dozed	_____	24. sheepish	_____
5. soared	_____	25. surrounds	_____
6. hives	_____	26. Horton	_____
7. shout	_____	27. thirty	_____
8. thorns	_____	28. vision	_____
9. those	_____	29. pharynx	_____
10. haste	_____	30. third base	_____
11. perhaps	_____	31. goiter	_____
12. shorter	_____	32. terror	_____
13. perused	_____	33. thousand	_____
14. unversed	_____	34. contour	_____
15. mother	_____	35. shortcake	_____
16. consumed	_____	36. varied	_____
17. mirage	_____	37. defies	_____
18. potions	_____	38. discussed	_____
19. overt	_____	39. shorthand	_____
20. Tarzan	_____	40. muttered	_____

Complete Assignment 5-3.

The Affricate Consonants

Pronunciation Guide

/tʃ/   as in "chair"   /tʃɛr/
/ʤ/   as in "jar"   /ʤɑr/

The **affricate** manner of production involves a combination of the stop and fricative manners. For this reason, affricates are obstruents. Both English affricates are considered to have a palatal place of articulation. During production of the two affricates, the articulation begins as an alveolar stop. The tongue tip contacts the posterior alveolar ridge; there is a corresponding increase in intraoral pressure in the oral cavity. However, when the breath stream is released (voiced or voiceless), the air is forced through the constriction formed by the tongue and palate, creating a turbulent noise. (The constriction is similar to that formed during production of the palatal fricatives /ʃ/ and /ʒ/, that is, palatal, or palatoalveolar.)

/tʃ/, /ʤ/

Description

/tʃ/   voiceless, palatal affricate
/ʤ/   voiced, palatal affricate

Sample Words

/tʃ/	/ʤ/
chick	jelly
righteous	adjoin
nature	injure
crutch	badger
chimney	Jake
hatchet	refrigerate
wretched	generous

Minimal Pairs

/tʃ/	/ʤ/		/tʃ/	/ʤ/
etch	edge		chin	gin
batch	badge		cherry	Jerri
match	Madge		cheap	jeep
rich	ridge		chalk	jock
H	age		choke	joke

Allographs

	/tʃ/		/ʤ/
Grapheme	*Example*	*Grapheme*	*Example*
ch	check	j	joke
tch	witch	g	gem
t	nature	gg	exaggerate
te	righteous	d	educate
ti	question	dg	lodge
		di	soldier

Discussion Although English has only two phonemic affricates, different languages possess others, such as /ts/. This affricate combines the voiceless alveolar stop /t/ and the voiceless alveolar fricative /s/. The phonemes /t/ and /s/ do appear together in some English words and phrases such as "cats" /kæts/ and "let's go" /lɛtsgoʊ/. In these contexts, /ts/ is not a distinct phoneme. It is actually the result of the phoneme /t/ plus the morpheme /s/. (In these contexts, /s/ is used as a plural morpheme in "cats" and as a contraction in "let's.") Be sure not to confuse these two phonemes with the fricatives /ʃ/ and /ʒ/.

Practice Exercises

EXERCISE 5.4 – THE AFFRICATE CONSONANTS

A. Indicate the words below that have /tʃ/ or /ʤ/ in their transcription. Write the correct phoneme next to the word.

____ bon voyage	____ fantasia	____ cabbage
____ barrage	____ touches	____ exertion
____ arrange	____ pasture	____ sabotage
____ charming	____ nitrogen	____ gender
____ vulture	____ riches	____ glacier
____ mushroom	____ charade	____ eject
____ gerbil	____ rigid	____ unchained

B. For each item, create as many real words (or proper names) as possible by placing one of the following fricatives or affricates in the blank. Write your answers to the right of each item. More than one answer is possible for each item.

$$/f, v, θ, ð, s, z, ʃ, ʒ, h, tʃ, ʤ/$$

1. /__ɛr/ _____
2. /__æt/ _____
3. /__oʊ/ _____
4. /__ɑrm/ _____
5. /__ɪn/ _____
6. /ri__/ _____
7. /bæ__/ _____
8. /bi__/ _____

C. For each item, select the word(s) that have the specified criterion in their transcriptions.

other	shrunk	none	jeans	hedge	churned	measure

1. Contains an initial voiced phoneme _____
2. Contains a fricative _____
3. Contains an affricate and a front vowel _____
4. Contains an affricate and a nasal _____

Continues

EXERCISE 5.4 (*cont.*)

5. Contains a palatal obstruent   _____

6. Contains an obstruent
   and a central vowel   _____

7. Contains a stop, nasal, and affricate   _____

8. Contains all voiced sounds   _____

D. Circle the words that represent real English words.

1. /skrʌntʃ/	5. /muʒd/	9. /ouðən/	13. /fæʃtɚ/
2. /pudʒɪ/	6. /kɪtʃən/	10. /dʒeɪd/	14. /gautʃt/
3. /tʃɔrz/	7. /moutʃ/	11. /hʌdʒ/	15. /dʒʌmpɪ/
4. /harʃɚ/	8. /ʃarm/	12. /tʃɜn/	16. /partʃt/

E. In the blanks, write each of the words using English orthography.

1. /tʃɜpt/ _____   9. /ʃurlɪ/ _____

2. /dʒʌŋk/ _____   10. /dʒɜzɪ/ _____

3. /tʃɪt tʃæt/_____ 11. /pɜtʃəs/_____

4. /wɪʃboun/_____   12. /tʃaklət/_____

5. /ədʒɔɪnd/_____   13. /mətʃur/_____

6. /matʃou/_____   14. /tʃʌmɪ/_____

7. /gəraʒ/ _____   15. /ædʒəteɪt/_____

8. /pæstʃɚ/_____   16. /dʒɛzəbɛl/_____

F. For each item below, correct any vowel or consonant transcription errors by
    marking out the incorrect IPA symbol and placing the correct symbol above
    it. If no error is present, so indicate by circling "no error."

1. major   /meɪʒɚ/   no error

2. March   /martʃ/   no error

3. jumped   /dʒʌmpt/   no error

4. Wichita   /wɪtʃita/   no error

5. wedged   /wɛdʒt/   no error

6. usher   /ʌʃɚ/   no error

7. sergeant   /sɜdʒənt/   no error

8. massage   /məsaʒ/   no error

9. gorge   /dʒɔrʒ/   no error

10. manger   /mændʒɚ/   no error

G. Transcription Practice
    Transcribe the following words using the IPA.

1. shocked _____   5. extra   _____

2. station _____   6. tangent _____

3. butcher _____   7. southern _____

4. knickers _____   8. necktie _____

Continues

9. corsage	_____	25. charming	_____
10. spirits	_____	26. sharpened	_____
11. vivid	_____	27. cashier	_____
12. shutter	_____	28. garbage	_____
13. excite	_____	29. orchids	_____
14. axon	_____	30. strengthen	_____
15. scoured	_____	31. exists	_____
16. carved	_____	32. ginger	_____
17. outshine	_____	33. thorny	_____
18. gender	_____	34. Egypt	_____
19. careless	_____	35. chow mein	_____
20. nurture	_____	36. perverse	_____
21. cashmere	_____	37. duchess	_____
22. chopping	_____	38. anxious	_____
23. cashbox	_____	39. mischief	_____
24. genders	_____	40. capture	_____

Complete Assignment 5-4.

The Approximant Consonants: Glides and Liquids

Pronunciation Guide

Glides

/j/   as in "yet"   /jɛt/   /w/   as in "wet"   /wɛt/

Liquids

/r/   as in "rip"   /rɪp/   /l/   as in "lip"   /lɪp/

The **approximants**, the last group of consonants to be discussed, fall into a manner of production quite different from the others already discussed. In some respects, these four phonemes behave both like vowels, and in other respects, like consonants. Even though these consonants are produced with an obstruction in the vocal tract, the articulators are only approximated during their production; the constriction in the vocal tract is less than that associated with the English obstruent consonants.

Because the approximants do not usually form the nucleus of a syllable, they cannot be categorized as vowels. (The phoneme /l/ may become syllabic in some contexts, however.) In a manner similar to vowels, all of the approximants are voiced, so their sound source originates in the larynx. Also, all approximants are produced with a closed velopharyngeal port.

Phoneticians have given various names to this group of consonants. The approximants have been termed *semivowels, frictionless continuants,* and *oral resonants.* The latter term will be used in this text to be consistent with the classification scheme already introduced. The approximants are generally subdivided into two groups: *glides* and *liquids.* These two subgroups will be examined individually in the next sections.

Glides, as their name suggests, involve a gliding motion of the articulators, in a manner similar to the production of a diphthong. For this reason, glides are often referred to as semivowels (although some individuals use this term to refer to *all* approximants). The duration of an approximant glide is shorter (faster) than the duration of a diphthongal glide. Glides are always prevocalic. The glides /j/ and /w/ are characterized by continued movement of the articulators throughout their production into the following vowel.

/j/

Description

/j/   voiced, palatal glide

Sample Words

/j/

your	feud
young	cured
yellow	mutate
Yale	onion
yes	fewer

Allographs

/j/

Grapheme	Example
y	yell
u	fuse
eu	feud
i	union

Discussion   The name for the phoneme /j/ is /jɑt/. /j/ is produced by raising the tongue blade toward the palate (see Figure 5.7). The tongue and lips are in a position similar to that for production of the vowel /i/. The articulators then glide away from the articulation for /j/ to the lip and tongue position necessary for production of the following vowel. The continual motion of the articulators is what characterizes this consonant as a glide. Because the articulators change while gliding from /j/ to the following vowel, a corresponding change occurs in relation to the resonance of the vocal tract.

To demonstrate the similarity in articulation for the glide /j/ and the vowel /i/, say the word "yam" /jæm/. Prolong the initial /j/ phoneme as you say the word. You should hear the phoneme /j/ being produced as you glide from /i/ to /æ/ (/iiiiæm/).

/w/

Description

/w/   voiced, labiovelar glide

Sample Words

/w/

when	swill
weed	Kuwait
quick	away
twins	penguin
square	quartz

Allographs

/w/

Grapheme	Example
w	we
wh	why
qu	quit
u	language

Discussion   The phoneme /w/ is characterized by its two simultaneous places of articulation, bilabial and velar. During the production of this phoneme, the lips become rounded, and at the same time, the back of the tongue approximates the soft palate. (Say a word beginning with /w/ and see for yourself.) In the production of this phoneme, the lips and tongue begin in the aforementioned position and continue their gliding movement into the following vowel. The beginning articulatory position for /w/ is quite similar to the position for the vowel /u/. Try saying the word "week" /wik/ by prolonging production of /w/. You should hear the glide /w/ being produced as you glide from /u/ to /i/ (/uuuuik/).

Some individuals differentiate between the voiced phoneme /w/ and the voiceless phoneme /ʍ/. The phoneme /ʍ/ is used by some speakers who pronounce the first two letters in words such as "when," "where," and "which" as "hw." For example, /ʍɛn/ would indicate a pronunciation of /hwɛn/ for "when." Although most speakers of American English do not distinguish between the voiced and voiceless /w/ in their speech habits, speakers in eastern New England, parts of Texas, and in the lower South do make a clear distinction between these two phonemes (Labov, Ash, & Boberg, n.d.). In this text, only the voiced /w/ will be adopted.

The term **liquid** is used to categorize the oral resonant consonants /r/ and /l/. Some phoneticians have categorized the liquids as semivowels and also as glides. The term liquid is in no way a reference to the way in which these phonemes are produced. Liquid is simply a general term that has been adopted by phoneticians to categorize these two phonemes.

/r/

Description

/r/   voiced, palatal liquid

Sample Words

/r/

red	car	rhesus	more
stress	fear	carrot	pure
brown	there	revolt	stork

Allographs

/r/

Grapheme	Example
r	rose
rr	barren
rh	Rhodesia

Discussion   The prevocalic phoneme /r/ can be produced in one of two ways, depending on the speaker. Both methods employ a double constriction in the vocal tract. The **retroflexed** articulation of /r/ involves raising the tip of the tongue and curling it back toward the alveolar ridge (or the anterior portion of the palate) as the back of the tongue creates a second velar constriction. The second method of producing /r/, the **bunched** articulation, involves lowering the tip of the tongue and raising (or bunching) the blade of the tongue so that it closely approximates the hard palate, while the tongue root forms a second pharyngeal constriction. The voiced breath stream is forced through the constrictions formed by either method. In both cases, the tongue does not touch the other articulator involved. Both articulations are commonly used by English speakers.

When /r/ occurs at the beginning of a word or syllable (prevocalic), it is always considered to be a consonant. In the final position of words (or syllables), /r/may become a vowel, as in the words "her" /hɝ/ or "murder" /mɝdɚ/. It is possible to consider final /ɝ/ (or /ɚ/) as a syllabic consonant. That is, "her" and "murder" could be transcribed as /hr̩/ or /mr̩dr̩/. In this manner, /r̩/ is the nucleus of the syllable and therefore becomes a syllabic.

In the case of r-colored vowels (postvocalic /r/), the final /r/ still serves as a consonant, that is, "hair" /hɛr/ or "fear" /fɪr/. Pronouncing "hair" or "fear" with a syllabic final consonant would change these one-syllable words into two-syllable words: /hɛr̩/ and /fɪr̩/.

In Southern and Eastern American dialects, the postvocalic /r/ in words is often deleted. Some examples (with possible pronunciations) include:

chair→	/tʃɛə/	horse→	/hɔəs/
feared→	/fɪəd/	tour→	/tʊə/

Notice that /r/ is produced as /ə/ in these contexts. This production lends a diphthongal quality to the vowel. Likewise, when the vowels /ɚ/ and /ɝ/ occur at the end of a word, they may lose their "r" quality. They will be produced without tongue retroflexion by some southern and eastern speakers.

The phenomenon of deleting postvocalic /r/ has been found to be related to a person's age and gender. There is a trend in the United States for younger southern and eastern speakers to restore the postvocalic /r/ in words (Hartman, 1985).

/l/

Description

/l/   voiced, alveolar liquid

Sample Words

/l/

lawn	jello
split	mulch
bowl	hollow
black	pistol
bottle	allure

Allographs

/l/

Grapheme	Example
l	lend
ll	ball

Discussion   The phoneme /l/ has two separate articulations depending on whether the phoneme occurs at the beginning or at the end of a syllable. For syllable-initial, or prevocalic, /l/ (as in "lip"), the tongue tip is raised in order to approximate the alveolar ridge. In this position, the back of the tongue remains low in the oral cavity, and the airstream is diverted over both sides of the tongue. This is the production for the so-called *light* /l/.

When /l/ occurs in the syllable-final position, especially after a back vowel (as in "pull"), almost the reverse occurs. The tongue tip is lowered, and the back of the tongue is raised to approximate the palate as the airstream passes over both sides of the tongue. This is the production for the velarized, or *dark*, /l/. This allophone of /l/ is transcribed as [ɫ]. Because the airstream for /l/ flows over the sides of the tongue (for both articulations), /l/ is classified as a **lateral** consonant.

In many words, postvocalic /l/ becomes a syllabic consonant. Examine the examples of syllabic /l/ below. Listen to each of the words so that you are comfortable with the use of this allophone. Note that syllabic /l/ is always velarized.

legalize	[ligɫaɪz]	bottled	[baɾɫd]
hobble	[habɫ]	hustle	[hʌsɫ]
cardinal	[kardn̩ɫ]	bundle	[bʌndɫ]

Practice Exercises

EXERCISE 5.5—THE APPROXIMANT CONSONANTS

A. Indicate which of the following words has an approximant in its transcription. Write the correct phoneme, that is, /w,j,r, or l/, next to the word.

___ awkward	___ reasoned	___ suede	___ jonquil
___ bellow	___ towered	___ fewer	___ screaming
___ quick	___ Jupiter	___ peril	___ barley
___ today	___ lazy	___ swiped	___ puny
___ torpedo	___ repaid	___ yawned	___ fired

B. Indicate with an "X" which of the following words have /j/ in their transcription.

___ tune	___ hood	___ choosy
___ jealous	___ piano	___ compute
___ putrid	___ maybe	___ usual
___ loop	___ jar	___ yours
___ skew	___ adjourn	___ daisy
___ keynote	___ Cupid	___ boysenberry

Continues

EXERCISE 5.5 (*cont.*)

C. Indicate with an "X" which of the following words have /w/ in their transcription.

____ awesome	____ why	____ warrior
____ well	____ awry	____ swept
____ stalwart	____ wrath	____ quirk
____ how	____ rowboat	____ borrowed
____ showed	____ reward	____ wrist
____ lower	____ Howard	____ wayward

D. Indicate with an "X" the words that have /r/ in their transcriptions.

____ lurk	____ surround	____ purchase
____ barter	____ rewritten	____ perfected
____ burgundy	____ tires	____ scorpion
____ unreal	____ fourth	____ flirtatious
____ guarded	____ spirited	____ grandiose
____ grasp	____ curvature	____ divert

E. Circle the words that represent real English words.

1. /ʤɛloʊ/	5. /ʤɑr/	9. /wʊln̩/	13. /swɪlz/
2. /blaɪð/	6. /sɝklz̩/	10. /pjaɪd/	14. /riwɝd/
3. /rɪljə/	7. /fjɝt/	11. /spjud/	15. /poʊləs/
4. /roʊlɚ/	8. /kwɔrld/	12. /wɑlʃat/	16. /fjunts/

F. In the blanks, write each of the words using English orthography.

1. /jɛloʊ/ _____	9. /lɪkwəd/ _____
2. /robʌst/ _____	10. /taɪld/ _____
3. /wɑrɪə/ _____	11. /kɚteɪld/ _____
4. /jɝnd/ _____	12. /kwɑrl̩/ _____
5. /bɪɾlz/ _____	13. /lʌkl̩/ _____
6. /graʊtʃt/ _____	14. /læʔn̩/ _____
7. /ripjut/ _____	15. /bʌkwit/ _____
8. /gwɑvə/ _____	16. /kwɛstʃən/ _____

G. For each item below, correct any vowel, diphthong, nasal, or stop consonant transcription errors by marking out the incorrect IPA symbol and placing the correct symbol above it. If no error is present, so indicate by circling "no error."

1. bowling	/boʊlɪŋ/	no error
2. wrongful	/wrɑŋfʊl/	no error
3. warbled	/wɑrbl̩d/	no error
4. pewter	/piuɾə/	no error
5. quandary	/qwɑndrɪ/	no error

Continues

6.	regional	/ridʒənl̩/	no error
7.	lawyer	/lɔjɚ/	no error
8.	flurries	/fl̩ɝiz/	no error
9.	fuming	/fjumɪŋ/	no error
10.	baloney	/bʌlounɪj/	no error

H. Transcription Practice

Transcribe the following two-syllable words, using the IPA.

1. quicksand _____
2. slouched _____
3. jury _____
4. acquaint _____
5. shoulder _____
6. slither _____
7. sergeant _____
8. skewer _____
9. cordial _____
10. useful _____
11. withdrew _____
12. worship _____
13. enshrined _____
14. fumed _____
15. luncheon _____
16. junior _____
17. unscathed _____
18. shrivel _____
19. Yankees _____
20. quarter _____
21. bugle _____
22. chisel _____
23. eunuch _____
24. Charles _____
25. belonging _____
26. rubric _____
27. unique _____
28. bequeathed _____
29. kayak _____
30. billiards _____
31. eyewash _____
32. lingual _____
33. quarreled _____
34. anguished _____
35. outward _____
36. rupture _____
37. shoe wax _____
38. quotient _____
39. strangler _____
40. allure _____

Complete Assignment 5-5.

Review Exercises

A. For the following words, determine whether a *tap* (ɾ), a *glottal stop* (ʔ), or *nasal plosion* (np) is found in its transcription. Fill in the blank with the appropriate answer. If none of these are apparent in the transcription, leave the answer blank.

_____ 1. writin'   _____ 6. certain

_____ 2. rudder   _____ 7. crater

_____ 3. about   _____ 8. winter

_____ 4. nutty   _____ 9. Martin

_____ 5. harden   _____ 10. sudden

B. Indicate with an "X" which of the following words or phrases have a syllabic consonant in their transcription.

_____ 1. wheel   _____ 6. pull

_____ 2. written   _____ 7. contagious

_____ 3. regal   _____ 8. that'll

_____ 4. Seton Hall   _____ 9. grab 'em by the neck

_____ 5. candles   _____ 10. hold 'er by the tail

C. For all of the consonant phonemes below, indicate their manner, place, and voicing.

	Manner	*Place*	*Voicing*
Example:			
/d/	stop	alveolar	voiced
/k/	_____	_____	_____
/r/	_____	_____	_____
/θ/	_____	_____	_____
/ŋ/	_____	_____	_____
/dʒ/	_____	_____	_____
/b/	_____	_____	_____
/ʃ/	_____	_____	_____
/j/	_____	_____	_____
/f/	_____	_____	_____
/n/	_____	_____	_____

D. Create at least two minimal pairs for the underlined phoneme so that they match the differing features given.

Differing Features

Example:

mit _____ pit, wit _____ voice   manner

1. <u>s</u>eed _____ voice   manner

2. co<u>p</u>e _____ voice   manner   place

3. <u>s</u>ome _____ place

4. z̲ip   _____   voice   place

5. b̲ag   _____   place   manner

E. Each of the following pairs of words differ by one phoneme. Determine how the phonemes differ in terms of manner, place, and/or voicing. Then, list the differing features for each pair given.

Differing Features

Example:

none-ton   _____voice, manner_____

1. sin-sing   _____

2. jaw-raw   _____

3. sue-shoe   _____

4. tin-tip   _____

5. clue-crew   _____

6. cop-mop   _____

7. choke-joke   _____

8. pet-met   _____

9. done-gun   _____

10. even-Eden   _____

11. Yale-rail   _____

12. late-lake   _____

13. fame-shame   _____

14. cat-cad   _____

15. pass-pad   _____

F. Identify the words that contain an affricate. If the word has an affricate, indicate the position in the word (pre-, post-, or intervocalic), and whether the affricate is voiced or voiceless.

Word	Transcribed Affricate	Voicing	Position in Word
Example:			
c̲harm	/tʃ/	voiceless	prevocalic
1. jester			
2. version			
3. itchy			
4. cash			
5. switched			
6. January			
7. regime			
8. mashing			
9. crush			
10. urgent			

G. Transcribe the underlined consonant allographs in the following words and indicate the appropriate voicing, place, and manner of articulation.

Word	Transcribed Phoneme	Voicing	Place	Manner
Example:				
<u>c</u>ab	/k/	voiceless	velar	stop
1. <u>c</u>elery				
2. bree<u>ch</u>				
3. <u>ph</u>ase				
4. w<u>r</u>eck				
5. ca<u>ll</u>				
6. me<u>th</u>od				
7. <u>y</u>es				
8. cru<u>d</u>e				
9. <u>ch</u>asm				
10. ed<u>g</u>e				
11. <u>w</u>alk				
12. cohe<u>s</u>ion				

H. Transcription Practice

Transcribe the following words, using the IPA.

1. birthmarks _____
2. conjuring _____
3. beachcomber _____
4. otherwise _____
5. George Bush _____
6. vatican _____
7. zinc oxide _____
8. handkerchief _____
9. expedite _____
10. foundation _____
11. admitted _____
12. thereafter _____
13. injunction _____
14. convergence _____
15. sabotage _____
16. physician _____
17. buttonhole _____
18. discouraged _____
19. evolved _____
20. indigent _____

21. cosmos _____
22. chimpanzees _____
23. discarded _____
24. prestigious _____
25. charming _____
26. Turkish bath _____
27. bothersome _____
28. jackknife _____
29. enzyme _____
30. tooth fairy _____
31. cherry pie _____
32. coauthor _____
33. hyacinth _____
34. enjoyment _____
35. pharmacist _____
36. unworthy _____
37. 100th _____
38. pasteurized _____
39. fidgety _____
40. Father's Day _____

I. Transcription Practice

Transcribe the following words (containing three syllables), using the IPA.

1. aorta _____
2. airliner _____
3. congealed _____
4. Caucasian _____
5. vocation _____
6. funeral _____
7. registered _____
8. yesterday _____
9. November _____
10. troublesome _____
11. upholstered _____
12. impudent _____
13. torrential _____
14. distribute _____
15. diaphragm _____
16. appetite _____
17. persevere _____
18. courageous _____
19. muscular _____
20. papyrus _____

21. sequential _____
22. portrayal _____
23. Thanksgiving _____
24. xylophone _____
25. artichoke _____
26. pigeonhole _____
27. Williamsburg _____
28. undergrowth _____
29. humorous _____
30. weariness _____
31. universe _____
32. ungathered _____
33. manuscript _____
34. obscurely _____
35. nucleus _____
36. quadrangle _____
37. harmonize _____
38. registrar _____
39. parboiled _____
40. structural _____

Complete Assignments 5-6 and 5-7.

Study Questions

1. What is a consonant? How do vowels and consonants differ?
2. Define the following terms:
   a. resonant
   b. nonresonant
   c. obstruent
3. Define the terms manner, place, and voicing.
4. Distinguish between prevocalic, postvocalic, and intervocalic consonants.
5. What is meant by the term *nasal plosion?*
6. What is a syllabic consonant? Which consonants can become syllabics in English? What are the rules that govern their usage?
7. What is the difference between a tap and a glottal stop?
8. Indicate the sound source for each of the following: vowels, stops, nasals, fricatives, affricates, and approximants.
9. Describe the actual ways in which the following consonant manners are produced: stops, fricatives, nasals, affricates, and approximants.

Assignment 5-1

Name _____

Stop consonant transcription.

Transcribe the following two- and three-syllable words.

1. deadbeat _____
2. darker _____
3. diode _____
4. packing _____
5. Vicky _____
6. backup _____
7. taboo _____
8. decoy _____
9. Cape Cod _____
10. tugboat _____
11. bedbug _____
12. bobcat _____
13. decode _____
14. doted _____
15. diaper _____
16. buckeye _____
17. dugout _____
18. tiptoe _____
19. beaded _____
20. khaki _____
21. co-op _____
22. edit _____
23. dittoed _____
24. tip top _____
25. guide dog _____

26. agape _____
27. go cart _____
28. goodbye _____
29. bagpiper _____
30. katydid _____
31. operate _____
32. terrier _____
33. peapod _____
34. boycotted _____
35. period _____
36. irrigate _____
37. gaiety _____
38. cataract _____
39. gadabout _____
40. carpeting _____
41. dedicate _____
42. barbaric _____
43. caterer _____
44. attitude _____
45. poetic _____
46. corrected _____
47. biotic _____
48. doorkeeper _____
49. bugaboo _____
50. corridor _____

Assignment 5-2

Name _____

Stop and nasal consonant transcription.

Transcribe the following two- and three-syllable words.

1. minute _____
2. windbag _____
3. cranky _____
4. mustard _____
5. coyness _____
6. downtime _____
7. condone _____
8. bookmark _____
9. tune-up _____
10. benign _____
11. magnet _____
12. bunker _____
13. curtain _____
14. negate _____
15. omit _____
16. kidney _____
17. pontoon _____
18. mundane _____
19. coward _____
20. pointing _____
21. inert _____
22. command _____
23. bumpkin _____
24. airman _____
25. tenant _____

26. animate _____
27. enduring _____
28. Canada _____
29. incarnate _____
30. ionic _____
31. entire _____
32. cantata _____
33. torpedoed _____
34. mitigate _____
35. pinto bean _____
36. piranha _____
37. bandana _____
38. motorcade _____
39. Montana _____
40. dignity _____
41. myopic _____
42. commando _____
43. accountant _____
44. pyramid _____
45. binary _____
46. nominate _____
47. mnemonic _____
48. dogmatic _____
49. interrupt _____
50. gabardine _____

Assignment 5-3

Name _____

Stop, nasal, and fricative consonant transcription.

Transcribe the following three- and four-syllable words.

1. succinctness _____
2. Alzheimer's _____
3. ambition _____
4. commercial _____
5. unsanctioned _____
6. decomposed _____
7. visionary _____
8. cathartic _____
9. admonish _____
10. systemic _____
11. ombudsman _____
12. redemption _____
13. Zambia _____
14. schematic _____
15. horrific _____
16. aversion _____
17. vehemence _____
18. Venetian _____
19. thoroughfare _____
20. orthodox _____
21. zucchini _____
22. xenophobe _____
23. fluorescent _____
24. excavate _____
25. symphonic _____

26. seventeenth _____
27. thereabouts _____
28. homeopath _____
29. understanding _____
30. uncertainty _____
31. vaporizer _____
32. thermometer _____
33. subconsciousness _____
34. sarcophagus _____
35. reservation _____
36. orthodontist _____
37. perversity _____
38. subdivision _____
39. weatherbeaten _____
40. unconvincing _____
41. chauvinism _____
42. innovative _____
43. impersonate _____
44. heterodyne _____
45. catechism _____
46. extortionist _____
47. disorganized _____
48. incandescence _____
49. criticism _____
50. conversation _____

Assignment 5-4

Name _____

Stop, nasal, fricative, and affricate consonant transcription.
Transcribe the following three and four-syllable words.

1. repackaged _____
2. compassion _____
3. digestive _____
4. confiscate _____
5. injury _____
6. membranous _____
7. Egyptian _____
8. geosphere _____
9. foundation _____
10. intersperse _____
11. maturate _____
12. exertion _____
13. effervesce _____
14. matchmaker _____
15. chimpanzee _____
16. astonish _____
17. gestation _____
18. omniscient _____
19. amateur _____
20. chastisement _____
21. advantaged _____
22. pasteurized _____
23. x-axis _____
24. disparage _____
25. educate _____

26. affectionate _____
27. contortionist _____
28. menagerie _____
29. moisturizing _____
30. notorious _____
31. pessimistic _____
32. North Dakota _____
33. unimportant _____
34. terrifying _____
35. punctuation _____
36. potassium _____
37. jurisdiction _____
38. pedagogy _____
39. participant _____
40. overshadow _____
41. homogenized _____
42. indigestion _____
43. damaged goods _____
44. thundershower _____
45. graduation _____
46. juxtaposing _____
47. photogenic _____
48. designation _____
49. sandwiches _____
50. pathologies _____

Assignment 5-5

Name _____

Stop, nasal, fricative, affricate, glide, and liquid consonant transcription.
Transcribe the following three- and four-syllable words.

1. quietly _____
2. wondrous _____
3. Hercules _____
4. cultural _____
5. koala _____
6. rebellious _____
7. quantify _____
8. subsequent _____
9. withering _____
10. aquarium _____
11. inquiry _____
12. curious _____
13. worldly _____
14. strategy _____
15. pressurized _____
16. puberty _____
17. symbolic _____
18. refusal _____
19. wonderfully _____
20. journalism _____
21. disgruntled _____
22. visualize _____
23. Yosemite _____
24. malicious _____
25. illustrious _____

26. glorified _____
27. flamboyant _____
28. chromium _____
29. extrapolate _____
30. employee _____
31. legalized _____
32. delinquency _____
33. accumulate _____
34. chlorinated _____
35. Asiatic _____
36. ballerina _____
37. quagmire _____
38. inflammable _____
39. legislation _____
40. futuristic _____
41. burglarize _____
42. slovenly _____
43. nonchalant _____
44. liquidate _____
45. infuriate _____
46. bureaucracy _____
47. exquisitely _____
48. acquittal _____
49. bulimia _____
50. ridicule _____

Assignment 5-6

Name _____

Transcribe the following geographic locations in IPA.

1. Bowling Green, Kentucky _____

2. Wheeling, West Virginia _____

3. Albuquerque, New Mexico _____

4. Tallahassee, Florida _____

5. Chattanooga, Tennessee _____

6. Joplin, Missouri _____

7. Honolulu, Hawaii _____

8. Anaheim, California _____

9. Thunder Bay, Ontario _____

10. Rochester, Minnesota _____

11. Prague, Czechoslovakia _____

12. Helsinki, Finland _____

13. Raleigh, North Carolina _____

14. Tijuana, Mexico _____

15. Omaha, Nebraska _____

16. Denton, Texas _____

17. Geneva, Switzerland _____

18. Istanbul, Turkey _____

19. Johannesburg, South Africa _____

20. Hiroshima, Japan _____

21. Antwerp, Belgium _____

22. Montreal, Quebec _____

23. Boise, Idaho _____

24. Boston, Massachusetts _____

25. Stockholm, Sweden _____

Assignment 5-7

Name _____

Transcribe the following.

1. curious savage
2. transmission fluid
3. terrible twos
4. lightning 'n' thunder
5. persuasive argument
6. apparent dilemma
7. algebra equation
8. legal document
9. implausible idea
10. perplexed child
11. veritable fortune
12. grapefruit juice
13. watermelon rind
14. Wuthering Heights
15. torrential downpour
16. Scranton, PA
17. very tranquil
18. butterscotch pudding
19. patchwork quilts
20. oxygen cycle
21. anxious parent
22. earthquake rumble
23. pasteurized milk
24. privileged character
25. punitive damages
26. pharyngeal inflammation

6

Connected Speech

The exercises in the previous chapters were designed so that you would learn to recognize all of the individual English speech sound segments and how to determine which IPA symbols best represent them. By now, you should feel fairly comfortable transcribing individual words using the correct IPA symbols for all the English phonemes. In Chapters 4 and 5, the words given in all of the examples and in all of the exercises were transcribed as isolated items, as if they were excised from a sentence. When a word is pronounced carefully as a single item, it is said to be spoken in its **citation form**. The identity of a word spoken in citation form may differ markedly from its identity in **connected speech**. Connected speech results from joining two or more words together in the creation of an utterance. In Chapter 5, some of the exercises involved transcription of items consisting of two words. However, these two-word utterances were transcribed as if each word was produced in citation form. The production of a particular utterance may vary drastically when comparing its citation form with its form in connected speech. In citation form, the word "him" would be transcribed as /hɪm/. The same word in connected speech might be transcribed as /əm/ as in the phrase "I caught him"—/aɪkɔt əm/. Also, in connected speech, the production of any particular utterance will most likely vary from speaker to speaker due to differences in dialect and speaking style.

In clinical practice, speech-language pathologists transcribe isolated words when administering phonological tests to their clients to determine which speech sounds are in need of remediation. More often than not, clinicians need to transcribe entire utterances as spoken by their clients. For example, after obtaining a language sample from a child, a clinician will need to analyze the utterances not only in terms of the specific syntactic (grammatical) structures being used, but also in terms of the particular phonemes the child is using correctly or incorrectly. To perform a thorough phonemic analysis of a client's speech patterns, the speech-language pathologist may need to transcribe entire utterances of connected speech.

There are several major issues that make transcribing connected or continuous speech much different from transcribing isolated words. In connected speech, the phonetic identity of words often changes. As already mentioned, the way a word sounds in citation form varies greatly from the way it might sound in a sentence. In connected speech, phonemes are eliminated and/or completely altered once words are strung together in an utterance. In addition, connected discourse is characterized by continuous changes in the stress, intonation and timing of phonemes, words, and complete sentences. Listening to, and transcribing, words in continuous discourse requires a lot of concentration. It takes a good ear to be able to hear the subtle nuances associated with connected speech. This chapter will focus on two major issues associated with the transcription of connected speech: (1) assimilation and (2) the suprasegmental aspects of speech.

Assimilation

In citation form, each word is spoken in a fairly deliberate manner. That is, the phonemes are pronounced quite carefully, keeping the inherent length of each phoneme fairly intact. Once words are produced in conversation, the deliberateness of speech disappears. Phonemes are not produced in a strictly serial order as we speak; the onset of one phoneme will occur before the previous one has been completely articulated. This often results in an overlapping of the individual phonemes of English. For instance, the utterance, "Where did you go?" might be produced as /wɛrʤəgoʊ/? The question, "What in the world are you going to do?" might be spoken as /wəʔn̩ðəwɜ˞ldəjəgʊnədu/? The syllable boundaries often become obscured in conversational, or casual, speech, even though listeners have little difficulty understanding what is being said. Also, notice that the quality of the vowels changes quite markedly in connected speech.

While we talk, it is necessary to overlap the production of the various phonemes to maintain the rapidity of connected speech. The overlapping of the articulators during speech production is termed **coarticulation**. Coarticulation is a time-efficient process; there is simply not enough time for the articulators to produce each phoneme in its intended isolated form. In addition, coarticulation makes connected speech easier for the speaker to produce. Speech would become quite laborious and slow, indeed, if each individual phoneme was produced in its full, isolated form in every syllable of every word.

An example of coarticulation can be found in the production of the word "soon." In this word, the lips are already rounded at the beginning of the word in anticipation of the rounded vowel /u/. That is, the normally unrounded phoneme /s/ becomes rounded due to the phonetic environment provided by the vowel. Say the word "soon," paying particular attention to the position of your lips for the phoneme /s/. This rounded version of /s/ is an allophone of the /s/ phoneme. Another example of coarticulation can be seen by examining the difference in the articulation of the phoneme /k/ in the words /kɪd/ "kid" and /kʊd/ "could." In /kɪd/, /k/ is produced further forward in the mouth (toward the palate) due to the phonetic environment provided by the front vowel /ɪ/. The /k/ in /kʊd/ remains toward the back of the mouth (toward the velum) because /ʊ/ is a back vowel. Thus, the two different productions of /k/ in the words "kid" and "could" are allophones of /k/.

It should be apparent (from the examples above) that a particular phoneme will be articulated differently if that phoneme is preceded or followed by a different sequence of consonants and vowels. Also, the effects of rapid continuous speech often will change the phonetic identity of phonemes. It is possible for a particular phonetic context to cause a phoneme to be replaced by a completely different phoneme. Sometimes it is even possible for the phonetic context to result in the complete deletion of a phoneme.

Examine the following utterance: /wʌz ʃi/ ("was she"). In conversation, this utterance is typically produced as /wʌʒ ʃi/. In this case, the /z/ phoneme is produced farther back in the mouth than normal due to the palatal fricative /ʃ/ found in the word "she." Notice that in this example, the change from /z/ to /ʒ/ (due to /ʃ/) occurs across the boundary between the two words. The process whereby phonemes take on the phonetic character of neighboring sounds is referred to as **assimilation**. Some phoneticians suggest that assimilation is brought about as a direct result of coarticulation during the production of connected speech (Calvert, 1986; Ohde & Sharf, 1992).

Some individuals support the notion that coarticulation and assimilation are two separate processes (MacKay, 1987), while others use the terms synonymously (Cruttenden, 2001). When viewed as separate processes, coarticulation would be defined as a change in the phonetic identity of a sound that results only in an allophonic variation of a phoneme, whereas assimilation would refer specifically to articulatory changes that result in the production of a completely different phoneme.

In this text, coarticulation will be viewed as the articulatory process whereby individual phonemes overlap one another due to timing constraints and simplicity of production. Assimilation will be viewed as the realized changes in the identity of phonemes brought about by coarticulation. The term assimilation will be used here to refer to *both* allophonic changes and phonemic changes brought about by phonetic environment.

There are of two basic forms of assimilation, regressive and progressive. **Regressive assimilation** occurs when the identity of a phoneme is modified due to a phoneme following it. This is also referred to as *right-to-left* or *anticipatory assimilation*. That is, the articulators anticipate the production of a phoneme occurring later in time. On the other hand, **progressive assimilation** occurs when a phoneme's identity changes as the result of a phoneme preceding it in time. This type of assimilation is also called *left-to-right* or *perseverative assimilation*. That is, the articulators persevere in their production of a particular phoneme and maintain a particular posture for a later phoneme.

Consider the utterance, "Would you like to go?" How might you say this utterance? One acceptable pronunciation of this utterance might be /wʊʤəlaɪktəgoʊ/? Notice that "would you" is transcribed as /wʊʤə/. The environment provided by the palatal glide /j/ of "you" alters the pronunciation of /d/ in the word "would," resulting in a right-to-left assimilation of /d/ to /ʤ/. In this case, the alveolar plosive /d/ becomes palatal, inducing articulation of the affricate /ʤ/. A similar example involves production of the word "question." This word can be pronounced one of two ways: /kwɛstʃən/ or /kwɛʃtʃən/. Notice that in the second example, the /s/ has been assimilated to /ʃ/ due to the palatal affricate /tʃ/ in the second syllable of the word. This is a clear demonstration of right-to-left assimilation.

Many of the assimilations brought about by phonetic environment are seen as a change in the *place of articulation* of a particular phoneme. Most of these assimilations are regressive; the phonemes become similar in place of articulation to later-occurring phonemes. All of the following examples demonstrate regressive assimilation resulting in a change in alveolar place of articulation (adapted from Cruttenden, 2001). Don't worry about memorizing these assimilatory changes. It is more important that you understand the process of assimilation and why it occurs.

change from /t/ → /p/
(alveolar to bilabial)
fat man → /fæp˺ mæn/
hat box → /hæp˺ bɑks/

change from /t/ → /k/
(alveolar to velar)
that guy → /ðæk˺ gaɪ/
spot clean → /spɑk˺ klin/

change from /d/ → /b/
(alveolar to bilabial)
bad boy → /bæb˺ bɔɪ/
road map → /roʊb˺ mæp/

change from /d/ → /g/
(alveolar to velar)
bad girl → /bæg˺ gɝl/
road kill → /roʊg˺ kɪl/

(Note: [˺] indicates an unreleased plosive)

change from /n/ → /m/
(alveolar to bilabial)
win more → /wɪm mɔr/
can play → /kæm pleɪ/
phone booth → /foʊm buθ/

change from /n/ → /ŋ/
(alveolar to velar)
tin cup → /tɪŋ kʌp/
mean guys → /miŋ gaɪz/
bacon grease → /beɪkŋ gris/

change from /s/ → /ʃ/
(alveolar to palatal)
misjudge → /mɪʃ ʤʌʤ/
cross check → /krɑʃʧɛk/
horse shoe → /hɔrʃ ʃu/

change from /z/ → /ʒ/
(alveolar to palatal)
was she → /wʌʒ ʃi/
those shoes → /ðoʒ ʃuz/
please share → /pliʒ ʃɛr/

change of alveolar /s , z, t, or d/ + /j/ → /ʃ, ʒ, ʧ, or ʤ/
(alveolar to palatal)

Miss **U**niverse → /mɪʃunəvɚs/	(/s/ + /j/ → /ʃ/)
free**ze y**our toes → /friʒɚtoʊz/	(/z/ + /j/ → /ʒ/)
I'll be**t y**ou → /aɪlbɛʧə/	(/t/ + /j/ → /ʧ/)
I rea**d y**our book → /aɪrɛʤɚbʊk/	(/d/ + /j / → /ʤ/)

Progressive, or left-to-right, assimilation occurs when the plural morpheme /s/ is pronounced as /z/ when it follows a voiced phoneme, for example, /dɑgz/ "dogs" or /ɑrmz/ "arms." In these examples, the voiced phoneme has a left-to-right (progressive) effect on the following /s/ phoneme, causing it to be produced as /z/. Similarly, production of the past tense morpheme "ed" is produced as /t/ when preceded by a voiceless phoneme, for example, /wɑkt/ "walked." Note the effect of progressive assimilation brought about by the /k/ phoneme.

Another example of progressive assimilation occurs when a nasal phoneme follows a plosive with the same place of articulation as in /hæpm̩/ "happen." In this case, the place of articulation of the plosive is preserved in production of the nasal, that is, left-to-right, assimilation (see Cruttenden, 2001).

Elision

In English, it is common for phonemes to be eliminated during production due to particular phonetic contexts. For example, the word "exactly" may be spoken as /əgzæklɪ/. Notice that the /t/ has been eliminated in this particular pronunciation. Omission of a phoneme during speech production is called **elision**. Another example of elision occurs in the word "camera." It is not uncommon for speakers to pronounce this word as /kæmrə/ as opposed to /kəmɚə/. Note that in /kæmrə/, an entire syllable has been deleted, or *elided*.

Elision often results as a historical process as a language develops over time. Elision also occurs as a result of coarticulation associated with connected speech. In addition, elision is found to occur across word boundaries due to certain phonetic environments. Examine the words and phrases (along with their transcriptions) in Table 6.1 to see the resultant elision brought about by effects of phonetic context.

EXERCISE 6.1

Examine each of the following utterances and their transcriptions. Indicate, in the blank, the phoneme that has been elided.

1. lengths   /lɛŋks/   ____
2. friendship   /frɛnʃɪp/   ____
3. countess   /kaʊnəs/   ____
4. bands   /bænz/   ____
5. kept quiet   /kɛpkwaɪət/   ____
6. I caught her.   /aɪkɔɾɚ/   ____
7. word of mouth   /wɝɾəmaʊθ/   ____
8. Where did he go?   /wɛrdɪɾigoʊ/   ____

TABLE 6.1   Examples of Elision

Utterance	Transcription	Elided Phoneme
aptly	/æplɪ/	/t/
hunter	/hʌnɚ/	/t/
con'tracts (verb)	/kəntræks/	/t/
asthma	/æzmə/	/ð/
fifths	/fɪfs/	/θ/
glands	/glænz/	/d/
kept busy	/kɛpbɪzɪ/	/t/
used to	/juztu/	/d/
cracked nuts	/kræknʌts/	/t/
cup of tea	/kʌpəti/	/v/
What's his name?	/wətsəzneɪm/	/h/
I want to go home.	/aɪwɑnəgohoʊm/	/t/
I caught them.	/aɪkɔɾəm/	/ð/
Give me that.	/gɪmɪðæt/	/v/

Epenthesis

In connected speech, additional phonemes are sometimes inserted in words during their production. The addition of a phoneme to the production of a word is termed **epenthesis**. Epenthesis can be the result of factors related to (1) coarticulation, (2) variation in production, or (3) speech disorders.

In terms of coarticulation, the glides /j/ and /w/ may sometimes *seem* to appear between two adjacent vowels, either in the same word or in two different words. For example, it may seem that the glide /j/ is inserted after a front vowel (or diphthong) in words such as "Leo" → /lijoʊ/, "Ohio" →/ohaɪjoʊ/ or "we own" → /wijoʊn/. Similarly, it may seem that the glide /w/ is inserted after a back vowel, as in the words "cooing" → /kuwɪŋ/, "going" → /goʊwɪŋ/, or "to each" → /tuwiʧ/. In these examples, the tongue is gliding in transition from one vowel nucleus to another. The addition of these "transitional" phonemes often result as "native speakers correctly pronounce their own language" (MacKay, 1987, p. 147).

Epenthesis sometimes occurs in words in which a nasal consonant precedes a voiceless fricative. In the words "tense" → /tɛnts/, "lengths" → /lɛŋkθs/, and "Amsterdam" → /æmpstɚdæm/, it may appear that a homorganic voiceless stop is added during production, even though the stop does not actually occur in the word. These added phonemes are the result of physiological constraints on the articulators (due to coarticulation) when producing the phoneme sequence of nasal + fricative, that is, /ns/(tense), /ŋθ/ (lengths), and /ms/ (Amsterdam).

Due to individual speaking style or dialectal variation, some speakers do not make a true distinction in production of words such as "chance"/"chants" or "tense"/"tents." For these individuals, both productions would be identical and therefore would be transcribed the same, that is, /ʧænts/ or /tɛnts/. However, many speakers *do*, in fact, make a clear distinction between the two pronunciations of these words, that is, /ʧæns/-/ʧænts/ or /tɛns/ - /tɛnts/. You will have to listen carefully during transcription to determine whether a speaker is actually inserting a stop following the nasal in these contexts.

Other examples of epenthesis occur in the idiosyncratic or dialectal production of certain words. For instance, the words "elm" and "film" are pronounced by some individuals (including my father) as /ɛləm/ and /fɪləm/. Also, some speakers in the southern and eastern United States insert the phoneme /j/ before /u/ in words such as "Tuesday" → /tjuzdeɪ/ or "due" → /dju/. Speakers in the East also sometimes insert an /r/ at the end of some words that normally end with schwa, for example, "soda" → /soʊdɚ/ or "Cuba" → /kjubɚ/.

Finally, epenthesis is sometimes observed in individuals with disordered speech patterns. For instance, some children with phonological disorders will insert /ə/ in the middle of a consonant blend. Examples include "break" → /bəreɪk/ and "glad" → /gəlæd/. Schwa insertion is also prevalent in the speech of some deaf individuals.

EXERCISE 6.2

Examine each of the following words and their corresponding transcriptions. Indicate with an "X" the transcriptions that illustrate epenthesis.

	word	transcription	
1.	noon	/nuən/	____
2.	pants	/pænts/	____
3.	choose	/tʃjuz/	____
4.	friends	/frɛndz/	____
5.	lamb	/læm/	____
6.	straw	/strɔr/	____
7.	rinse	/rɪns/	____
8.	milk	/mɛlk/	____
9.	clam	/kəlæm/	____
10.	Wednesday	/wænzdeɪ/	____

Metathesis

The transposition of sounds in a word is known as **metathesis**. Metathesis can occur as a result of a "slip of the tongue," personal speaking style, dialectal variation, or a speech disorder. Some examples include:

"elephant" → /ɛfələnt/	"spaghetti" → /pəsgɛɾɪ/
"ask" → /æks/	"cinnamon" → /sɪmənən/
"realtor" → /rilətɚ/	"animal" → /æmɪnl̩/

Vowel Reduction

Another issue commonly encountered when transcribing connected speech involves the phenomenon called **vowel reduction**. Often, the full form (full weight) of a vowel (such as /æ/) becomes more like the mid-central vowel /ə/ when spoken in connected speech. Compare the following transcriptions of the utterance "I can go."

/aɪ kæn goʊ/	*citation form with full vowel /æ/*
/aɪ kən goʊ/	*casual form with reduced vowel /ə/*

The first transcription would be indicative of very careful pronunciation, as if all three words were spoken in isolation. Contrast the citation form with the second transcription, the more casual form. Notice that the vowel /æ/ has been reduced to /ə/. In other words, the articulation of the vowel shifted from low-front to mid-central. In this case, the tongue does not meet the true articulatory target for /æ/ in the low front portion of the mouth. Instead, the body of the tongue remains towards the center of the oral cavity. You have already experienced vowel reduction in certain isolated words such as "feasible." When transcribing this word, it would be possible to transcribe the second vowel with /ɪ/ as in /fizɪbl̩/ or with /ə/ as in /fizəbl̩/, depending on the pronunciation. In the second transcription, the /ɪ/ vowel reflects reduction to /ə/.

What causes vowel reduction? In connected speech, there is often not time for the articulators to achieve their target positions because speech occurs so rapidly. Therefore, the articulators adopt new positions that are still acceptable to the ear. These vowel reductions are not considered to be "bad," "lazy," or "sloppy" articulations. They are simply considered to be the product of connected speech. Below is a list of words, demonstrating the process of vowel reduction. Each word is transcribed twice, first using a particular vowel in its full form, and second, using the reduced vowel form. Notice that the two pronunciations for each word are acceptable depending upon the way a person might say the words.

Examples of Vowel Reduction

	Full Vowel	Reduced Vowel
to**morrow**	/tumɑroʊ/	/təmɑroʊ/
de**cide**	/disaɪd/	/dəsaɪd/
tri**bunal**	/traɪbjunl̩/	/trəbjunl̩/
ob**scene**	/ɑbsin/	/əbsin/
ex**cel**	/ɛksɛl/	/əksɛl/
do**mestic**	/domɛstək/	/dəmɛstək/

The following six words pairs are comprised of words sharing the same morpheme. Note the difference in pronunciation between the vowels (in bold) in each pair. The first word in each pair has a vowel with full weight, that is, not reduced. The second word of each pair has the reduced form of the vowel. In each pair, the change in vowel form from full to reduced is due to a change in primary word stress *away from the syllable* in question.

transform	/træns'fɔrm/	concept	/'kɑnsɛpt/
transformation	/trænsfɚ'meɪʃən/	conception	/kən'sɛpʃən/
excrete	/ɛks'krit/	impose	/ɪm'pouz/
excretory	/'ɛkskrətɔrɪ/	imposition	/ɪmpə'zɪʃən/
sequence	/'sikwɛns/	condemn	/kən'dɛm/
sequential	/sə'kwɛnʃəl/	condemnation	/kɑndəm'neɪʃən/

Each of the following word pairs demonstrates more than one vowel undergoing a change in vowel quality. Examine each pair in order to see the changes from the full to the reduced vowel form, or vice versa.

demon	/'dimən/	geometry	/dʒi'ɑmətri/
demonic	/də'mɑnək/	geometric	/dʒiə'mɛtrək/
metabolism	/mə'tæbəlɪzm̩/	parameter	/pə'æmərɚ/
metabolic	/mɛtə'bɑlɪk/	parametric	/pɛrə'mɛtrək/

EXERCISE 6.3

Transcribe each of the following word pairs, paying attention to the changes in vowel quality (for the bold letters) inherent in their pronunciations.

Example:

valid   /vælɪd/

validity   /vəlɪdɪɾɪ/

1. miracle   _____
   miraculous   _____
2. accuse   _____
   accusation   _____
3. authorize   _____
   authority   _____
4. demolish   _____
   demolition   _____
5. mechanical   _____
   mechanistic   _____

In connected speech, several English monosyllabic words undergo a change in pronunciation when compared to the way they might be spoken in isolation. The change in pronunciation of these words is brought about by vowel reduction associated with changes in word stress. An example can be demonstrated with the pronunciation of the word "as," as in the phrase, *as soon as possible* (/əz sun əz pɑsəbl̩/). The reason for this change in the pronunciation of "as" (from /æz/ to /əz/) is due to the fact that, in isolation, the word "as" could be spoken as a stressed monosyllable. In connected, casual speech, it would rarely be stressed. The change in the pronunciation of "as" demonstrates a shift from what is called the *strong form* of the word (/æz/) to the *weak form* of the word (/əz/). Table 6.2 provides a list of some of these monosyllabic English words, both in their strong and weak forms. The strong form would indicate the word has been stressed. In conversational speech, these words rarely receive stress. For example, the word "the" is rarely pronounced with full stress on the vowel, as in /ðʌ/. More commonly, the pronunciation would be unstressed, that is, /ðə/.

TABLE 6.2 Examples of Strong and Weak Forms of Some English Monosyllabic Words (adapted from Cruttenden, 2001)

Strong (Stressed) Form		Weak (Unstressed) Form(s)
a	/eɪ/	/ə/
an	/æn/	/ən/, /n̩/
and	/ænd/	/ən/, /ənd/, /n̩/
are	/ɑr/	/ɚ/
as	/æz/	/əz/
but	/bʌt/	/bət/
can	/kæn/	/kən/
does	/dʌz/	/dəz/, /əz/
for	/fɔr/	/fɚ/
had	/hæd/	/həd/, /əd/
has	/hæz/	/əz/
her	/hɝ/	/ɚ/
him	/hɪm/	/ɪm/, /əm/, /m̩/
his	/hɪz/	/ɪz/, /əz/
of	/ʌv/	/əv/, /ə/
than	/ðæn/	/ðən/
to	/tu/	/tə/
will	/wɪl/	/l̩/
you	/ju/	/jə/

EXERCISE 6.4

Transcribe each phrase twice: first in citation form and then in casual form.

Example:

bigger than me   /bɪgɚ ðæn mi/   /bɪgɚ ðən mi/

1. your mother   _____   _____
2. right and left   _____   _____
3. food for thought   _____   _____
4. What will they do?   _____   _____
5. Thank him.   _____   _____
6. as big as   _____   _____
7. of mice and men   _____   _____
8. What is her name?   _____   _____

The following examples help to demonstrate pronunciation changes inherent in continuous speech. Compare the first transcription, the citation form of each utterance, with the second transcription, the more casual pronunciation. Keep in mind that the examples given are only *one* possible way of saying each utterance in connected speech. Pay particular attention to the inherent vowel reduction, as well as the assimilation, associated with the more casual form. Note the use of the double bar symbol in the transcriptions below. It is used to represent punctuation marks in transcription of connected speech. The double bar /‖/ replaces semicolons, periods, and question marks.

What has your brother done with my cat and dog ?
/wʌt hæz jɔr brʌðɚ dʌn wɪθ maɪ kæt ænd dɑg‖/
/wətʃɚbrəðɚdʌnwɪθmaɪkæʔn̩dɔg‖/

When does the train arrive with her luggage?
/wɛn dʌz ðʌ treɪn əraɪv wɪθ hɝ lʌgədʒ‖/
/wɛnzðətrenəraɪvwɪðəlʌgədʒ‖/

I am going to tell his sister that she should get out of my way.
/aɪ æm goʊɪŋ tu tɛl hɪz sɪstɚ ðæt ʃi ʃʊd gɛt aʊt ʌv maɪ weɪ‖/
/əmgʊnətɛlɪzsɪsɾɚ ðətʃiʃədgɛtaʊɾəmaɪweɪ‖/

Did you eat yet? I could eat a horse.
/dɪd ju it jɛt‖ aɪ kʊd it eɪ hɔrs‖/
/dɪdʒəitjɛt‖aɪkədiɾəhɔrs‖/

What in the world are you going to do about it?
/wʌt ɪn ðə wɝld ɑr ju goʊɪŋ tu du əbaʊt ɪt‖/
/wəʔn̩ðəwɝldəjəgʊnəduəbaʊɾət‖/

Complete Assignment 6-1.

EXERCISE 6.5

Transcribe the following utterances, first in citation form, and then in casual form.

1. I bet you I can help them get out of that mess.

   _____

   _____

2. I caught you cheating on that test. I am going to tell the teacher.

   _____

   _____

3. What is his reason for not being able to come to the party?

   _____

   _____

4. What's the matter with Thelma? Let me see if I can cheer her up.

   _____

   _____

5. What did you do to your car? I should be able to get it going.

   _____

   _____

Suprasegmental Aspects of Speech

Examine the following statement: "In order to get good grades, you will have to study harder." Say this sentence out loud, pronouncing it carefully and deliberately, stressing each word as if it existed in isolation, that is, "In-order-to-get-good-grades-you-will-have-to-study-harder." Pronouncing the sentence in this manner makes it sound quite robotic and unnatural. The pronunciation is mechanical and monotonous, showing no emotional content whatsoever. Now say the sentence a couple of times in a more natural manner. What do you notice about your production of the sentence now? Did the sentence have any particular characteristics that stood out? Say the sentence again, listening carefully. Perhaps you noticed that certain words received more emphasis, or stress, than others. You also may have noted that some of the words in the sentence were spoken faster than others. Additionally, you may have observed that you varied the pitch or intonation of your voice as you uttered the sentence.

In contrast with isolated words, connected speech is characterized by continual modifications or alterations in stress, in the timing of words, and in intonation. It is these alterations that give connected speech its natural characteristic rhythm. Stress, timing, and intonation variations do not affect solely the individual speech sound segments of words. These modifications span entire syllables, words, phrases, and sentences. For this reason, stress, timing, and intonation are generally referred to as the **suprasegmental** aspects of speech production. The prefix *supra-* means *above, beyond,* or *to transcend.* Therefore, the suprasegmental features of speech go beyond or transcend the boundaries of the individual speech sound segment or phoneme, affecting an entire utterance.

Stress Revisited

The preceding discussion should not imply that isolated words are immune from the effects of the suprasegmental features of speech. In Chapter 2, the importance of identifying word stress for purposes of phonetic transcription was discussed. As you recall, a stressed syllable in a word is generally spoken with more articulatory force, resulting in a syllable that is louder, longer in duration, and higher in pitch than an unstressed syllable. Word stress is a suprasegmental feature of speech because entire syllables are stressed, not just individual phonemes. Your transcription practice in the previous chapters has helped you to clearly understand the importance of being able to identify the syllables with primary stress in any word. During transcription, you know when to accurately use /ə/ versus /ʌ/ and /ɚ/ versus /ɝ/. Without this knowledge, it would not be possible to transcribe English accurately using the IPA.

In Chapter 2, we were concerned only with identifying primary stress in words. It is time to turn our attention to the other degrees of word stress. Multisyllabic words have syllables with more than one degree or level of stress. For instance, the word "pretense" has two levels of stress: primary and secondary. This word would be transcribed as /ˈpriˌtɛns/. Note that the IPA symbol for indicating secondary stress is a small mark below and to the left of the syllable receiving secondary stress. The following two-syllable words each have two levels of stress.

ˌmainˈtain	ˌtranˈscend	ˈvalˌue
ˌinˈclude	ˌalˈthough	ˈproˌnoun
ˌtranˈscribe	ˈeˌgo	ˈcouˌpon
ˌsarˈdine	ˈmoˌped	ˈpayˌroll

EXERCISE 6.6

The following words have two levels of stress, primary and secondary. Mark each syllable's stress pattern accordingly, using the appropriate IPA symbols for stress.

1. intense	5. teabag	9. erode
2. falsehood	6. frostbite	10. handshake
3. Lucite	7. obese	11. react
4. rosette	8. entree	12. household

Not all multisyllabic words have syllables with both primary and secondary stress. Some multisyllabic words have only one (primary) stressed syllable. When the nucleus of the other syllable(s) contains either /ə/, /ɚ/, /m̩/, /n̩/ or /l̩/, (or sometimes /ɪ/ and /ʊ/ when produced in a reduced form), the syllable is said to be unstressed. We already know that /ə/ and /ɚ/ are never found in a syllable receiving primary stress. According to Carrell and Tiffany (1960), the schwa vowel is referred to as an indefinite vowel because it is more of a "murmur" than a full vowel. Its indefinite status makes it a nonprominent nucleus, so much so that it receives no stress at all. The following bisyllabic words have only one stressed syllable (marked appropriately). The other syllable is unstressed.

ˈriddle	ˈperson	surˈround
ˈbutton	ˈzebra	preˈtend
ˈmelon	ˈhappy	conˈtain
ˈmanage	seˈdate	reˈmind

Note that when /ɪ/ is the nucleus of a final open syllable (as in "happy") or the nucleus of the syllable /ɪŋ/, it is unstressed (and lax) as well.

EXERCISE 6.7

The following bisyllabic words have only one syllable that receives stress; the other syllable is unstressed. Mark the stressed syllable using the correct IPA symbol for primary stress.

1. leopard	5. murky	9. scary
2. sweater	6. anoint	10. naked
3. rhythm	7. magnet	11. extreme
4. contend	8. belief	12. parade

The following three-syllable words have only one stressed syllable:

conˈtagious	baˈloney	aˈlerted
ferˈocious	ˈcalendar	ˈconstable
aˈversion	ˈterrible	ˈshivering
conˈcession	beˈhavior	ˈinterval

The following four-syllable words also have only one stressed syllable:

ˈliteracy	ˈpassionately	volˈuminous
ˈdefinitely	ˈknowledgeable	chroˈnology
ˈspeculative	chryˈsanthemum	couˈrageously
ˈpersonable	toˈgetherness	exˈperience

EXERCISE 6.8

The following three- and four-syllable words have only one stressed syllable. Mark each one correctly using the IPA symbol for primary stress.

1. measuring	5. courageous	9. sorority
2. statistics	6. Germany	10. fraternity
3. laryngeal	7. unbearable	11. Albuquerque
4. warranted	8. Canadian	12. dysphonia

Now contrast the following three- and four-syllable words that each have syllables with primary and secondary stress (in addition to unstressed syllables).

ˌplanˈtation   ˌreimˈburse   ˌmorˈphemic

ˈinterˌnet   ˌtranˈsistor   ˈtantaˌmount

ˌtranˈscription   ˌMonˈtana   ˈpeneˌtrate

ˈsaxoˌphone   ˈtermiˌnate   ˈzodiˌac

ˈmandaˌtory   ˌparaˈplegia   disˈcriminˌate

ˈrepliˌcate   ˌeduˈcation   ˈgeneralˌize

EXERCISE 6.9

The following three- and four-syllable words have two levels of stress (in addition to some unstressed syllables). Mark primary and secondary stress using the appropriate IPA symbols.

1. myopic
2. cyberspace
3. architect
4. idea
5. citation
6. circumstance
7. bacteria
8. effervescent
9. alimony
10. communicate
11. elevator
12. Indiana

Complete Assignment 6-2.

Sentence Stress

In addition to word stress, each sentence a speaker produces also has inherent **sentence stress**. Examine the following: Cheryl drove to school. Say this sentence aloud in a natural manner, the way you might say it while conversing with a friend. In this manner, you may have noticed that the last word in the sentence tends to stand out or have more emphasis. Say the sentence again, and see if you notice the emphasis on the last word, Cheryl drove to ˈschool. Many sentences and phrases are spoken with the primary emphasis or stress on the last word. Examine the following phrases and sentences. Listen for the emphasis on the final word. Notice the words that receive primary stress, especially in the last two examples.

> I like his ˈstyle.
> Bill and Jane went ˈhome.
> If I get ˈcaught, I will get in ˈtrouble.
> In order to get good ˈgrades, you will have to study ˈharder.

Phrases and sentences do not always end with a stressed word. Certain words in a sentence will usually receive emphasis or stress depending on (1) the level of importance of that word in the sentence and (2) the speaker's intent of the message being conveyed. Words that contain salient information in a sentence are called **content words**. Content words generally include nouns, verbs, adjectives, and adverbs. The less important words in a sentence—including pronouns, articles, prepositions, and conjunctions—are called **function words**. Content words tend to (but not always) receive sentence stress; function words usually do not receive stress. In the sentence, "Cheryl drove to school," the content words are "Cheryl," "drove," and "school." Although "school" tends to receive stress when this sentence is produced in a neutral manner, it would be possible to stress the other content words, depending on the speaker's intent. When the final word of the sentence, "school," is stressed, the speaker denotes the location to which

Cheryl drove—she drove to school, not the library. Compare these variations of the sentence:

Cheryl ʹdrove to school.   ʹCheryl drove to school.

What is the speaker's intent in each of these sentences? In the first sentence, the speaker stressed the word "drove" to indicate Cheryl's mode of transportation; Cheryl drove to school, she did not walk. In the second sentence, the speaker stressed the word "Cheryl" to indicate that Cheryl, not her brother Ethan, drove to school. Notice that in each case, stress was placed on a content word.

Examine the following statements as spoken by two different customers in a restaurant. Each customer has a different message to convey to the waiter:

Sentence: *Intent:*
Customer #1: I want ʹiced coffee.   I don't want *hot* coffee.
Customer #2: I want iced ʹcoffee.   I don't want iced *tea*.

The customers' intent in the two statements is completely different. In the first instance, sentence stress is used to indicate the temperature of the coffee desired; sentence stress is used to contrast between *iced* and *hot* coffee. In the second sentence, sentence stress is used to contrast between the type of beverage the patron desires—*coffee* or *tea*. The use of sentence stress to indicate a speaker's particular intent is termed *contrastive stress*.

Examine the stress shifts in the following statements. In each case, the speaker uses stress contrastively to indicate the particular intent desired.

Sentence: *Intent:*
Sheila purchased a new red sedan.   *Doug* didn't buy the car.
Sheila **purchased** a new red sedan.   Sheila didn't *sell* the car.
Sheila purchased a **new** red sedan.   Sheila didn't buy a *used* car.
Sheila purchased a new **red** sedan.   Sheila didn't buy the *green* car.
Sheila purchased a new red **sedan**.   Sheila didn't buy the *SUV*.

EXERCISE 6.10

<u>Underline</u> the word in each of the following sentences that would receive primary sentence stress, based upon the given intent.

Example:

Intent: I didn't buy pants.

Sentence: I bought a <u>shirt</u> last week.

1. Intent: We did not go to a play last night.
   Sentence: Carol and I went to a matinee.

2. Intent: David doesn't live on West Brooklyn.
   Sentence: My neighbor David lives at 4555 East Brooklyn Avenue.

3. Intent: Sam doesn't care for taffy.
   Sentence: Flo ate the taffy from the circus.

4. Intent: Jason and Andrea talked to their grandmother.
   Sentence: Jason and Andrea did not get a chance to talk to their uncle.

5. Intent: They liked Mrs. Harlan's husband.
   Sentence: The third graders really liked Mr. Harlan.

EXERCISE 6.11

Listen to each of the following sentences on the audio CD. <u>Underline</u> the word that is given primary sentence stress. Then, write the intent of the utterance on the blank line.

Example:

> Mary had a little <u>lamb</u>.
> <u>She didn't have a goat.</u>

1. The girl's name was Chris.

   _____

2. Jared only forgot to get the toothpaste at the store.

   _____

3. Why did they walk to the playground?

   _____

4. Why did they walk to the playground?

   _____

5. Mark got a new blue bike for his birthday.

   _____

6. Mark got a new blue bike for his birthday.

   _____

7. Mark got a new blue bike for his birthday.

   _____

Sentence stress also plays an important role in distinguishing the *type* of information being presented by a speaker. When conversing with someone, the conversation usually volleys back and forth between the two participants. Two types of information are provided during a conversation, **given information** and **new information**. When people converse, each person will typically provide new information to the conversation, adding to the given (old) information previously discussed. For instance, a friend might ask, "What did you have for lunch?" Your reply might be, "I had a hamburger and french fries for lunch." *Hamburger* and *french fries* would be considered new information since this is your addition to the conversation. Since these words provide new information to the listener, these words would typically be stressed. The phrases "I had a . . ." and "for lunch" would be given information since the information refers back to prior conversation; these phrases would not receive stress. Suppose your friend responds, "Oh, I only had a cheeseburger." In this case *cheeseburger* would be the new information in the dialog; it would correspondingly receive stress.

Examine the following conversation between Sally and Jane. They are discussing Sally's most recent purchase. As you read the dialogue, it is easy to see that each participant's response advances the conversation:

Sally: You got a new purse.
Jane: Yeah, I got it at the mall.
Sally: Which mall?
Jane: The one downtown.

Sally: Which store?

Jane: Oh. I got it at Green's.

Sally: Was it expensive?

Jane: It was on sale.

Sally: Was it more than fifty dollars?

Jane: It was only twenty!

Sally begins the conversation by asking about Jane's new *purse*. Sally would probably stress the word purse since she was asking specifically about that item. When Jane replies, she states where she bought the purse. In doing so, Jane would have emphasized the word *mall*. Sally then asks Jane "*Which* mall" (emphasizing *which* since she wishes to know the location of the shopping center). Jane gives her the location by replying, "The one downtown." Sally asks Jane "*Which* store," and Jane replies, emphasizing *Green's* since it is the name of the store. As the conversation ensues, each participant stresses or emphasizes the new information she wishes to convey. Of course neither participant is consciously stressing these words; it happens as a result of knowing how sentence stress is utilized in conversation. The use of sentence stress (as well as other suprasegmental features) is behavior that is the direct consequence of learning language and being familiar with the way language operates in conversation. Below is a duplication of Sally and Jane's conversation. New information is presented in boldface.

Sally: You got a new **purse**.

Jane: I got it at the **mall**.

Sally: **Which** mall?

Jane: The one **downtown**.

Sally: Which **store?**

Jane: Oh. I got it at **Green's**.

Sally: Was it **expensive**?

Jane: It was on **sale**.

Sally: Was it more than **fifty dollars?**

Jane: It was only **twenty**!

Actually, if you reread the above conversation, saying only the new information (bold words) you would have a very good understanding of the conversation!

EXERCISE 6.12

The following dialogue is between a waitress and a customer in a restaurant. Circle the words in the dialogue that are stressed in order to convey new information.

Waitress: Would you like something to drink?

Customer: Lemonade, please. I would also like to order.

Waitress: Would you like an appetizer?

Customer: No, thank you.

Waitress: Would you like to hear about our specials?

Continues

EXERCISE 6.12 (*cont.*)

Customer:	Please.
Waitress:	We have grilled salmon and fettuccine alfredo.
Customer:	I'll have the fettuccine.
Waitress:	Would you like our house dressing on your salad? It's Italian.
Customer:	I would like to have blue cheese, please.
Waitress:	I'll also bring out some fresh rolls.
Customer:	Thank you.
Waitress:	You're welcome.

When marking sentence stress in transcription, you will first need to identify the word(s) that receive sentence stress. Then, you will need to identify the other content words in the utterance. The word(s) receiving primary sentence stress will be marked with the traditional IPA symbol (ˈ) preceding the syllable that normally receives word stress. The stressed syllables of the other content words will be marked using the IPA symbol for secondary stress (ˌ). For example, the sentence, "I want iced coffee" would be marked for sentence stress in the following manner (depending on the speaker's intent):

ˌI want ˈiced ˌcoffee. (I want cold coffee.)

ˌI want ˌiced ˈcoffee. (I do not want tea.)

Now contrast the following sentence pairs:

The **boys** *jumped into the pool.*
The ˈboys ˌjumped into the ˌpool.

I'll be married in September.
ˈI'll be ˌmarried in Sepˌtember.

The boys **jumped** *into the pool.*
The ˌboys ˈjumped into the ˌpool.

*I'll be **married** in September.*
ˌI'll be ˈmarried in Sepˌtember.

The boys jumped into the **pool**.
The ˌboys ˌjumped into the ˈpool.

*I'll be married in **September**.*
ˌI'll be ˌmarried in Sepˈtember.

Foreign speakers who are seeking help in learning English as a second language may have trouble with English stress patterns, both in words and in sentences. Word stress is not predictable in English as in other languages. It is quite difficult for new users of English to learn to use stress patterns correctly. Improper use of word and sentence stress makes English quite difficult to understand.

Hearing-impaired individuals with a severe or profound hearing loss may experience difficulties producing stress patterns correctly because their auditory channel is diminished. One common characteristic of "deaf speech" is incorrect placement of stress on function words, because the rules of stress placement are not fully understood. A speaker who stresses function words has speech patterns that appear unintelligible to normal hearing listeners because they are not accustomed to hearing this type of spoken stress pattern.

EXERCISE 6.13

Mark sentence stress for each of the following items using the appropriate IPA notation. Each sentence will be spoken by two different speakers. Pay attention to differences in stress between the two speakers. You will need the optional audio CD for this exercise.

Example:

      a. The ˌcow ˌjumped over the ˈmoon.

      b. The ˌcow ˈjumped over the ˌmoon.

1. a. Steve's roommate is from Minneapolis.
    b. Steve's roommate is from Minneapolis.

2. a. Tim went skydiving on Saturday.
    b. Tim went skydiving on Saturday.

3. a. The answer on the exam was "false."
    b. The answer on the exam was "false."

4. a. Mary's birthday is next Tuesday.
    b. Mary's birthday is next Tuesday.

5. a. I'd like a steak for dinner.
    b. I'd like a steak for dinner.

6. a. I went to New York City to see some plays.
    b. I went to New York City to see some plays.

7. a. My professor shaved his mustache.
    b. My professor shaved his mustache.

8. a. I need potatoes from the store.
    b. I need potatoes from the store.

Intonation

It is often difficult to talk about sentence stress without addressing the topic of intonation, another suprasegmental feature of speech. Because stress involves changes in voice pitch, speakers continually modify the fundamental frequency of their voice while speaking in order to stress particular words in an utterance. The modification of voice pitch is known as **intonation**. A speaker's intonation pattern cues a listener as to the type of utterance being spoken, that is, a statement of fact, a question, an exclamation, and so forth. When someone asks a question requiring a yes/no answer, voice pitch generally rises at the end of the utterance. Intonation is also responsible, at least in part, for indicating a speaker's particular mood.

Consider the short sentence, "I did." This statement can be spoken in several ways, depending upon the speaker's intent and the corresponding intonation pattern. For instance, "I did" could be spoken as a casual, matter-of-fact reply to the question, "Did you read the paper today?" The statement could be spoken with emphasis on the word "did" in response to the never-ending parental question, "Have you cleaned your room yet?" In response to "Who ate the pie?", a speaker would probably emphasize the word "I." With each change in speaker intent, there would be a corresponding change in the intonation applied to the utterance. Note that in each version of the utterance, there is both a change in sentence stress *and* a corresponding increase in the fundamental frequency of the voice.

The change in fundamental frequency that span the length of a meaningful utterance is called an **intonational phrase**. An intonational phrase may consist of an entire sentence, a phrase, or simply one word. Long sentences will usually have more than one intonational phrase. Intonational phrases in longer sentences are signaled by a slight pause in the utterance (indicated in writing with a comma, hyphen, or semicolon). Below are several utterances comprised of one, two, and three intonational phrases.

One intonational phrase:	**Two intonational phrases:**
Yes!	*You took my umbrella, didn't you?*
I want to go home.	*I got a blue scarf, not a red one.*

Three intonational phrases:
The boys, who ate the candy, got sick.
Pete, my best friend, took me to the ball game.

There are two intonational phrases in the accusation, "You took my **umbrella, didn't** you?" The words in bold type would most likely have the highest voice pitch. Say the sentence out loud, paying particular attention to the changes in the pitch of the voice. You will notice that the highest voice pitch occurs on the words "umbrella" and "didn't." Similarly, in the sentence "The boys, who ate the candy, got sick," there are three distinct intonational phrases (separated by commas). You should notice that the highest voice pitch occurs on the words, "boys," "candy," and "sick."

The syllable that receives the greatest pitch change in any particular intonational phrase is called the **tonic syllable** (Ladefoged, 2001) or **nuclear syllable** (Fudge, 1984). Likewise, the emphasis given to this syllable is referred to as the **tonic accent** or the **nuclear accent**. Each intonational phrase is characterized by only one tonic accent. In the question, "Are you done?," the tonic accent would fall on the final word "done." The tonic accent would be located on the second syllable of the word "confused" in the statement, "He was confused," because word stress is normally found on the second syllable of that word. In the sentence, "You took my umbrella, didn't you?," the tonic accent is on the second syllable of umbrella (um'brella) in the first intonational phrase, and the first syllable of didn't ('didn't) in the second intonational phrase.

The tonic accent most often is located at the end of an intonational phrase (Ladefoged, 2001). However, when a speaker uses contrastive stress to draw attention to a particular word in an utterance, the tonic accent would be located on the stressed syllable. Compare the two pronunciations of the following sentence.

It won't rain *today*.
It *won't* rain today.

In the first example, the tonic accent would be located on the last syllable of the utterance ("It won't rain to'day"). In the second example, the tonic accent would be located on the second word ("It 'won't rain today").

Intonational phrases are characterized by the *direction* of their pitch change; they are generally classified as falling or rising. If a waiter asks you, "Would you like some soup?" you would hear a rise in intonation at the end of the question, because "soup" carries the tonic accent. If a waiter states, "We have two special soups tonight," you would probably not hear a rising intonation pattern. The voice pitch would most likely fall at the end of this statement.

Falling Intonational Phrases

Falling intonational phrases accompany complete statements and commands and are indicative of the finality of an utterance (Jones, 1963). In the sentence, "The boys went home" (spoken as an unemotional statement), the voice pitch falls throughout the utterance. There is a general fall, or declination, in the pitch of the voice over the length of most neutrally spoken statements. Some other examples of falling intonational phrases would be evident in utterances such as the following:

I guess.   That should do it.   It's time to go.

A scheme, adopted by phoneticians to represent the changes in voice pitch in an intonational phrase, is to use a line drawing indicating both the pitch levels and the direction of the change in voice pitch. For example, the sentence "The boys went home" would be diagrammed as:

The boys went home.   *Unemotional Statement*

Notice that the line ends lower than where it began, signifying the difference between the voice pitch at the beginning and at the end of the utterance.

If this sentence was spoken as a matter-of-fact, declarative statement, emphasis would be given to the final word "home" (The boys went **home**). There would be a steady voice pitch throughout the intonational phrase up to the tonic accent, *home*. Beginning on the tonic accent, the voice pitch would rise and fall within the same tonic syllable. This pattern is appropriately termed a *rise-fall intonational phrase*. "The boys went home" (spoken as a declarative statement) would be diagrammed as:

The boys went home.   *Declarative Statement*

Note in this example that the rise-fall in the voice pitch on the tonic accent is displayed over the *vowel* of the tonic syllable.

Most declarative statements in English have a similar intonation pattern. That is, the utterance begins on a medium voice pitch and continues at that level until the tonic accent is reached. At that point, the voice pitch is raised and the voice then falls to a level lower than the voice pitch used to begin the utterance. This rise-fall pattern usually occurs within the same tonic syllable. Other examples of this intonation pattern include:

I play the trombone.   My mother drove to Detroit.

I saw her at the circus.   Let's go swimming.

If the intent of the utterance was such that one of the other content words was emphasized, the intonation would change accordingly, that is:

I play the trombone.   My mother drove to Detroit.

Rise-fall intonational phrases also are typical in utterances comprised of Wh-questions. Wh-questions are those that begin an utterance with the words "where," "what," "why," "when," "which," and "how." Examples include:

Why did you go?   What's your favorite color?

Where is your friend?   When did you arrive?

One last example of the rise-fall pattern is often found in utterances that express an element of surprise. The rise and fall can occur over several syllables or may to occur in only one-syllable utterances. Examples include the following:

Really???   I can?!?   Wow!!!

Yes!!   I think so!   No!!

Rising Intonational Phrases

Rising intonational phrases (typical of questions and incomplete thoughts) usually indicate some uncertainty on the speaker's part (Jones, 1963; Pike, 1945). As previously indicated, yes/no questions have a rising intonation pattern. The extent of the rise in voice pitch depends upon the speaker's intent. For instance, the question, "Are you coming?" spoken curiously, could be diagrammed as:

Are you coming?   *Curious Question*

If spoken more emphatically, the question would be diagrammed as:

Are you coming?   *Emphatic Question*

Rising intonational phrases also are common when reciting a list of items. For example:

My favorite colors are red, blue, and green.

Richie, Darren, and William came along.

Notice the expected falling intonation at the end of these utterances.

Now examine the following incomplete utterances:

When I got to work, . . .

If she saved her money, . . .

Gary went to the bank . . .

These utterances indicate to a listener that the speaker's thoughts are not fully expressed; there is more information to be provided. These rising intonation patterns are characteristic of nonfinal intonational phrases situated in longer utterances. Examine the same three utterances in a completed sentence, paying careful attention to the intonation pattern of each. The first intonational phrase is characterized by a rising intonation pattern, and the second intonational phrase of each is characterized by a rise-fall:

When I got to work, I became ill.

If she saved her money, she'd be rich!

Gary went to the bank to make a withdrawal.

The first phrase in these examples also could be pronounced with a fall-rise intonation pattern. (This pattern is still considered to have an overall rise.)

When I got to work, I became ill.

If she saved her money, she'd be rich.

Gary went to the bank to make a withdrawal.

The examples given above only represent some of the more common intonation patterns seen in American English. In addition, the various examples given are only suggestions of the way the utterances could be spoken. It would be possible to pronounce any of the examples in a variety of ways. If you recall, the earlier example, "I did," was used as an example of an utterance that could be spoken differently, depending on a speaker's intent. Let's return to this phrase as a way to review several intonation patterns possible for one utterance.

Question:	Reply:
"Did you get the mail?"	I did.
"Who ate the last cookie?"	I did.
"Are you sure you studied?"	I did.
"Take out the trash!"	I did.
"You left your keys on the table."	I did?
"Did you know you left your headlights on?"	I did?
"Did you know you got an 'A' on the exam?"	I did?

EXERCISE 6.14

Indicate whether the intonational phrases in the following utterances are generally rising or falling. Circle the appropriate response.

Example:

Are you ready?	Rising	Falling
1. When will you leave?	Rising	Falling
2. Is your brother home?	Rising	Falling

Continues

EXERCISE 6.14 (cont.)

3. I need to go the library.	Rising	Falling
4. What's your favorite season?	Rising	Falling
5. Did you get paid yet?	Rising	Falling
6. The dog ran away.	Rising	Falling
7. Sophie is my oldest friend.	Rising	Falling
8. How did you know about that?	Rising	Falling
9. Honest?!?	Rising	Falling
10. I'm sure!!!	Rising	Falling

Tempo

Tempo is the term used to describe the durational aspect of connected speech. Because timing, or duration of articulatory events, affects entire utterances, tempo also is considered to be a suprasegmental feature of speech. Obviously, the overall rate of speech plays a role in determining the tempo of speech. For adults, the average speech rate is on the order of approximately 5 to 5.5 syllables per second (Calvert, 1986). Tempo also is determined by the duration of individual phonemes and the duration of pauses located between syllables, words, phrases, and sentences.

Duration of Individual Phonemes

Each of the phonemes in English, when spoken in isolation, has an inherent duration. As a rule, diphthongs have a greater duration than vowels, and vowels have a greater duration than the consonants. Among the consonants, the glides and liquids have the greatest duration; the stop consonants have the shortest duration. The duration of any individual phoneme will change once placed in connected speech. For instance, you already know that the stressed syllable of a word is longer in duration than an unstressed syllable. Obviously, the syllable is lengthened due to the increased duration of its individual phonemes.

The inherent length of individual phonemes also varies depending upon phonetic context. For instance, vowels preceding voiceless consonants are shorter than vowels preceding voiced consonants. That is, the vowel /u/ in "loose" is shorter than /u/ in the word "lose." Vowels in open syllables also are longer than vowels in closed syllables. Compare the length of the vowel /i/ in the words "beet" and "bee." The IPA uses a colon to indicate that a phoneme has been lengthened. Therefore, in the preceding examples, the words "loose" and "lose" could be transcribed as [lus] and [lu:z], respectively. Similarly, the words "beet" and "bee" could be transcribed as [bit] and [bi:].

In connected speech, the final phoneme of one word and the initial phoneme of the following word may oftentimes be the same, as in "Yes, Susie." Say this phrase aloud. You will notice that there is really no break in the production of the two /s/ phonemes. Instead, you most likely hear a prolonged /s/ phoneme. This phrase would be transcribed /jɛs:uzɪ/ using the colon diacritic to indicate the lengthened /s/ phoneme. Note that the syllable boundary disappears due to the prolonged /s/. Some other examples of this phenomenon include:

but, Terry	[bʌt:ɛrɪ]	with them	[wɪð:ɛm]
bad day	[bæd:eɪ]	call Linda	[kɑl:ɪndə]
men know	[men:oʊ]	Miss Smith	[mɪs:mɪθ]

EXERCISE 6.15

Select the one word from each pair that would have the longer vowel. Transcribe that word using the diacritical marking [:].

Example:

key   keep   _[ki:]_

1. peace peas _____
2. leave leaf _____
3. rude root _____

4. spa spot _____
5. lack lag _____
6. toot too _____

EXERCISE 6.16

Transcribe the following utterances, using the [:] diacritic where appropriate.

Example:

kite tail   _[kaɪt:eɪl]_

1. rice soup _____
2. cotton netting _____
3. big guns _____
4. patched tires _____
5. tail light _____
6. calm morning _____
7. bar room _____
8. rock candy _____
9. leaf fire _____
10. push Sherri _____

Pauses and Juncture in Connected Speech

When discussing connected speech, we tend not to think about the lapses or pauses that occur between words, phrases, and sentences. As normal listeners, you have learned to interpret these lapses to indicate a pause in the flow of speech. What do these pauses mean to a listener? A pause may simply indicate that the speaker is taking a breath. Pauses may also indicate hesitations on the part of a speaker as in the following, "Her name was . . . um . . . um . . . , oh, I remember . . . Leslie."

Pauses also are important in alerting a listener to a speaker's particular intent and meaning. They are used in conversation to indicate the presence of a new thought or to emphasize a particular point. Examine the utterance, "I want to go to the movies, but I don't have any money." The comma, which separates the two clauses, marks a pause in the utterance when it is said aloud. The speaker pauses because two ideas are being presented. The speaker needs to emphasize the importance of each idea, especially the latter. Similarly, there would be a pause at each of the commas in the utterance, "I need to buy shampoo, tissue, bath soap, and deodorant," signaling the identity of each of the items. Recall that each comma also indicates the beginning of a separate phrase, with an accompanying change in intonation.

Juncture is the term used to indicate the way in which syllables and words are linked together in connected speech. **External juncture** is the term given to a pause that connects two intonational phrases. (That is, the connecting pause is external to the phrase.) The IPA symbols / | / and / || / are used to mark external juncture in connected speech. These symbols replace the commas, semicolons, and periods that mark the juncture on the printed page. The single bar IPA symbol / | / is used to indicate the presence of a short pause (represented in print as a comma). As you recall, longer pauses, represented in print by a period or semicolon, would be represented with a double bar / || /. The sentence, "Yes, I would like to go, but I can't," would be transcribed as /jɛs|aɪ wʊd laɪk tə goʊ|bət aɪ kænt || /.

When transcribing connected speech, it sometimes becomes necessary to indicate the presence of a pause between words in the same intonational phrase because the transition between syllables may become blurred. Consider the utterances, "I scream" and "ice cream." They share an identical phoneme string—/aɪskrim/. To indicate the pause between "I" and "scream" in the first utterance, a /+/ diacritic is used, that is, /aɪ + skrim/. The syllables /aɪ + skrim/ are said to have **open internal juncture** because there is a pause between the syllables. The transcription of the second utterance, /aɪskrim/ has no pause between the two syllables. Therefore, /aɪskrim/ has **close internal juncture**. No special symbols are needed to indicate close internal juncture because there is no pause between the syllables. Another example of open and close internal juncture occurs with the utterances, *night rate* —/naɪt + reɪt/ and *nitrate* — /naɪtreɪt/.

EXERCISE 6.17

Use the diacritical markings [|] and [||] to indicate external juncture in the following utterances. All punctuation marks have been omitted.

Example:
[When I'm sleepy | I go to bed ||]

1. I want hot dogs ice cream and cotton candy
2. They left didn't they
3. The family who lived next door moved away
4. What is her problem
5. My uncle the dentist is 34 years old

Complete Assignments 6-3 and 6-4.

Review Exercises

A. For each of the following pronunciations, indicate the phonemic change that occurred as a result of assimilation. Also indicate the change in place in articulation.

Example:	pronunciation	phoneme change	change from alveolar to:
bad boy	[bæb:ɔɪ]	b/d	bilabial
1. can make	[kæm:eɪk]		
2. How's your mother?	[haʊʒɚ mʌðɚ]		
3. gin game	[dʒɪŋ geɪm]		
4. lead pipe	[lɛb paɪp]		
5. has shaken	[hæʒ ʃeɪkn̩]		
6. red gown	[rɛg gaʊn]		

B. Transcribe each of the following items after eliding the indicated phoneme.

Example:	elided phoneme	transcription
aptly	/t/	/æplɪ/
1. bends	/d/	
2. winter	/t/	
3. land mine	/d/	
4. can of worms	/f/	
5. counter	/t/	
6. twelfths	/θ/	
7. What's her problem?	/h/	
8. wept loudly	/t/	

C. Transcribe each of the following utterances, first in citation form, and then in casual form.

1. I want to go home.

   _____

   _____

2. Let me see your book.

   _____

   _____

3. Could you move a little to the right?

   _____

   _____

4. Did John ever get paid?

   _____

   _____

5. Why did she leave so early?

   _____

   _____

6. It is raining cats and dogs.

_____

_____

7. When are you going to leave?

_____

_____

8. You have got to be kidding!

_____

_____

9. Who is going to rake the leaves tonight?

_____

_____

10. I want to wax my truck tomorrow morning.

_____

_____

D. Rewrite each of the following in English orthography (citation form).

1. /ʤɛvəgoɾəðəsɝkəs ‖/

_____

2. /wɛndədʃilivdʒɔrdʒə‖/

_____

3. /maɪsɪsɾəgɑɾənubɔɪfrɛnd ‖/

_____

4. /gɪmɪədeɪətutədəsaɪd ‖/

_____

5. /aɪmgʊnəhæftəseɪnoʊfənaʊ ‖/

_____

6. /aɪθɪŋkɪtsgʊnəreɪniðətədeɪətəmɑroʊ ‖/

_____

7. /wʊʤəɛvəθɪŋkəduənðætfəmi ‖/

_____

8. /dujəθɪŋkðətsuzn̩tʊkənʌfəvəm ‖/

_____

9. /əmʃəðətðɛrgʊnəteljəwəʧənɪdtəduət ‖/

_____

10. /traɪəzimaɪt│hi ʤəst kʊdənt du wət ʃi wɑnəd ‖/

_____

E. Indicate primary and secondary stress, where appropriate, in each of the following three- and four-syllable words. Keep in mind that some syllables in the words are unstressed. Use a dictionary to help identify any syllable boundaries of which you are unsure.

1. courageous
2. terrified
3. majestic
4. asthmatic
5. Plexiglas
6. plurality
7. mandatory
8. clandestine
9. flamboyant
10. creation

11. computation
12. cranberry
13. bulletin
14. surrendered
15. semantics
16. colonial
17. mercenary
18. independent
19. October
20. ballerina

F. 1. Transcribe the following word pairs. Be sure to indicate primary and secondary stress with the appropriate symbols.

2. Compare your vowel transcriptions in each pair (for the vowels represented by the bold letters). If vowel reduction results when going from the first to the second word, place an "X" in the "reduced" column. If your transcription indicates a change from a reduced vowel to the full form of the vowel, place an "X" in the "full" column.

		reduced	full
Examples:			
valid	validity		
/ˈvælɪd/	/vəˈlɪdɪɾi/	X	
1. **o**rigin	**o**riginate		
2. micr**o**scope	micr**o**scopy		
3. arist**o**crat	arist**o**cracy		
4. strat**e**gy	strat**e**gic		
5. m**a**niac	m**a**niacal		
6. homog**e**nous	homog**e**neous		
7. par**a**lyze	par**a**lysis		
8. fel**o**ny	fel**o**nious		

9. perspire   perspiration

_____

10. rep**e**at   rep**e**titious

_____

G. Indicate with an "X" whether the following utterances have an overall rising or falling intonation contour.

		Rising	Falling
1.	I got a sweater for my birthday.	_____	_____
2.	Are you happy?	_____	_____
3.	The girls had spaghetti for supper.	_____	_____
4.	Are you positive?	_____	_____
5.	When you're finished, go to bed.	_____	_____
6.	Were you late for work today?	_____	_____
7.	Let me get back to you.	_____	_____
8.	Did you buy a new CD?	_____	_____
9.	What do you mean?	_____	_____
10.	Is that your idea of a joke?	_____	_____

H. Use the diacritical markings [|] or [||] to indicate external juncture for each of the following utterances. All punctuation marks have been omitted.

1. If I want your help you'll be the first to know
2. Maybe I will maybe I won't
3. They bought a new house didn't they
4. The girls who went swimming all got a cold
5. I can't really make up my mind
6. I scream you scream we all scream for ice cream
7. When are you leaving on vacation
8. Are your cousins coming for a visit or not
9. Do you have ants in your pants
10. I quit my job but only when I was sure I could get another

I. Transcribe each of the following utterances in casual form, indicating a lengthened phoneme [ː] where appropriate. Also use the diacritical markings [|] or [||] to indicate external juncture where appropriate.

Example:

Did you have a good day?

[dɪdʒəhævəgʊdːdeɪ ||]

1. I caught my cat Tom by the tail.

_____

2. Which shampoo did you buy at the store?

_____

3. Would you put the white tablecloth on the table, please?

   _____

4. Mom might take me shopping, if I get good grades.

   _____

5. Have you finished taping the TV special yet?

   _____

6. With them, it's hard to tell what they are thinking.

   _____

7. Please give me your phone number before you leave.

   _____

8. Clem made a home run at the big game last Tuesday.

   _____

9. Teddy and Farrell love to play outside with the water sprinkler.

   _____

10. I won't take any more of the junk Ken hands out.

    _____

J. Each of the following sentences will be spoken by two different speakers. Transcribe each of the utterances in casual form. Be sure to use single bar or double bar diacritics to indicate external juncture.

1. Why can't you ever act your age?

   _____

   _____

2. Why, oh why did I ever leave Iowa?

   _____

   _____

3. When did they say their flight was?

   _____

   _____

4. I will probably go home tomorrow, or the day after.

   _____

   _____

5. Where did she ever get an idea like that?

   _____

   _____

6. You have got to be pulling my leg.

   _____

   _____

7. My friends, S.B. and Dale, are going to pick me up at 3:00.

_____

_____

8. Why did you repaint the barn already?

_____

_____

9. They are going to tell you what you need.

_____

_____

10. Did she take two of them? Nah, she took four.

_____

_____

Study Questions

1. What is coarticulation, and what is assimilation? What is the difference between these two processes?

2. What is the difference between regressive and progressive assimilation? What are other terms that could be used to represent the same processes?

3. Define the following processes associated with connected speech:

   a. elision   b. epenthesis   c. metathesis

4. Describe the process of vowel reduction.

5. What is the cause of the change in the casual pronunciation of the following words?

   "was shared" → /wʌʒ ʃɛrd/   "tan car"   → /tæŋ kɑr/
   "bat girl"   → /bæk gɝl/   "would you" → /wʊd ʒu/

6. What is the difference between a syllable that receives secondary stress and a syllable that is unstressed? What is the difference in the way these levels of stress are marked?

7. How is sentence stress marked?

8. What is the difference between given and new information?

9. What is a content word? What is a function word?

10. Define the terms *intonation* and *intonational phrase.*

11. When you would observe: (1) a rising intonational phrase and (2) a falling intonational phrase.

12. How does phonetic environment affect vowel duration?

13. What is the difference between internal and external juncture?

14. What is the difference between open and close internal juncture?

15. What role do pauses play in connected speech?

Assignment 6-1

Name _____

Transcribe each of the following utterances, first in citation form, and then in casual form. Only the casual form will be presented on the CD.

1. I bet you that you are going to win the race.

    _____

    _____

2. We really have to study tonight for the phonetics test.

    _____

    _____

3. Tell Sherry that she will have to go to the store to get some bacon and eggs.

    _____

    _____

4. My friend Caroline is having a party on the third of next month.

    _____

    _____

5. Bob can always finish his homework when he gets home.

    _____

    _____

6. Let me think about your answer for a minute.

    _____

    _____

7. We have just got to clean the house tomorrow.

    _____

    _____

8. Don't forget to pick up our cleaning on the way to work.

    _____

    _____

9. I am going to miss you when you move to the country.

    _____

    _____

10. Please share those ideas with the rest of the group.

    _____

    _____

Assignment 6-2

Name _____

Indicate primary and secondary stress (where appropriate) for the following words.

1. stethoscope
2. zoology
3. synchronized
4. latitude
5. execute
6. conversion
7. voyager
8. triangle
9. nomadic
10. infinite
11. fluoridate
12. December
13. detonate
14. vulcanize
15. bronchitis

16. automate
17. symmetrical
18. stupendous
19. flirtatious
20. distribute
21. chlorinate
22. magazine
23. openness
24. kitchenette
25. gullible
26. flamingo
27. evasive
28. caravan
29. modernize
30. comprehend

Assignment 6-3

Name _____

Each of the following items will be spoken by two different speakers. Transcribe the following utterances in casual form. Be sure to use single bar and/or double bar diacritics to indicate external juncture. Also use the lengthening diacritic [:] when appropriate.

1. You can lead a horse to water, but you can't make him drink.

2. I am not sure we have those shoes in your size; they only come in sizes seven, eight and one-half, or nine.

3. That man said he would drive around back to pick up his packages.

4. My professor remembered to bring in the model of the larynx; it was really helpful.

5. When you are finished typing the paper, remember to come over so we can celebrate.

6. Miss Smith thinks that her cousin, Neil, will be coming over for a visit today.

7. My niece Sarah's favorite colors have always been magenta, turquoise, and chartreuse.

8. Don't tell her I told you, but Jeannene said she has always been neutral when it comes to that topic.

9. If you stay a little while longer, I'll give you a piece of that terrific carrot cake.

10. Now, remember, the game begins sharply at 4:30. Don't forget to bring your bat and glove.

Assignment 6-4

Name _____

Rewrite each of the following questions in English orthography. Then write your answer to each one in both IPA and in English orthography.

1. /ðə nʌmbɚ əv deɪz wɪtʃ əkɚ ɪn ə lip jɪr ɪz .... ‖ /

_____

_____

2. /ðə sɪɾi ɪn wɪtʃ ðə statʃu əv lɪbɚɾi ɪz loʊkeɾəd ɪz noʊn æz ...... ‖ /

_____

_____

3. /kardiɔləʤɪsts ˌdəmətɔləʤɪsts ˌænəsθiziɔləʤɪsts ænd nɚɔləʤɪsts ar al taɪps əv ...... ‖ /

_____

_____

4. /wɛn ju meɪk ə lɔŋ dɪstəns foʊn kal ˌðə fɚst θri nʌmbɚz ju daɪl̩ ar rəfɚd tu æz ðə ...... ‖ /

_____

_____

5. /əsum ju səksɛsfʊli fɪnɪʃ jɔr frɛʃmən jɪr əv kaləʤ ˌju wɪl rətɚn jɔr sɛkənd jɪr æz ə ...... ‖ /

_____

_____

6. ðə neɪm əv ðə halɪdeɪ wɛn tʃɪldrən goʊ trɪk ɔr trɪɾɪŋ ɪz noʊn æz .... ‖ /

_____

_____

7. /əv ælʤəbrə ˌhɪstɚi ˌʤiɔɡrəfi ˌænd saɪkɔləʤi ˌðə sʌbʤɛkt wɪtʃ ɪnvalvz ðə stʌdi əv mæθəmætɪks ɪz .... ‖ /

_____

_____

8. /ðə sɛkənd mʌnθ əv ɛni kæləndɚ jɪr ɪz .... ‖ /

_____

_____

9. /wɛn ju æd ðə nʌmbɚz twɛni θri plʌs əlɛvən təgeðɚ ˌðə rəzʌlt ikwəlz .... ‖ /

_____

_____

10. /ə træfɪk saɪn wɪtʃ ɪz ʃeɪpt laɪk ən aktəgan ɪz kamənli rəfɚd tu æz ə .... ‖ /

_____

_____

Assignment 6-4 (cont.)   Name _____

11. /ðə sɪzn̩ əv ðə jɪrl wɛn ðə livz ʧeɪnʤ ðɛr kʌlə˞ ɪz juʒəlɪ kɑld .... ‖ /

_____

_____

12. /ðə skwɛr rut əv eɪɾɪ wʌn ikwəlz .... ‖ /

_____

_____

13. /ɪf ju mɪks ðə kʌlə˞z blu ænd jɛlou təgɛθə˞ ju ʃʊd gɛt .... ‖ /

_____

_____

14. /eɪprəl ʃaʊə˞z most ɔfən brɪŋ meɪ .... ‖ /

_____

_____

15. /ðə pɑrt əv ðə tʌŋ ʤʌst bəhaɪnd ðə tɪp ɪz kɑld ðə .... ‖ /

_____

_____

Clinical Phonetics

The purpose of this chapter is to introduce you to the application of phonetics in a clinical setting. The focus of the book thus far has been to acquaint you with the process of transcribing typically developing speech patterns (at least what is considered to be typical in Standard American English). As future clinicians, you will be faced with the task of evaluating a client's articulatory behavior to determine whether that client is in need of intervention. Therefore, you should have a good understanding of the process of typical speech-language development. In addition, you will need to know how to evaluate your client to determine whether there is a problem with speech-language production. Ultimately, if the client is in need of intervention, you will need to know how to generate a plan for treatment. These topics will be briefly introduced in this chapter. However, a thorough discussion of these topics is beyond the scope of this text. This material will be covered in other courses in your curriculum that focus on phonological development and disorders.

Overview of the Clinical Process

The terms **articulation disorder** and **phonological disorder** both have been used by hearing and speech professionals to characterize a client who experiences difficulty with speech production. Prior to the 1970s, the term articulation disorder was routinely used to indicate that a client had a problem in coordinating the articulators in correct production of certain phonemes. During the 1970s, considerable research in the area of phonology changed the way speech-language pathologists viewed speech sound errors. Speech production was no longer thought of simply in terms of the role the speech organs played during the articulation of phonemes. Instead, phoneme production began to be described by the phonological rules that govern the combination and order of phonemes in words. Today, a child with problems related to the rules that dictate the use of sounds in words is said to have a phonological disorder.

The distinction between the terms articulation disorder and phonological disorder for describing speech sound errors is still unclear and is still debated by some hearing and speech professionals. Elbert and Gierut (1986) suggested the use of the term articulation disorder to refer to children who only have a problem in producing a few phonemes, or whose speech errors are tied to the motoric aspects of speech production. The term phonological disorder would be reserved for a child with multiple speech sound errors, ultimately involving the sound system of a language. To avoid confusion between these two terms, some professionals use the term phonological disorder to include all disorders involving speech sound production. In this text, the term phonological disorder will be used in this manner.

To evaluate the speech production capabilities of your clients in a clinical setting, you will need to administer one or more tests to assess articulatory competency. The results of testing will ultimately help determine the therapeutic approach you select for your clients. One method commonly used to analyze the speech production abilities of a client is to administer a standardized articulation test. A standardized test is one that has been given to a test group comprised of hundreds or thousands of individuals so that average test scores can be determined. The standard group may be comprised of (1) a group of all "normal" people, (2) a representative sample of individuals from the general population, or (3) a group of people with a particular disorder. An individual's test behavior may then be compared to the behavior of a particular group to determine how that person performed on the test. Standardized articulation tests attempt to systematically identify the correct/incorrect usage of speech sounds in a child's repertoire by having the child name pictures of objects with which they are familiar. Consonants and consonant clusters (and sometimes vowels) are evaluated in various positions of words to determine whether the individual phonemes of English can be produced correctly in differing phonetic contexts. Transcription should be attempted face-to-face with the client as the test is performed. The session also should be recorded so that transcription of items missed during testing may be completed once the client has departed. The client's responses are then compared to the normative data collected from the standard group to determine whether the child's speech behavior is age appropriate.

Another method of speech evaluation involves obtaining a spontaneous, connected speech sample from the client. This is often done by engaging the client in conversation about hobbies, favorite activities, or a favorite TV show or movie. With very young children, connected speech samples may be obtained while children describe pictures in a book or while they play with toys. The spontaneous, connected speech samples also are tape-recorded, and words from the speech sample are transcribed. The transcriptions are then analyzed for age-appropriate behavior.

If testing reveals that a child has a phonological disorder, the transcriptions are subjected to analysis to catalog the specific errors the client displays. Evaluation may take several different forms. One method involves the evaluation of articulation errors, or **misarticulations**, on a phoneme-by-phoneme basis. Errors that are present in a child's speech are then categorized as errors of substitution, omission, distortion, and/or addition. A **substitution** error involves the replacement of one phoneme by another. For example, if a child produces the word "hello" as /hɛwoʊ/, the error would be classified as a substitution. This would be written as a w/l ("w for l") substitution. An example of an **omission** error would be the production of the word "big" as /bɪ/. A **distortion** would involve the production of an allophone of the intended phoneme. For instance, a dentalized production of /s/ in production of the word "sit," that is, [s̪ɪt] (which sounds like /θɪt/), would be considered a distortion. This type of distortion is commonly referred to as a "lisp." Addition errors, which are generally less common, involve the insertion of an extra phoneme in a word. One example of an **addition** is the placement of /ə/ in the word "cat"—/kætə/. This addition error is an example of epenthesis.

Analyzing speech errors phoneme-by-phoneme is an appropriate method of evaluation, especially for a child who displays only a few phonemic errors. Should a child have several misarticulations, it may be more efficient to evaluate the client's speech in terms of error patterns that may be present. For example, speech patterns may be examined in terms of errors involving the manner, place, and/or voicing of misarticulated phonemes.

Suppose you just evaluated a 6-year-old child using a picture naming task, and you transcribed the following responses for seven of the words presented:

Picture	*Child's Production*
stove	/toʊb/
bird	/bʊd/
bath	/bæt/
sun	/tʌn/
zipper	/dɪpʊ/
blue	/bu/
drum	/dʌm/

A phoneme-by-phoneme analysis would reveal several errors, including the following:

omission	/s/	(stove)		
	/l/	(blue)		
	/r/	(drum)		
substitution	d/z	(zipper)	ʊ/ɚ	(zipper)
	t/θ	(bath)	ʊ/ɝ	(bird)
	t/s	(sun)	b/v	(stove)
distortions	none			
additions	none			

Because there are several different types of errors, it would be difficult to summarize them in terms of substitutions, omissions, and so forth. However, if the errors are scrutinized in terms of manner, place, and voicing, a clearer picture of this child's speech patterns emerges. Examine the errors above, and you will see that the child routinely replaces stops for fricatives in several of the words. The child also omits the fricative /s/ in the word "stove." Additionally, the liquids /l/ and /r/ are omitted in the words "blue" and "drum," respectively. All substitutions involved correct voicing patterns; voiced stops replaced voiced fricatives, and voiceless stops replaced voiceless fricatives. In relation to place of articulation, this child substituted one labial phoneme for another in the word "stove," that is, b/v, and substituted alveolar phonemes for alveolars and interdentals (in the words "sun," "zipper," and "bath").

From this extremely limited speech sample, it appears that this child has problems producing the fricative and liquid manners of production. This pattern would not be immediately evident had the errors been evaluated individually, that is, phoneme by phoneme. The observed pattern of misarticulations could then be used as a starting point in planning treatment for this child.

An alternative approach for examining the patterns of children's speech errors is to perform a distinctive feature analysis of the misarticulated phonemes. (See Chapter 2 for a discussion of distinctive features.) Treatment would then focus on correct production of features in error, with the idea that once a feature is learned, the child will be able to generalize correct production to other phonemes containing that feature.

A completely different approach to the assessment of errors in children's speech is to examine the phonological processes the child is using. To understand the concept of phonological processes, it is important to turn our attention to the process of typical phonological development in children.

Typical Phonological Development

Over the past 60 years, many studies have attempted to delineate the order of phoneme acquisition in typically developing children (Poole, 1934; Prather, Hedrick, & Kern, 1975; Smit, Hand, Freilinger, Bernthal, & Bird, 1990; Templin, 1957; Wellman, Case, Mengert, & Bradbury, 1931). These developmental studies all examined a large number of children in order to answer the basic question, "What is the age at which children typically develop and master English speech sounds?" Without this knowledge, it would be impossible to know whether a child is developing speech in a typical manner.

When comparing the findings from different developmental phonological studies, it becomes apparent that the ages cited for typical development of individual speech sounds vary (see Table 7.1). For instance, according to Sander (1972), /r/ is mastered by the age of 6;0 (meaning 6 years; 0 months). However, the research of Smit and colleagues indicates that /r/ is not mastered until the age of 8;0. The disparity in findings between developmental studies is common and may be due to several factors. These factors may include (1) differences in the socioeconomic status of the children being examined, (2) differences in the number of subjects being studied, and (3) the way in which a speech sample is obtained by the experimenter. For example, children's speech productions may be obtained spontaneously (in response to questions asked by the experimenter or by naming pictures or objects) or by imitating words spoken by the examiner.

Another methodological discrepancy between developmental phonology studies may be related to the way in which sound mastery is defined. **Mastery** is usually defined as the age at which a particular phoneme is produced with some degree of accuracy (usually from 75 to 100 percent). The actual percentage of mastery may vary from study to study, depending upon the researcher's own definition of the term. Sander (1972) suggested that phoneme development in children be viewed not only in terms of sound mastery, but also in terms of "customary production." **Customary production** is defined as the age at which a particular phoneme is produced with greater than 50 percent accuracy, in at least two word positions (Sander, 1972). Sander defined mastery as the age at which 90 to 100 percent correct production of a phoneme occurs in all word positions (i.e., at the beginning, in the middle, and at the end of words). In this manner, developmental data can be presented for each phoneme in English as a range in age from customary production (greater than 50 percent correct production) to mastery (at least 90 percent correct).

Using the concept of customary production, Sander reanalyzed phonological development data from two studies conducted several years earlier, that is, Wellman and colleagues (1931) and Templin (1957). In their study, Wellman and colleagues evaluated spontaneous and imitated speech samples from 204 children, aged 2 to 6 years. Likewise, Templin examined spontaneous and imitated speech samples from 480 children between the ages of 3 and 8. Both studies reported phonemic development in terms of 75 percent sound mastery for sounds in the initial, medial, and final positions of words. Sander's analysis of these two studies is presented in Table 7.1. His data reflects (1) the age at which children were able to correctly produce a particular phoneme 51 percent of the time (customary production in at least two word positions) and (2) the age at which production was at a 90 percent correct production level (mastery).

Smit and colleagues (1990) more recently examined phoneme development in 997 children between the ages of 3 and 9, by using a picture naming task. Smit

TABLE 7.1 Developmental Phonological Data from Sander (1972) and Smit, Hand, Freilinger, Bernthal, and Bird (1990). Data are presented as years and months. For example, 6;0 means 6 years and 0 months.

	Sander (1972)		Smit and colleagues (1990)			
			75% mastery		90% mastery	
Phoneme	>50% customary production	90% mastery	Girls	Boys	Girls	Boys
m	<2;0	3;0	≤3;0	≤3;0	3;0	3;0
p	<2;0	3;0	≤3;0	≤3;0	3;0	3;0
h	<2;0	3.0	≤3;0	≤3;0	3;0	3;0
w	<2;0	3;0	≤3;0	≤3;0	3;0	3;0
b	<2;0	3;0	≤3;0	≤3;0	3;0	3;0
n	<2;0	3;0	≤3;0	≤3;0	3;6	3;0
k	2;0	4;0	≤3;0	≤3;0	3;6	3;6
d	2;0	4;0	≤3;0	≤3;0	3;0	3;6
g	2;0	4;0	≤3;0	≤3;0	3;6	4;0
t	2;0	6;0	≤3;0	≤3;0	4;0	3;6
f	2;6	4;0	≤3;0	3;6	3;6–5;6	3;6–5;6
j	2;6	4;0	3;6	3;6	4;0	5;0
ŋ	2;0	6;0	5;6	6;0	7;0–9;0	7;0–9;0
r	3;0	6;0	6;0	5;6	8;0	8;0
l	3;0	6;0	4;6	6;0	5;0–6;0	6;0–7;0
s	3;0	8;0	3;0	5;0	7;0–9;0	7;0–9;0
tʃ	3;6	7;0	4;0	5;0	6;0	7;0
ʃ	3;6	7;0	4;0	5;0	6;0	7;0
z	3;6	8;0	5;0	6;0	7;0–9;0	7;0–9;0
dʒ	4;0	7;0	4;6	4;0	6;0	7;0
v	4;0	8;0	4;0	4;6	5;6	5;6
θ	4;6	7;0	5;6	6;0	6;0	8;0
ð	5;0	8;0	4;0	5;6	4;6	7;0

and colleagues defined mastery as 90 percent correct phoneme usage in the initial and final positions of words for the children they examined in their study. They also presented developmental data for 75 percent correct phoneme production. Interestingly, Smit and her colleagues found some differences between girls and boys in terms of their phonological development; girls less than 6 years of age tended to develop some phonemes earlier than boys in the same age group. Therefore, the data from their study is presented separately for boys and girls in Table 7.1, both for 75 percent and 90 percent mastery.

EXERCISE 7.1

Examine the findings from the two studies displayed in Table 7.1. Answer the following questions:

1. Which manners of articulation do children appear to develop first?
2. Which places of articulation do children appear to develop first?
3. Which manners of articulation still appear to be problematic for typical 5-year-old children?
4. For which manner of articulation do children first use voiceless/voiced pairs?

EXERCISE 7.2

Compare the two studies in Table 7.1 by examining the columns indicating *90% mastery* of phoneme production. For which phonemes do Smit and colleagues suggest *later* development (i.e., greater than one year difference), when compared to the data given by Sander? For which phonemes do Smit and colleagues suggest *earlier* development (i.e., greater than one year difference)?

Although the findings from these two studies differ, upon close inspection of the data, certain similarities emerge. The similarities include:

1. Ninety-percent mastery of several phonemes occurs by the age of 3 years. The mastery of all English phonemes may not be complete until a child is at least 7 to 9 years of age.
2. In relation to manner of articulation, the nasal and stop consonants are acquired first, followed, in order, by the glides, fricatives, liquids, and affricates.
3. In relation to place of production, sounds produced in the front of the mouth (e.g., labial and alveolar) are usually developed first, followed by velar and palatal articulations.

Developmental speech sound studies all focused on segmental (phoneme-by-phoneme) acquisition. A more recent method used in the analysis of the phonological development of children is to examine production in terms of underlying patterns or processes children may use in the production of speech sounds. Stampe (1969) proposed a theory of **natural phonology** that supports the idea that young children are born with innate processes necessary for the production of speech. Because young children are not capable of producing adult speech patterns, they often simplify the adult form. These simplifications are termed **phonological processes**. As children mature, they learn to suppress these processes. When this happens, children then are able to produce the more appropriate adult form of the articulation.

If only segmental development is considered, a child who is not capable of producing a certain phoneme may be viewed as not having that sound in his or her phonetic inventory. When viewed in terms of phonological processes, the child may be using a phonological process that results in the deletion of that sound. Adults may have difficulty understanding the speech patterns of a young child with whom they are not familiar. This is often not due to missing sounds in the child's phonetic repertoire; it is most likely due to the fact that adults are not accustomed to the simplifications, or processes, being produced by the child (Hodson & Paden, 1991).

Phonological Processes

Many phonological processes are found to occur in the speech patterns of typically developing children. These processes can be divided into three general categories: **syllable structure processes, substitution processes** and **assimilatory processes** (Ingram, 1976). Some of the more common processes associated with these subdivisions are presented below and are summarized in Table 7.2. Developmental data (the age when specific processes are suppressed) in the following sections are from Grunwell (1987). Pay particular attention to the examples given in terms of their phonetic transcription.

TABLE 7.2   Examples of Some Common Phonological Processes of Children

Syllable Structure Processes	Example Word	Production
weak syllable deletion	surprise	/praɪz/
final consonant deletion	look	/lʊ/
reduplication	baby	/bibi/
cluster reduction	clean	/kin/

Substitution Processes		
stopping	sand	/tænd/
fronting	kite	/taɪt/
deaffrication	jump	/ʒʌmp/
gliding	lake	/weɪk/
vocalization	bird	/bʊd/

Assimilatory Processes		
labial assimilation	put	/pʊp/
alveolar assimilation	mine	/naɪn/
velar assimilation	garden	/gɑrgn̩/
prevocalic voicing	cop	/gɑp/
devoicing	ride	/raɪt/

Syllable Structure Processes

These processes, as a group, affect the production of syllables so that they are simplified, usually into a consonant-vowel (CV) pattern (Ingram, 1976). CV patterns are among the first syllable types to be used in the speech patterns of developing infants.

Weak Syllable Deletion

Weak syllable deletion, or simply syllable deletion, is a phonological process that involves the omission of an unstressed (weak) syllable either preceding or following a stressed syllable. This process may persist until a child is nearly 4;0. It is also common in some adult productions (Hodson & Paden, 1991).

Examples:

telephone → /tɛfon/	probably → /prɑblɪ/ or /prɑlɪ/
tomato → /meɪɾo/	above → /bʌv/
paper → /peɪp/ or /peɪ/	yellow → /jɛl/

EXERCISE 7.3

Indicate with an "X" the transcriptions that are examples of weak syllable deletion.

Examples:

	Intended Word	Transcription
___	please	/piz/
X	elephant	/ɛfənt/
___	1. yes	/ɛs/
___	2. baby	/beɪ/
___	3. banana	/nænə/
___	4. mama	/mə/
___	5. today	/deɪ/
___	6. milk	/mɪk/
___	7. mitten	/mɪt/
___	8. lady	/di/
___	9. scissors	/sɪ/
___	10. juice	/ʤu/

Final Consonant Deletion

Final consonant deletion effectively reduces a syllable to a CV pattern, that is, to an open syllable. Typically developing children begin to use most consonants in the coda (final) position of words by the time they reach the age of 3 years, 0 months (3;0). Therefore, this process is generally suppressed completely by age 3;6.

Examples:

bake → /beɪ/	mouse →/maʊ/
cat → /kæ/	coat → /koʊ/
mom → /mɑ/	nice → /naɪ/

EXERCISE 7.4

Which of the following words could be affected by final consonant deletion? Indicate those words with an "X" and then transcribe the word in IPA, applying the process of final consonant deletion.

Examples:

shoe	___	_____
foot	_X_	/fʊ/

away	1. ___	_____
cup	2. ___	_____
through	3. ___	_____
clown	4. ___	_____
bread	5. ___	_____
say	6. ___	_____
phone	7. ___	_____
black	8. ___	_____
stop	9. ___	_____
go	10. ___	_____

Reduplication

Reduplication involves the repetition of a syllable of a word. Total reduplication involves a repetition of an entire syllable, as in "mommy" → /mɑmɑ/. Partial reduplication involves repetition of just a consonant or vowel, as in "bottle" → /bɑdɑ/ (Lowe, 1996). Reduplication is common in the early speech development of some children. It is generally suppressed before 2;6.

Other examples:

daddy → /dædæ/ or /dɑdɑ/   doggy → /dɑdɑ/
baby → /beɪbeɪ/   movie → /mumu/

EXERCISE 7.5

For the words given, indicate with an "X" the transcriptions that indicate the process of reduplication.

___ 1.	wagon	/wægə/	___ 4.	pencil	/pɛpɛ/
___ 2.	children	/dɪdɪ/	___ 5.	water	/wɑwɑ/
___ 3.	jacket	/dækɪ/	___ 6.	yellow	/jɛdo/

Cluster Reduction

Cluster reduction results in the deletion of a consonant from a consonant cluster (adjacent consonants in the same syllable). If the cluster contains three consonants, one or two of the consonants may be deleted, as in "spray" → /preɪ/ or /reɪ/. Cluster reduction may persist until approximately 4;0.

Other examples:

snow → /noʊ/	play → /peɪ/	stripe →/traɪp/, /taɪp/, or /raɪp/
green → /gin/	plump → /plʌp/	help → /hɛp/

EXERCISE 7.6

For the words given, indicate with an "X" the transcriptions that indicate the process of cluster reduction.

___	1. blue	/bu/		___	6. stop	/tɑp/
___	2. spot	/spɑ/		___	7. crayon	/keɪɑn/
___	3. stripe	/raɪp/		___	8. milk	/mɪk/
___	4. path	/pæt/		___	9. wish	/wɪs/
___	5. spring	/rɪŋ/		___	10. grape	/geɪp/

Substitution Processes

Substitution processes involve the replacement of one class of phonemes for another. For instance, the phonological process known as **stopping** involves the substitution of a stop for a fricative or affricate. Similarly, the process known as **fronting** involves the substitution of an alveolar phoneme for a velar or palatal articulation.

Stopping

As just mentioned, stopping involves the substitution of a stop for a fricative or an affricate. This is a commonly occurring process because stops are acquired before most fricatives in typically developing speech (see Table 7.1). The substitution is usually for a stop produced with the same, or similar, place of articulation:

fricative/affricate		substituted stop
/s,ʃ, ʧ, θ/	→	/t/
/z, ʒ, ʤ, ð/	→	/d/
/f/	→	/p/
/v/	→	/b/

Sometimes children produce a stop for a fricative or affricate along with a change in voicing, for example, /sɪp/ → /dɪp/. The change in voicing is a phonological process called *prevocalic voicing* and will be discussed in more detail below. Stopping of fricatives and affricates may continue for some phonemes until 4;0 or 5;0.

Examples:

sake → /teɪk/ (voiceless alveolar fricative → voiceless alveolar stop)

zoo → /du/ (voiced alveolar fricative → voiced alveolar stop)

fat → /pæt/ (voiceless labiodental fricative → voiceless bilabial stop)

think → /tɪŋk/ (voiceless dental fricative → voiceless alveolar stop)

ship → /tɪp/ (voiceless palatal fricative → voiceless alveolar stop)

Jane → /deɪn/ (voiced palatal affricate → voiced alveolar stop)

Note: The last two examples ("ship" and "Jane") demonstrate not only stopping, but also a more forward place of production of the affected consonant phoneme. That is, place of production shifted from palatal to alveolar in both cases. This process is called fronting and is discussed in the next section.

EXERCISE 7.7

Place an "X" in front of the following transcriptions that represent an example of the process of stopping.

____ 1. shoe → /zu/   ____ 6. comb → /goʊm/

____ 2. thank → /tæŋk/   ____ 7. summer → /tʌmɚ/

____ 3. raisin → /weɪzn̩/   ____ 8. yellow → /wɛloʊ/

____ 4. march → /mɑrt/   ____ 9. bath → /bæt/

____ 5. shave → /seɪv/   ____ 10. shop → /tɑp/

Fronting

It is common for young children to substitute velar and palatal consonants with an alveolar place of articulation. This substitution process is commonly referred to as *fronting*. The alveolar substitutions typical of fronting are given below:

velar		alveolar		palatal		alveolar
/k/	→	/t/		/ʃ/	→	/s/
/g/	→	/d/		/ʧ/	→	/ts/
/ŋ/	→	/n/		/ʒ/	→	/z/
				/ʤ/	→	/dz/

Fronting usually disappears in typically developing children's speech by the age of 2;6 to 3;0.

Examples:

cat → /tæt/ (voiceless velar stop → voiceless alveolar stop)

wash → /wɑs/ (voiceless palatal fricative → voiceless alveolar fricative)

juice → /dzus/ (voiced palatal affricate → voiced alveolar affricate)*

chip → /tsɪp/ (voiceless palatal affricate → voiceless alveolar affricate)*

get → /dɛt/ (voiced palatal stop → voiced alveolar stop)

cookie → /tʊtɪ/ (voiceless velar stop → voiceless alveolar stop)

match → /mæt/ (voiceless palatal affricate → voiceless alveolar stop)

*The affricates /ts/ and /dz/ are not phonemes of English, but may occur in disordered speech patterns, as in these examples.

Note: The pronunciation of /mæt/ for "match" displays both fronting and stopping of the final phoneme:

"match" /mætʃ/ → /mæts/ (fronting, i.e., palatal /tʃ/ → alveolar /ts/)

and

/mæts/ → /mæt/ (stopping, i.e., affricate /ts/ → stop /t/)

EXERCISE 7.8

Place an "X" in front of the following transcriptions that are indicative of fronting.

_____ 1. candy → /gændɪ/   _____ 6. ridge → /rɪd/

_____ 2. rake → /reɪt/   _____ 7. fishing → /fɪʃɪŋ/

_____ 3. bring → /brɪn/   _____ 8. paper → /teɪpɚ/

_____ 4. clown → /kraʊn/   _____ 9. goose → /dus/

_____ 5. brush → /brʌs/   _____ 10. sing → /tɪŋ/

Deaffrication
Deaffrication occurs when a child substitutes a fricative for an affricate.

Examples:
chip → /ʃɪp/   (voiceless, palatal affricate → voiceless, palatal fricative)
matches →/mæʃəz/   (voiceless, palatal affricate → voiceless, palatal fricative)
juice → /ʒus/   (voiced, palatal affricate → voiced, palatal fricative)
ridge → /rɪʒ/   (voiced, palatal affricate → voiced, palatal fricative)
ledge → /lɛz/   (voiced, palatal affricate → voiced, alveolar fricative)

Note: The last example, that is, ledge → /lɛz/, demonstrates two substitution processes: (1) deaffrication and (2) fronting. In addition to the substitution of the fricative for an affricate, that is, /dʒ/ → /ʒ/ (deaffrication), the palatal /ʒ/ is produced as the alveolar /z/ (fronting).

Suppose a child produced the word "June" as /dun/. How many substitution processes are occurring in this production? If you answered "three," you are correct. A change from /dʒ → d/ involves deaffrication, fronting, and stopping. Study this example to make sure you understand the three processes that are occurring:

"June" /dʒun/ → /ʒun/   (deaffrication)
/ʒun/ → /zun/   (fronting)
/zun/ → /dun/   (stopping)

EXERCISE 7.9

Place an "X" in front of the following transcriptions that are indicative of de-affrication.

_____ 1. shake → /seɪk/   _____ 6. gem → /ʧɛm/

_____ 2. choose → /tsuz/   _____ 7. witch → /wɪʃ/

_____ 3. brush → /brʌt/   _____ 8. chalk → /sɔk/

_____ 4. Jack → /ʒæk/   _____ 9. chase → /ʃeɪs/

_____ 5. mesh → /mɛs/   _____ 10. bridge → /brɪdz/

Gliding

This substitution process involves a substitution of the glides /w/ or /j/ for the liquids /l/ and /r/. **Gliding** is common in children displaying typical developmental patterns as well as in those with phonological disorders. This process is overused in cartoons to depict characters with disordered speech patterns, for example, /wæbɪt/ for "rabbit." This phonological process is seen in children as young as 2;0, and may persist until a child is 5;0 or older.

Examples:

red → /wɛd/   blue → /bwu/

look → /wʊk/ or /jʊk/   carrot → /kɛwət/

green → /gwin/   hello → /hɛjoʊ/

like → /jaɪk/   grow → /gwoʊ/

EXERCISE 7.10

Place an "X" in front of the following transcriptions that are indicative of gliding.

_____ 1. soap → /woʊp/   _____ 6. yes → /wɛs/

_____ 2. leaf → /wif/   _____ 7. loop → /wup/

_____ 3. ring → /jɪŋ/   _____ 8. grow → /gwoʊ/

_____ 4. lazy → /jeɪzɪ/   _____ 9. laugh → /jæf/

_____ 5. rice → /laɪs/   _____ 10. free → /fli/

Vocalization

Vocalization, or **vowelization**, involves the substitution of a vowel for postvocalic /l/ or /r/. Vocalization is especially common in words with /əl/ (or syllabic /l̩/), /ɚ/, and /ɝ/. The vowels commonly substituted include /ʊ/, /ɔ/, and /o/ (or /oʊ/).

Examples of vocalization:

		substitution
tiger → /taɪgʊ/		ɚ → ʊ
turn → /tɔn/		ɝ → ɔ
third → /θʊd/		ɝ → ʊ
deer → /dɪʊ/		r → ʊ
hair → /hɛʊ/		r → ʊ
help → /hɛʊp/		l → ʊ
milk → /mɪʊk/		l → ʊ
meal → /mioʊ/		l̩ → oʊ
little → /wɪɾoʊ/		l̩ → oʊ

Note that the last example (little → /wɪɾoʊ/) demonstrates both vocalization and gliding.

EXERCISE 7.11

Place an "X" in front of the following transcriptions that are indicative of vocalization.

____ 1. middle → /mɪdo/	____ 6. belt → /bɛʊt/
____ 2. lamp → /wæmp/	____ 7. bottle → /bɔɾo/
____ 3. answer → /ænsʊ/	____ 8. curtain → /kʊʔn̩/
____ 4. Kirk → /kɔk/	____ 9. bark → /bɑk/
____ 5. could → /kɔd/	____ 10. fair → /fɛʊ/

Complete Assignment 7-1.

Assimilatory Processes

Assimilatory processes involve an alteration in phoneme production due to phonetic environment (see Chapter 6 for a review of assimilation). Assimilatory processes involve labial, velar, nasal, and/or voicing assimilation. The assimilation in any of these instances may be either progressive or regressive. These processes are not present in all typically developing children. When they occur, they usually disappear before the age of 3. The assimilation processes associated with consonant production are also referred to as *consonant harmony*.

Labial Assimilation
Labial assimilation occurs when a nonlabial phoneme is produced with a labial place of articulation. This is due to the presence of a labial phoneme elsewhere in the word.

Example:

    book → /bʊp/   (progressive assimilation)

(In this case, the nonlabial /k/ is produced with a labial articulation due to the presence of the /b/ phoneme at the beginning of the word.)

mad → /mæb/   (progressive assimilation)
cap → /pæp/   (regressive assimilation)
swing → /ɸwɪŋ/   (regressive assimilation)

/ɸ/ is a voiceless bilabial fricative, a phoneme found on the IPA chart, but not common to English. To produce this phoneme, place your lips together and blow out so air escapes (but don't whistle). Pretend you are softly blowing out a candle. (Don't push air from the glottis, otherwise you will produce /h/.) Say the word "whew." The initial phoneme is a bilabial, voiceless fricative. When producing the word "swing" as /ɸwɪŋ/, the alveolar fricative /s/ undergoes labial assimilation due to the presence of /w/.

EXERCISE 7.12

Place an "X" in front of the words that correctly indicate the process of labial assimilation.

____ 1. pie → /baɪ/   ____ 6. boat → /boʊp/
____ 2. tap → /pæp/   ____ 7. train → /preɪn/
____ 3. frog → /frɑk/   ____ 8. peg   → /pɛb/
____ 4. lip → /lɪb/   ____ 9. cause → /pɔz/
____ 5. numb → /mʌm/   ____ 10. big → /bɪb/

Alveolar Assimilation

Alveolar assimilation occurs when a nonalveolar phoneme is produced with an alveolar place of articulation due to the presence of an alveolar phoneme elsewhere in the word.

Examples:

time → /taɪn/   (progressive assimilation)
neck → /nɛt/   (progressive assimilation)
shut → /sʌt/   (regressive assimilation)
bat → /dæt/   (regressive assimilation)

EXERCISE 7.13

Place an "X" in front of the words that correctly indicate the process of alveolar assimilation.

____ 1. pig → /tɪg/   ____ 6. knife → /naɪs/
____ 2. pat → /tæt/   ____ 7. that   → /zæt/
____ 3. short→ /sɔrt/   ____ 8. phone → /soʊn/
____ 4. Tom→ /mɔm/   ____ 9. vat   → /væp/
____ 5. tune→ /dun/   ____ 10. hard → /kɑrd/

It is not always easy to determine whether a child's speech productions are a result of assimilation or of a substitution process. For instance, a child who produces the word "cat" as /tæt/ might be using alveolar assimilation or may be fronting the /k/ phoneme. To determine whether a child is using assimilatory processes, it is necessary to evaluate several productions from the child's speech sample. In this manner, a particular phonological pattern may emerge. Examine two different children's productions of the following six words. What phonological pattern do you see?

	child #1		*child #2*
kite	/taɪt/	kite	/taɪt/
dog	/dɑd/	dog	/dɑd/
should	/sʊd/	should	/sʊd/
push	/pʊs/	push	/pʊʃ/
go	/doʊ/	go	/goʊ/
bike	/baɪt/	bike	/baɪk/

Child #1's productions of "kite," "dog," and "should" could be suggestive of either alveolar assimilation or fronting. However, productions of the words "push," "go," and "bike" reflect only fronting, because no alveolar phonemes exist in these words. Therefore, this child appears to be using the process of fronting. Contrast this pattern with child #2 who only mispronounces the first three words, words with alveolar phonemes. Child #2 appears to be using alveolar assimilation.

Velar Assimilation

Velar assimilation occurs when a nonvelar phoneme is produced with a velar place of articulation due to the presence of a velar phoneme elsewhere in the word.

Examples:

cup → /kʌk/	(progressive assimilation)
gone → /gɔŋ/	(progressive assimilation)
take → /keɪk/	(regressive assimilation)
doggy → /gɑgɪ/	(regressive assimilation)

EXERCISE 7.14

Place an "X" in front of the words that correctly indicate the process of velar assimilation.

_____	1. turkey → /kɜ˞kɪ/	_____	6. ring → /wɪŋ/
_____	2. kill → /gɪl/	_____	7. bang → /gæŋ/
_____	3. mouse → /maʊp/	_____	8. shook → /ʃʊg/
_____	4. grass → /kræs/	_____	9. cap → /kæk/
_____	5. fake → /keɪk/	_____	10. brag → /græg/

Voicing Assimilation

There are two types of voicing assimilation. The first type, **prevocalic voicing,** involves voicing of a normally unvoiced consonant. This occurs when the consonant precedes the nucleus of a syllable. That is, the unvoiced consonant assimilates to the (voiced) nucleus.

Examples:

> pig → /bɪg/   (regressive assimilation)
>
> cup →/gʌp/   (regressive assimilation)

Another type of voicing assimilation involves the **devoicing** of syllable-final voiced phonemes that either precede a pause or silence between words, or occur at the end of an utterance. That is, the final phoneme "assimilates to the silence" following the word (Ingram, 1976, p. 35).

Examples:

> bad → /bæt/   (regressive assimilation)
>
> hose → /hos/   (regressive assimilation)

EXERCISE 7.15

Indicate whether the transcriptions of the following words indicate prevocalic voicing (P) or devoicing (D). Write P or D in the blanks. If neither process is demonstrated, leave the item blank.

____	1. pear → /bɛr/		____	6. gone → /kɔn/
____	2. led → /lɛt/		____	7. train → /dreɪn/
____	3. fair → /vɛr/		____	8. flag → /flæk/
____	4. card → /kɑrt/		____	9. shoe → /ʒu/
____	5. high → /haɪt/		____	10. chair → /ʃɛr/

Complete Assignments 7-2 and 7-3.

As demonstrated in some of the examples above, phonological processes may occur individually or in combination in the speech patterns of children. For example, the pronunciation of the word "little" as /wɪɾo/ suggests two processes, gliding and vocalization. Pronunciation of the word "spoon" as /pu/ would be the result of cluster reduction as well as final consonant deletion. Also, as pointed out previously, more than one process may affect the pronunciation of any one phoneme, as in "June" → /dun/ (deaffrication, stopping, and fronting).

Not all of the processes outlined above necessarily occur in the speech patterns of all typically developing children. The processes that are most common in typical children's speech include weak syllable deletion, final consonant deletion, gliding, and cluster reduction (Stoel-Gammon & Dunn, 1985). Also, suppression of a particular process does not happen all at once. Suppression may initially occur for only certain phonemes in a class. For instance, children who demonstrate stopping may suppress the process for /f/ and /s/ before they suppress it for the fricatives /v, z, ʃ, ð, and θ/ and also for the affricates /ʧ/ and /ʤ/ (Grunwell, 1987). Although most phonological processes disappear in the speech patterns of typically developing children by the age of 4 (Hodson & Paden, 1991), some processes disappear earlier.

Let us return to the previous example that showed the results of the articulation test from our fictitious 6-year-old child. Now, the errors will be considered in terms of the phonological processes that this child has not yet suppressed.

picture	child's production	phonemic change	phonemic process(es)
stove	/toʊb/	st → t; v → b	cluster reduction; stopping
bird	/bʊd/	ɝ → ʊ	vocalization
bath	/bæt/	θ → t	stopping
sun	/tʌn/	s → t	stopping
zipper	/dɪpʊ/	z → d; ɚ → ʊ	stopping; vocalization
blue	/bu/	bl → b	cluster reduction
drum	/dʌm/	dr → d	cluster reduction

Upon analysis of the child's responses, it now becomes evident that the child is still using the following phonological processes:

stopping

cluster reduction

vocalization

This child would be considered to have a phonological disorder because these phonological processes typically disappear by the age of 6. In this case, treatment would be indicated, and it would focus on the reduction of these processes.

Children with Phonological Disorders

Children with phonological disorders often display the same types of phonological processes as typically developing children. However, as indicated in the above example, the processes may be suppressed later than typically observed. Stoel-Gammon and Dunn (1985) compared eight studies that had investigated children with disordered phonology. The pooled data from these eight studies revealed phonological error patterns for 128 children, ranging in age from 2;7 to 13;0. The results of this comparison revealed several processes common to many children with phonological disorders. These processes included:

cluster reduction

weak syllable deletion

final consonant deletion

stopping

velar and palatal fronting

voicing processes

labial, nasal, and velar assimilation

liquid simplification (a combination of gliding and vocalization)

Of these processes, the most consistently used by the children with disorders included cluster reduction, stopping, and liquid simplification. These specific processes are among those consistently seen in typically developing children as well.

Children with disordered phonology also display several processes not usually found in the speech of typically developing children. These processes are called **idiosyncratic processes** (Stoel-Gammon & Dunn, 1985). Several idiosyncratic processes include (from Stoel-Gammon & Dunn, 1985):

1. *Glottal replacement*—the substitution of a glottal stop for another consonant.

   pick → /pɪʔ/; butter → /bʌʔʊ/ (with vocalization) ; lip → /ʔɪp/

2. *Backing*—the substitution of a velar stop consonant for consonants usually produced more anterior in the oral cavity. Backing usually involves alveolars and palatals; however, labial sounds may be affected.

   time → /kaɪm/; zoom → /gum/; push → /pʊk/

3. *Initial consonant deletion*—the omission of a single consonant at the beginning of a word.

   cut → /ʌt/; game → /eɪm/

4. *Stops replacing a glide*—the substitution of a stop for a glide.

   yes → /dɛs/
   wait → /beɪt/

5. *Fricatives replacing a stop*—the substitution of a fricative for a stop.

   sit → /sɪs/
   doll → /zɔl/

EXERCISE 7.16

For each of the given transcriptions, fill in the blank with the name of the appropriate idiosyncratic process just described. There may be more than one answer for each item.

Example:

    cat →/kæʔ/   glottal replacement

1. chairs → /ɛrz/ _____
2. letter → /lɛsɚ/ _____
3. witch → /dɪʧ/ _____
4. tape → /keɪp/ _____
5. bunny → /ʌʔɪ/ _____
6. bad → /gæʔ/ _____

So far in this chapter, phonological problems in children have been discussed in terms of what a particular child *cannot* do instead of what a child *can* do. That is, analyses have been performed to examine the errors in a child's speech sound system. The child's system is then compared with a developmental standard in order to determine what is "missing" or "wrong" in the child's speech sound repertoire. The standard could be a developmental norm that looks at typical mastery of particular phonemes at certain ages (Smit et al., 1990, for example). Another approach would be to compare a child's errors to an adult standard, as is typically done in a phonological process analysis.

A clinician who compares a child's phonological abilities to some existing standard is performing a *relational analysis*. That is, a child's error patterns are related to correct production by other children of the same age or compared to what is expected in adulthood. By performing only a relational analysis, it may not be possible to analyze what part of the child's phonological system is functional. To determine the functional aspect of a child's phonological system, it is important to perform an *independent analysis*. In this approach, the child's sound system is evaluated independently with no reference to a given standard. An independent analysis explains the phonetic system the child uses and the phonological patterns the child *is* capable of producing with that system. It is important to be able to evaluate a child's intact phonological system to determine how it contributes (or fails to contribute) to overall communication effectiveness (speech intelligibility.) Since relational and independent analyses provide different information, both are performed when evaluating a child's phonological abilities.

Velleman (1998) promotes a "do-it-yourself" independent analysis that is useful in cataloging a child's phonological system. The analysis is called "do-it-yourself" because it utilizes nonstandardized worksheets or checksheets that are developed by the clinician in order to inventory the phonological system of a child. In this type of analysis, the child's speech sample can come from both administration of standardized phonological tests (naming pictures) and/or from elicitation of spontaneous speech (e.g., telling a story). The clinician then takes the recorded sample and transcribes each word the child produces. Some of the information the clinician can gather from such an independent analysis includes:

1. A complete inventory of the individual consonants and vowels the child produces.

2. An inventory of syllable shapes used by the child; i.e., whether a child produces open and/or closed syllables and consonant clusters at the beginning and/or end of syllables.

3. The combination of consonants (C) and vowels (V) the child uses to produce various syllable types; i.e., CV, VC, CVC, CCVC, CVCC, etc.

4. The word shapes the child produces; i.e., the number and types of syllables in a word. (That is, can a child produce only one-syllable words, or can he or she also produce two-, three-, and four-syllable words?)

5. The stress patterns the child produces in bisyllabic and multisyllabic words with varying stress patterns; e.g., lion, giraffe, elephant, orangutan.

This type of analysis is important because the child's sound system is evaluated not just in terms of the phonemes that are produced correctly relative to the adult model, but it is also analyzed independently, as a functional system in its own right in terms of phoneme production in words varying in phonetic composition, stress, and number of syllables. In other words, phonemes are identified without consideration of what is phonemic or contrastive in the target language, but rather which consonants and vowels are used contrastively in particular contexts in the child's system.

Analysis of a child's phonological system at more than one level is termed *nonlinear phonology*. That is, the child's phonological system is evaluated by looking at sound patterns at various levels including words, syllables, segments, and features. In this manner, phonological structure can be viewed in a hierarchical manner (i.e., nonlinear) by utilizing tree diagrams to show the relationships between the differing levels. These tree diagrams are similar to those introduced in Chapter 2 to illustrate syllable structure in words. Only now, there are more branches in the trees.

Utilizing this nonlinear approach, the phonological structure of the word "window" is presented in Figure 7.1. Note the hierarchical arrangement of the various levels, or tiers, labeled "word tier," "syllable tier," "onset-rhyme tier," "CV tier," "segment tier," and "feature tier." In nonlinear phonology, segments are further divided into a set of hierarchically arranged features known as *feature geometry*. For our purposes, the feature tier will be described in terms of manner, place, and voicing (after Stoel-Gammon, 1996).

How does nonlinear phonology help in remediation of children with phonological problems? A simple example may help answer this question. Your client may produce the word "cat" as /kae/. At first glance, it appears that she may have problems producing the final /t/ phoneme. However, does she really have problems with final /t/, or does she generally have problems producing final consonants in all CVC words? Since nonlinear phonology looks at phoneme production at several levels, the answer may become more evident by analyzing the client's speech sample and looking for patterns of production across a number of words. If it is determined that the child cannot produce final consonants in words, it could be considered a "constraint" on a particular tier of her phonological system, whereas the absence of /t/ in "cat" but the presence of other consonants in coda position would be a constraint on a different tier. Nonlinear phonology emphasizes the fact that all levels or tiers are connected hierarchically to each other and the interactions between segments and syllables can be observed by

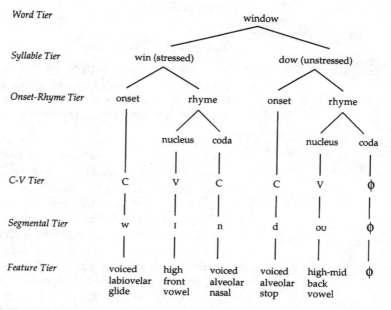

FIGURE 7.1 Hierarchical structure of the word "window."

diagramming the client's phonological system. In order for your client's phonology to improve, therapy will need to consider what constraints exist and how remediation aimed at different tiers would improve her ability to produce the adult pattern.

Complete Assignments 7-4 and 7-5.

Allophonic Transcription of Speech

If a child demonstrates the process of gliding, pronouncing "red" as /wɛd/, phonemic transcription would be adequate in capturing the production on paper. However, systematic phonemic transcription will not always suffice in transcribing disordered speech patterns. Systematic narrow (allophonic) transcription may be necessary to adequately represent a client's speech pattern on paper.

Consider the speech patterns of a child who has a cleft palate and has problems with nasal emission, that is, air escaping through the nasal cavity. Systematic phonemic transcription of the child's production of the word "smile," /smaɪl/, would not indicate the occurrence of nasal emission. A systematic narrow transcription of this word, [s̃maɪl], reveals that nasal emission occurred during production of /s/. (The symbol [˜] represents an allophone of [s], [s] with nasal emission.)

In the last chapter, you were introduced to some symbols used in the transcription of the suprasegmental aspects of speech. These diacritical markings included those for timing of phonemes [ː] and juncture [|, ||]. In the following section, several diacritics will be introduced as they relate to allophonic variants of speech associated with (1) changes in place of articulation, (2) stop consonant production, (3) nasality, and (4) the sound source. Some of the allophonic variants demonstrated result from progressive assimilation, others result from regressive assimilation. Only some of the more commonly used diacritics will be discussed below. The diacritic markings adopted in this text are from the 1993 revision of the IPA (updated 1996). Refer to Figure 2.1 for the complete list of the 1996 IPA diacritics.

Place of Articulation

There are several IPA diacritics that are used to indicate allophonic variants related to changes in place of articulation of consonants and vowels. Some of these changes occur as a result of assimilation processes. Others occur as a result of dialect, speaking style, or phonological disorder.

Front/Back [k̟] [t̠]
When a phoneme is produced with the tongue more forward in the oral cavity than normal, the symbol [₊] is used. For instance, the narrow transcription of the word "key" would be [k̟i] because the /k/ (normally produced with the body of the tongue in the velar region) is produced closer to the palate due to the environment provided by the front vowel /i/ (regressive assimilation).

When a phoneme is produced with the tongue farther back than normal, the symbol [₋] is used. When the alveolar stops /t/ or /d/ precede /r/, their place of articulation becomes postalveolar (closer to the palate) because /r/ is a palatal phoneme. Some examples include "true" [t̠ru] and "dry" [d̠raɪ] (regressive assimilation). Because of the backed articulation of these consonants, the words "true" and "dry" may appear to sound like /tʃru/ and /dʒraɪ/, respectively.

EXERCISE 7.17

Place an "X" by the words that have a correct transcription using the diacritics [₊] and [_].

1. ____ good [gʊd]   3. ____ drop [d̲rɑp]   5. ____ keep [k̟ip]
2. ____ kiss [k̟ɪs]   4. ____ clam [k̲læm]   6. ____ comb [koʊm̟]

Advanced, Retracted Tongue Position [₋ᵥ, ₋]

These two symbols are used to indicate a variation in tongue position associated with vowel production. The change would involve the front/back dimension. For example, a retracted production of /æ/ would be transcribed as [æ̠], indicating that the vowel is farther back than would be expected, but not so far back as to result in the production of the vowel /ɑ/. Similarly, an advanced production of /ɑ/, that is, [ɑ̟], would be farther forward than normal, but not enough to result in production of /æ/. Make sure you use the symbols [₊] and [₋] to transcribe differences in vowel advancement and the symbols [₊] and [_] for changes in consonant advancement.

Raised, Lowered Tongue Position [₊, ꜜ]

These diacritics are placed beneath a vowel when there is a change in the height dimension associated with that vowel. The change in tongue height may be the result of a particular dialectal pronunciation of a vowel or as a result of a speech disorder. The symbol [₊] indicates that a vowel is produced with the body of the tongue raised more than expected for that particular vowel. For instance, if an adult attempts to produce the vowel /ɛ/, but raises the tongue higher than expected (but not so high as to produce /ɪ/), the transcription would be [ɛ̝]. Likewise, production of /ʊ/ with a lowered tongue position would be transcribed as [ʊ̞], as long as the production does not result in articulation of the vowel /o/.

EXERCISE 7.18

Examine each of the following vowels and their transcriptions. Then indicate which vowel would result if the articulation were slightly higher, lower, advanced, or retracted (depending on the diacritic used).

Example:

vowel produced:	resultant vowel is closer to:
[i̞]	/ɪ/
[ɑ̟]	/æ/

1. [ɛ̠] ____   5. [ʊ̟] ____
2. [æ̟] ____   6. [ɛ̝] ____
3. [o̝] ____   7. [i̞] ____
4. [o̞] ____   8. [ʊ̟] ____

Labialization [k̃]

A consonant that is not normally produced with lip rounding may become rounded in the presence of certain phonemes, for example, /u/, /ʊ/, or /w/. This phenomenon can be seen in the initial consonantal phoneme of "quick," "good," "zoo," and "rude." The additional articulation of lip rounding, associated with consonant production, is called **labialization**. The diacritic commonly used for labialization is a "w" placed to the right of the normally unrounded phoneme as in [k̃wɪk], [g̃ʊd], [z̃u], and [r̃ud]. Keep in mind that [k̃] is an allophone of the phoneme /k/, and [z̃] is an allophone of /z/, and so forth. That is, lip rounding does not result in the creation of a *different* phoneme. The transcriptions [k̃wɪk], [g̃ʊd], [z̃u], and [r̃ud] represent regressive, or right-to-left, assimilation, because the normally rounded phoneme follows the phoneme undergoing assimilation.

EXERCISE 7.19

Transcribe the words below, using the [ᵂ] diacritic if the initial phoneme is labialized due to the phonetic environment. If the word does not have a labialized initial phoneme, leave the item blank.

Examples:

swim	[s̃wɪm]
wood	_____*_____

1. hood   _____
2. shock   _____
3. roof   _____
4. thin   _____
5. wool   _____
6. plus   _____
7. sweet   _____
8. dune   _____

*(/w/ is already a labialized consonant)

Labiodental Articulation [ɱ], [m̪]

In words in which the nasal consonants /m/ or /n/ are followed by /f/, the place of articulation is altered, due to the influence of the labiodental place of articulation for /f/ (regressive assimilation). Although English does not have a labiodental nasal phoneme, other languages do. The IPA symbol for this phoneme is /ɱ/. Because English does not make use of /ɱ/ phonemically, this assimilation may be considered an allophonic variant, not a phonemic change. Words in which this labiodental nasal occurs (depending on an individual speaker's pronunciation) include "comfort" /kʌɱfɚt/, "conference" /kɑɱfrəns/, "unfair" /əɱfɛr/, "emphasis" /ɛɱfəsəs/, and "symphony" /sɪɱfəni/. The symbol /m̪/ (which indicates dentalization) also may be used to transcribe labiodental assimilation.

EXERCISE 7.20

Transcribe the following words using /ŋ/ where appropriate. If not appropriate, leave the item blank.

1. inferential   _____
2. sphinx   _____
3. Memphis   _____
4. perform   _____
5. unfriendly   _____
6. camphor   _____
7. sunflower   _____
8. pharynx   _____
9. identify   _____
10. kinfolk   _____

Dentalization [t̪]

In the phonetic context of /θ/ or /ð/, alveolar consonants may become produced with the tongue tip farther forward than normal. This process is termed **dentalization**. For example, the /n/ in the word "ninth" becomes dentalized; it now has a dental articulation brought about by the final phoneme /θ/. It would be possible to transcribe this word as [naɪn̟θ], given that the articulation is more forward than usual. However, when an alveolar phoneme is produced with a dental articulation, the symbol [̪] is used instead, for example, [naɪn̪θ]. Other words with dentalized alveolars include "filth" [fɪl̪θ] and "month" [mʌn̪θ]. These examples show regressive or right-to-left assimilation.

The effect of dentalization crosses word boundaries as well. For instance, in the phrase "with Terry," the /t/ becomes dentalized, that is, [wɪθt̪ɛrɪ]. Notice that the plosive /t/ is released between the teeth. This is an example of progressive or left-to-right assimilation.

EXERCISE 7.21

Transcribe the following utterances, using the diacritic [̪] when necessary. Leave the item blank if it is not necessary to use the diacritic.

1. anthem   _____
2. moth   _____
3. either   _____
4. bathroom   _____
5. math time   _____
6. wealth   _____
7. rhythm   _____
8. panther   _____

The dental diacritic [̪] also may be used in transcription of disordered speech when alveolar fricatives are dentalized—that is, when the tip (apex) of the tongue is placed just behind the upper front teeth (anterior to the alveolar ridge). Examples include /s̪ut/ for "suit," /mɪs̪/ for "miss," and /z̪ibrə/ for "zebra." This type of speech production is sometimes referred to as a *frontal lisp*. Some individuals transcribe this particular speech production as a /θ/ for /s/, or a /ð/ for /z/ substitution, that is, /θut/, /mɪθ/, or /ðibrə/. It is suggested that the correct transcription for this particular production should be [s̪] or [z̪], not /θ/ or /ð/, as long as its articulation retains a sibilant quality (Hodson & Paden, 1991).

Lateralization [sˡ], [ɬ], [ɮ], [ꞵ], [ɮ]

A lateralized production of the fricatives /s/ or /z/ occurs when the constricted airflow is diverted over the sides of the tongue, instead of being able to flow centrally. To produce a lateralized /s/, place your tongue in position for the initial phoneme in the word "let." Now, holding your tongue in place, try to produce an /s/ phoneme. Notice how the air flows over the sides of the tongue because it cannot escape anteriorly. This lateral production of /s/ or /z/ is sometimes referred to as a *lateral lisp*.

The IPA diacritic for a lateralized phoneme is a raised /l/, placed to the right of the indicated phoneme, as in [jɛsˡ]. There are other IPA symbols specifically used for transcription of a lateral fricative. These symbols are [ɬ] for a lateralized /s/, and [ɮ] for a lateralized /z/, as in "yes" [jɛɬ] or "zoo" [ɮu]. The symbols /ꞵ/ and /ɮ/ have been adopted more recently for lateral /s/ and /z/, when airflow is directed both laterally and centrally (Duckworth, Allen, Hardcastle, & Ball, 1990).

Velarization [ɫ]

Velarization occurs when the alveolar consonant /l/ is produced in the velar region of the vocal tract. This production of /l/ is said to be "dark," or velarized. An example of velarization occurs with the phoneme /l/ in the words "ball" and "eagle." In "ball," the /l/ is produced in the velar region of the vocal tract because it follows the production of /ɑ/, a low back vowel. In the word "eagle," because the consonant /g/ is a velar articulation, the articulation of /l/ becomes velar. The diacritic commonly used for velarization is a tilde through the middle of the phoneme, as in [bɑɫ] and [igɫ]. This is another demonstration of progressive or left-to-right assimilation. The velarized [ɫ] is found in all occurrences of syllabic [l̩]. Keep in mind that [ɫ] and [l̩] are two different allophones of /l/.

Another example of velarization is produced when the nasal /n/ occurs before the velar consonants /k/ or /g/, as in the words "long," "pink," and "tango." It is too difficult to pronounce these words without velarizing the /n/ and producing it as /ŋ/. Try saying these words without the /ŋ/ phoneme, that is, /lɔng/, /pɪnk/, and /tængoʊ/. You will agree that these words are easier to pronounce as /lɔŋ/, /pɪŋk/, and /tæŋgoʊ/. In essence, the phoneme /ŋ/ is actually an allophone of /n/, which occurs only as a result of velarization (regressive assimilation).

EXERCISE 7.22

Place an "X" next to the words that would have a velarized /ɫ/ in their transcriptions.

1. ____ lake
2. ____ mingle
3. ____ loop
4. ____ beagle
5. ____ shoulder

6. ____ liked
7. ____ angle
8. ____ scald
9. ____ ladle
10. ____ bile

Stop Consonant Production

In Chapter 5 you learned that stop consonants are comprised of an articulatory closure, an increase in intraoral pressure, and a release burst at one of three points of articulation: bilabial, alveolar, or velar. The manner in which stop consonants are produced (released, unreleased, aspirated, unaspirated) also varies as a function of phonetic environment, regardless of the original place of articulation.

Unreleased Stops [p̚]

An **unreleased** stop consonant is one that has no audible release burst associated with it. Unreleased stops occur quite often in English at the ends of words as in "leak," "put," "map," "hog," and "red." Contrast the production of the word "stop" first by releasing the final /p/ and then by not releasing it. The transcription of the unreleased production would be [stɑp̚]. Likewise, contrast the two productions of the word "bid," that is, [bɪd̚] and [bɪd]. When two voiceless stop consonants occur one after the other in the same syllable, the first one is not released, as in the words "stacked" [stæk̚t] and "reaped" [rip̚t].

Aspiration of Stops [pʰ]

Aspiration is often defined as a burst of air associated with the production of voiceless stop consonants (Calvert, 1986; MacKay, 1987). This definition may be somewhat misleading, because all stop consonants have a noise burst associated with their production. Aspiration involves the production of a frictional noise (similar to the glottal phoneme /h/) following the release of a voiceless stop and preceding the following vowel. There is, in a sense, a second burst of noise associated with voiceless stops. Keep in mind that aspiration occurs only in the presence of the voiceless stop consonants /p/, /t/, and /k/. Although there is an audible release burst associated with voiced stops, aspiration (the second frictional noise) is absent.

Aspiration occurs most often in released voiceless stops in the initial position of *stressed* syllables. Examples of aspiration occur in the words: "pass" [pʰæs], "torn" [tʰɔrn], "kiss" [kʰɪs], "atone" [ətʰoʊn], and "repay" [rəpʰeɪ]. Released voiceless stops at the ends of words may be aspirated as well, as in "leap" [lipʰ], "snake" [sneɪkʰ], and "right" [raɪtʰ]. Aspiration does *not* occur when a voiceless stop follows the fricative /s/, as in "spoon," "scat," or "stood."

Unaspirated [p⁼]

The symbol [⁼] is placed above and to the right of unaspirated voiceless stops, those that do not have a second burst. Unaspirated stops are most common when they occur immediately following the fricative /s/ as in the words "spin" [sp⁼ɪn] or "escape" [əsk⁼eɪp˺]. Although stops may be unaspirated, they may still be released. Both of the unaspirated stops in "spin" and "escape" are released.

EXERCISE 7.23

Place an "X" next to each of the following words that contain an unaspirated phoneme.

1. ____ slack   5. ____ excuse
2. ____ praised   6. ____ surprise
3. ____ scorn   7. ____ stripe
4. ____ despite   8. ____ smooth

EXERCISE 7.24

Place an "X" next to the words that are possible transcriptions for the words given, using the diacritics for unreleased, unaspirated, and aspirated productions. If a transcription is given that is not possible for a particular word, correct it.

Examples:

X	licked	[lɪk˺tʰ]	
____	cap	[kæp˺]	_____ [kʰæp˺] _____
1. ____	skunk	[sk⁼ʌŋkʰ]	_____
2. ____	snacked	[snæk˺tʰ]	_____
3. ____	target	[tɑrgət˺]	_____
4. ____	brave	[bʰreɪv]	_____
5. ____	toga	[tʰougʰə]	_____
6. ____	guarded	[gɑrdəd˺]	_____
7. ____	person	[pɝsʰən]	_____
8. ____	carefully	[kʰɛrfʊlɪ]	_____
9. ____	slope	[sl⁼oup˺]	_____
10. ____	great	[gʰreɪtʰ]	_____

Nasality

Several diacritcs are used in narrow transcription to indicate changes in nasality associated with speech production. These include nasalization, nasal emission, and denasality.

Nasalization [æ̃]

Oral phonemes sometimes become nasalized in the presence of nasal phonemes. This process is called **nasalization**. For example, the word "mean" has a vowel surrounded by two nasal phonemes. The velum lowers during the production of the initial consonant /m/ and remains lowered throughout the word (for articulatory efficiency), because the final phoneme /n/ also is a nasal. The result is a nasalized vowel, represented by the IPA notation [mĩn]. Note the use of the tilde over the nasalized sound. The following words also have nasalized vowels due to the nasal environment provided by /m/, /n/, or /ŋ/: "hang," "in," "mom," and both vowels in "roomy" and "any." The effects of nasalization can also be seen across word boundaries as in "When Amy left . . ." [wɛnẽɪmɪlɛft . . .] or "can only" [kænõʊnlɪ]. Note that nasalization can be regressive, progressive, or a combination of both (as in the word "mom").

In the transcription of disordered speech, this diacritic is also used to indicate the presence of excessive nasality associated with the production of non-nasal phonemes. This condition is known as **hypernasality**. Hypernasality is usually due to improper velopharyngeal closure, as in cleft palate speech. Hypernasality also may extend throughout an entire production of a word or an utterance.

Some deaf individuals also display hypernasality in their speech. In fact, deaf speech is often described as sounding "nasal." The problem in this case is not a physical one, since there is no structural deviation in the speech organs associated with velopharyngeal closure. Improper use of nasality is more likely due to faulty learning associated with the hearing loss. The auditory cues associated with nasality are difficult for deaf individuals to hear (Erber, 1983). Without having an appropriate auditory model of how oral versus nasal consonants should sound, it is difficult for deaf individuals to use nasality correctly.

EXERCISE 7.25

Place an "X" next to the words that are transcribed correctly using the diacritic for nasalization.

1. ____ mean   [m̃in]   4. ____ string   [strĩŋ]
2. ____ boon   [bũn]   5. ____ slam   [s̃læm]
3. ____ muddy   [mʌdĩ]   6. ____ thong   [θã̃ŋ]

Nasal Emission [˜]

Nasal emission is the audible escape of air through the nares due to improper velopharyngeal closure. Airflow may escape through the velopharyngeal port itself or may escape through a cleft in the palate or velum. Individuals with cleft palate often exhibit nasal emission during the production of stops and fricatives. The diacritic [˜] is used when nasal emission accompanies a phoneme that is *not* normally nasalized. Examples include "snail" [s̃neɪl], "nice" [naɪs̃], "zoo" [z̃u], and "pie" [p̥aɪ]. Keep in mind that nasal emission is not the same as nasalization. Nasalization of speech results when the velum is lowered in production of oral sounds, resulting in nasal resonance. Nasal emission is a process in which air escapes through the nares.

Denasality [˜]

Another condition related to nasality is **denasality**, also known as **hyponasality**. Denasality results when the nasal phonemes /m, n, and ŋ/ are produced without nasalization. Denasality is most often associated with the speech patterns of a person with a cold or upper respiratory infection. The utterance, "My name is Matt" would sound like "By dabe is Batt," when spoken denasalized. Using the diacritic [˜] to indicate denasality, the above utterance would be transcribed as [m̃aɪ ñeɪm̃ ɪz m̃æt]. Children who do not have a cold, but consistently sound like they do, should probably be evaluated by a physician to determine whether a structural abnormality exists that may interfere with the production of nasal phonemes.

Sound Source

This group of diacritics indicates a change in the manner of vocal fold vibration during the production of consonants and vowels. These changes include voicing, devoicing, whistled articulation, and breathy articulation.

Voicing [t̬]

This diacritic is used when a voiceless phoneme is produced with partial voicing. A good example of voicing occurs when using the tap [ɾ] in the transcription of words such as "better" [bɛɾɚ] and "kitty" [kɪɾɪ]. In these words, the voiceless /t/ becomes partially voiced due to the voiced environment provided by the surrounding phonemes. However, the assimilation does not result in production of the voiced phoneme /d/. Some people use the diacritic for voicing instead of a tap when transcribing words such as "better" [bɛt̬ɚ] or "kitty" [kɪt̬ɪ]. Another example of partial voicing may occur in some pronunciations of the words "pester" [pɛs̬tɚ], "mister" [mɪs̬tɚ], and "Leslie" [lɛs̬lɪ].

EXERCISE 7.26

Transcribe the following words, using the diacritic for voicing instead of a tap (when necessary).

1. kettle _____   4. attempt _____

2. written _____   5. baton _____

3. water _____   6. battled _____

Devoicing [r̥]

In certain phonetic environments, phonemes that are normally voiced, become less voiced. This phenomenon is known as *devoicing*. Phonemes that become devoiced still have some voicing associated with them; they are not completely voiceless. The concept of devoicing is not really new to you. Recall that a word such as "ladder" is transcribed with the tap /ɾ/, indicating devoicing of the /d/ phoneme. You may recall that this assimilation results when /t/ or /d/ is intervocalic.

Devoicing also occurs when one of the approximants /w, l, r, or j/ follows a voiceless consonant. Examples include "pray" [pɹ̥eɪ], "few" [fju], "clip" [kl̥ɪp], and "queen" [kw̥in]. Devoicing also may occur across word boundaries as in "thank you" [θæŋkju].

Words ending with a voiced fricative or affricate may become devoiced if silence follows the word, that is, if they are at the end of an utterance (Cruttenden, 2001). Examples include [bæʤ̥], [wʌz̥], and [lʌɣ̥]. In connected speech, when a word that ends with a voiced fricative is followed by a word that begins with a voiceless consonant, the fricative also may become devoiced (Cruttenden, 2001). For instance, the phrase "has seen" may be pronounced as [həz̥ sin]. Other examples include "of course" [əɣ̥kɔrs], "she's sorry" [ʃiz̥ sɑɪ], and "I've passed" [aɪɣ̥pæst].

EXERCISE 7.27

Using the diacritic for devoicing [̥], transcribe the following utterances.

1. pewter   _____
2. clearly   _____
3. he's stubborn   _____
4. bathe Pam   _____
5. he does   _____
6. Ridge Street   _____
7. I lose   _____
8. they've played _____

Whistled Articulation [̘]

Fricatives are sometimes characterized as having a "whistled articulation." This is especially true of the /s/ phoneme. A whistled articulation occurs when the apex of the tongue directly contacts the back of the upper central incisors. The resulting production can be described as a "whistling" /s/ or also as "effeminate" speech. This speech error is sometimes referred to as a *dental lisp* (Ohde & Sharf, 1992). To produce a whistled /s/, say the word "withstand," paying particular attention to your production of the /s/ following the /θ/ phoneme, that is [wɪθʂ̟tænd] (progressive assimilation).

Breathy Voice [V̤]

When the vocal folds do not make sufficient contact during voicing, audible air may escape through the glottis. This condition results in a breathy voice quality. You may recognize this vocal quality as the "sexy voice" stereotype, portrayed by movie actresses such as Marilyn Monroe. Causes of breathiness include growths, such as polyps or nodules, on the vocal folds. Some deaf speakers also display breathiness due to improper valving of air by the vocal folds, as air flows through the glottis from the lungs. Because the vocal folds do not always make sufficient contact to ensure adequate subglottal pressure, air wastage occurs. The IPA diacritic [̤] is used beneath specific phonemes that are produced with a breathy voice quality. If an entire utterance is breathy, it may be transcribed by using the symbol [V̤] preceding and following the breathy utterance. For example:

{V̤ aɪ hævə nɑʤl̩ ɑn maɪ voʊkl̩ foldz V̤}

Note the use of the braces, and not brackets, when transcribing an alteration in voice quality. This notation scheme is part of an extension to the IPA, called the **VoQS** (voice quality symbols). This extension was developed in order to provide speech pathologists with a more in-depth system of transcribing disorders associated with voice production, such as breathiness or hoarseness (Ball, Esling, & Dickson, 1995).

It is beyond the scope of this text to describe other conditions of the larynx that result in an alteration of voice quality. This material will be covered in coursework examining voice production (most likely at the graduate level). However, the entire VoQS notation system is given in Figure 7.2 for your inspection.

Complete Assignments 7-6 and 7-7.

The extIPA

During the late 1970s and early 1980s, a British group of phoneticians and speech-language pathologists convened in an attempt to create and systematize a set of diacritics for the transcription of disordered speech. These professionals formed what is called the Phonetic Representation of Disordered Speech (PRDS) group. Then, in 1989, the International Phonetic Association Congress convened in Kiel, Germany, to revise the International Phonetic Alphabet. This was the first major revision to the IPA in 50 years. The purpose of this landmark revision was to make the IPA more representative of world languages and also to account for new theories in phonetics.

Suggestions from the PRDS and from other phoneticians and speech-language pathologists resulted in the formation of a new extension to the IPA, entitled the **extIPA**. The extIPA was adopted in 1994 by the International Clinical Phonetics and Linguistics Association (ICPLA) as the official set of diacritics to be used in the transcription of disordered speech. The complete set of extensions to the IPA is located in Figure 7.3. You will notice that you are already familiar with several of these symbols. The extIPA introduces several new terms that are defined below, using descriptions from Duckworth and colleagues (1990).

lateral + central fricative—a fricative produced with both a lateral and a central airstream as in the production of some lateral lisps

nareal fricative—production of a nasal phoneme, /m, n, ŋ/, with accompanying nasal emission due to velopharyngeal incompetency.

percussive—a stop produced by striking together two articulators, such as the cutting edges of the teeth

dentolabial—a phoneme produced when the lower lip contacts the upper teeth

linguolabial—a phoneme produced when the tongue contacts the upper lip

labioalveolar—a phoneme produced by contacting the alveolar ridge with the lower lip

labial spreading—an abnormal degree of lip spreading associated with the production of a phoneme

reiterated articulation—an articulation that is repeated, as in stuttering

velopharyngeal friction—the production of a frictional noise, or "snort," at the velopharyngeal port, due to velopharyngeal incompetency

VoQS: Voice Quality Symbols

AIRSTREAM TYPES

Œ	oesophageal speech	И	electrolarynx speech
Ю	tracheo-oesophageal speech	↓	pulmonic ingressive speech

PHONATION TYPES

V	modal voice	F	falsetto
W	whisper	C	creak
V̰	whispery voice (murmur)	V̰	creaky voice
V̤	breathy voice	C̰	whispery creak
V!	harsh voice	V!!	ventricular phonation
V̰!!	diplophonia	V̰!!	whispery ventricular phon.
V̩	anterior or pressed phonation	W̱	posterior whisper

SUPRALARYNGEAL SETTINGS

L̝	raised larynx voice	L̞	lowered larynx voice
Vᴼᴱ	labialized voice (open round)	Vʷ	labialized voice (close round)
V̹↔	spread-lip voice	Vᵛ	labio-dentalized voice
V̺	linguo-apicalized voice	V̻	linguo-laminalized voice
V˞	retroflex voice	V̪	dentalized voice
V̲	alveolarized voice	V̿ʲ	palatoalveolarized voice
Vʲ	palatalized voice	Vˠ	velarized voice
Vʁ	uvularized voice	Vˤ	pharyngealized voice
V̞ˤ	laryngo-pharyngealized voice	Vꟸ	faucalized voice
Ṽ	nasalized voice	V̊	denasalized voice
J̞	open jaw voice	J̝	close jaw voice
J̬	right offset jaw voice	J̌	left offset jaw voice
J̟	protruded jaw voice	Θ	protruded tongue voice

USE OF LABELED BRACES & NUMERALS TO MARK STRETCHES OF SPEECH AND DEGREES AND COMBINATIONS OF VOICE QUALITY

['ðɪs ɪz 'nɔˑməl 'vɔɪs {3V! 'ðɪs ɪz 'vɛɹi 'hɑˑʃ 'vɔɪs 3V!} 'ðɪs ɪz 'nɔˑməl 'vɔɪs wʌns 'mɔˑ {L̝1V! 'ðɪs ɪz 'lɛs 'hɑˑʃ 'vɔɪs wɪð 'loʊəd 'læɹɪŋks 1V!L̝}]

© 1994 Martin J. Ball, John H. Esling, B. Craig Dickson

FIGURE 7.2 The VoQS diacritic set. This chart first appeared in the *Journal of the International Phonetic Association* and is reproduced by permission of the International Phonetic Association.

extIPA SYMBOLS FOR DISORDERED SPEECH
(Revised to 1997)

CONSONANTS (other than those on the IPA Chart)

	bilabial	labiodental	dentolabial	labioalv.	linguolabial	interdental	bidental	alveolar	velar	velophar.
Plosive	p̪ b̪		p̟ ɓ	p̪ b̪	t̼ d̼	t̪ d̪				
Nasal			m̟	m̪	n̼	n̪				
Trill					r̼	r̪				
Fricative: central			f̟ v̟	f̪ v̪	θ̼ ð̼	θ̪ ð̪	ħ̪ ɦ̪			f̜ŋ
Fricative: lateral+central								ʪ ʫ		
Fricative: nareal	m̃							n̊̃	ŋ̊̃	
Percussive	ʷ ʷ					ʭ				
Approximant: lateral					l̼	l̪				

DIACRITICS

↔	labial spreading	ᶘ	strong articulation	f̬	�.
͏	dentolabial	v̼	weak articulation	v̥	ᵔm denasal
͏	interdental/bidental	n̪	reiterated articulation	p\p\p	ṽ nasal escape
=	alveolar	t̪	whistled articulation	s̫	s̃ velopharyngeal friction
͏	linguolabial	d̼	sliding articulation	θs	p↓ ingressive airflow
					!↑ egressive airflow

CONNECTED SPEECH

(.)	short pause
(..)	medium pause
(...)	long pause
f	loud speech [{f laʊd f}]
ff	louder speech [{ff laʊdə ff}]
p	quiet speech [{p kwaɪət p}]
pp	quieter speech [{pp kwaɪətə pp}]
allegro	fast speech [{allegro fɑːst allegro}]
lento	slow speech [{ lento sloʊ lento}]
crescendo, ralentando, etc. may also be used

VOICING

ˬ	pre-voicing	ˬz
ˬ	post-voicing	zˬ
(˳)	partial devoicing	(z̥)
(˳	initial partial devoicing	(z̥
˳)	final partial devoicing	z̥)
(ˬ)	partial voicing	(s̬)
(ˬ	initial partial voicing	(s̬
ˬ)	final partial voicing	s̬)
=	unaspirated	p=
ʰ	pre-aspiration	ʰp

OTHERS

(͜‿) indeterminate sound	(( )) extraneous noise ((2 sylls))
(V̱), (P̱l) indeterminate vowel, plosive, etc.	¡ sublaminal lower alveolar percussive click
(P̱l.vls) indeterminate voiceless plosive, etc.	‼¡ alveolar & sublaminal click ('cluck-click')
( ) silent articulation (ʃ), (m)	* sound with no available symbol

© 1997 ICPLA

FIGURE 7.3 The extension to the IPA (extIPA). This chart first appeared in the *Journal of the International Phonetic Association* and is reproduced by permission of the International Phonetic Association and the International Clinical Phonetics and Linguistics Association.

indeterminate sound—an unrecognizable phoneme during phonetic transcription; the unrecognizable sound is circled (the symbol in the extIPA chart is actually a typed circle)

silent articulation—a "mouthed" production of speech with no breath stream present

extraneous noise—speech or nonspeech noise that obliterates the intended phonetic transcription (this is marked with double parentheses)

Suggestions for Transcription

The complete set of combined diacritics from the revised 1996 IPA symbols, the extIPA, and from the VoQS seems extraordinarily overwhelming at first. The combined diacritic sets allow for the transcription of virtually all possible allophonic variants of English as well as most possible misarticulations of speech. Obviously, not all of these symbols would be used routinely in the transcription of disordered speech. This raises an interesting question. Which symbols should be used routinely when transcribing disordered speech? This is not an easy question to answer. Undoubtedly, every speech-language pathologist would have a different answer to this question. The most important consideration is the accuracy of the transcription being performed. It is not necessarily important to indicate normal allophonic variations of phonemes if they do not disrupt the production of speech. For instance, there would be no need to indicate nasalized vowels, as long as the nasalization was appropriate. If however, a client had inappropriate nasalization of speech, the appropriate diacritic [~] would then need to be indicated in the transcription.

When you begin transcribing both live and taped samples of your clients, there are several factors you will need to consider so that your transcriptions will be as accurate as possible. Keep in mind that your clients' speech patterns often will be difficult to understand. This means that a good tape-recording is necessary so that you will be able to replay the speech sample at a later time. However, no matter how good the recording is, certain phonemes may not be very audible on the tape. This is due to the fact that some English phonemes are naturally low in intensity. This is especially true of the voiceless fricatives /s/, /f/, and /θ/. This is one reason why it is extremely important for you to transcribe face-to-face during testing. Of course, wearing headphones (attached to your tape recorder) will aid in your transcription accuracy by reducing any background noise that might be present. Also, when you are performing a live transcription, you will be able to visually focus on the clients' articulators, especially in reference to lip rounding and tongue placement for certain phonemes. Although it is possible to videotape your clients' diagnostic session, facial features may not always be clearly represented because videotape only provides a two-dimensional view of the client. Another suggestion is to listen to the audiotape several times before attempting a transcription in order to become accustomed to the speech patterns of the client (Shriberg & Kent, 2003).

When listening to a taped sample of a client's speech, it will become immediately apparent that certain speech segments will be easier to transcribe than others. Begin with the speech segments of which you are sure. You also may want to transcribe phonemes first, adding the diacritics later. Ohde and Sharf (1992, pp. 351–352) offer several beneficial suggestions to help the clinician focus on speech patterns that are particularly difficult to transcribe. Their transcription techniques include the following:

1. Count the number of syllables in each produced utterance and determine if it agrees with the number in the target utterance.

2. Identify the vowels, diphthongs, or syllabic consonants that constitute the nucleus of each syllable, using the minimal contrasts of front-back, high-low, tense-lax, and rounded-unrounded to zero in on the vowel.

3. Transcribe the syllable nuclei you are certain of, leaving space for preceding and following consonants.

4. Determine whether each vowel nucleus is initiated and terminated by a consonant or consonant cluster and if a target consonant is deleted.

5. Identify the consonants, using manner, voicing, and place feature analysis to zero in on them, and transcribe those you are certain of.

6. Decide which features of the remaining consonants you are uncertain about and how they differ from the target consonants.

7. Transcribe the consonants, using appropriate diacritics to indicate deviations from targets, if necessary.

Review Exercises

A. For each of the words, create a production that demonstrates *weak syllable deletion*. Write your answer using the IPA.

Example:

about   /baʊt/

1. table ____		6. Denise ____
2. beside ____		7. turkey ____
3. carrot ____		8. dinner ____
4. pony ____		9. candy ____
5. basket ____		10. potato ____

B. Each of the following speech productions represent one type of *syllable structure process*. Match one of the processes given at the right to each transcription given.

Examples:

_b._ coat → /koʊ/   a. weak syllable deletion

_c._ kitty → /kɪkɪ/   b. final consonant deletion

                c. reduplication

                d. cluster reduction

____ 1. school → /kul/		____ 6. swing → /sɪŋ/
____ 2. candy → /kækæ/		____ 7. soap → /soʊ/
____ 3. lion → /laɪ/		____ 8. cookie → /kiki/
____ 4. mom → /mɑ/		____ 9. missed → /mɪt/
____ 5. running → /rʌn/		____ 10. water → /wɑ/

C. For each item, indicate whether the transcription indicates regressive (R) or progressive (P) assimilation.

Example:

_P_ cup → /kʌk/

____ 1. finger → /gɪŋgɚ/		____ 6. feather → /fɛvɚ/
____ 2. table → /peɪbl̩/		____ 7. pillow → /pɪboʊ/
____ 3. rabbit → /bæbɪt/		____ 8. mat → /mæp/
____ 4. map → /mæm/		____ 9. sip → /zɪp/
____ 5. park → /kɑrk/		____ 10. grab → /græg/

D. Each of the following transcriptions reflects some form of assimilation. Match the type of assimilation to each transcription given.

Example:

_P_ cup → /kʌk/   a. labial   d. prevocalic voicing

                b. velar   e. devoicing

                c. alveolar

____ 1. pan → /tæn/		____ 6. sunny → /zʌni/
____ 2. face → /veɪs/		____ 7. green → /grin/
____ 3. swim → /ɸwɪm/		____ 8. sack → /sæt/
____ 4. bad → /bæt/		____ 9. park → /kɑrk/
____ 5. numb → /mʌm/		____ 10. nag → /næk/

E. For each of the following, match the transcription to the appropriate substitution process being demonstrated. There may be more than one correct answer per item.

____ 1. mister → /mɪstʊ/   a. gliding
____ 2. yellow → /jɛwoʊ/   b. deaffrication
____ 3. matches → /mæʃəz/   c. vocalization
____ 4. cage   → /keɪʒ/
____ 5. reel   → /wiʊ/
____ 6. little → /jɪɾoʊ/
____ 7. choose → /ʃuz/
____ 8. press   → /pwɛs/

F. Match the transcriptions with the process being demonstrated. Each item has more than one correct answer.

____ 1. jumped → /dʌmpt/   a. fronting
____ 2. shampoo → /tæmpu/   b. stopping
____ 3. watch   → /wɑs/   c. deaffrication
____ 4. feet   → /bit/   d. prevocalic voicing
____ 5. said   → /dɛd/
____ 6. thicker → /dɪkɚ/
____ 7. shared → /zɛrd/
____ 8. chops   → /tɑps/

G. For each of the following words, apply the phonological process given and transcribe the resulting production.

Example:

lean   final consonant deletion   ____/li/____

1. sleep   cluster reduction   _____
2. brag   velar assimilation   _____
3. jar   stopping   _____
4. lemon   gliding   _____
5. bake   labial assimilation   _____
6. jelly   deaffrication   _____
7. above   weak syllable deletion _____
8. pine   alveolar assimilation   _____
9. came   fronting   _____
10. crow   prevocalic voicing   _____

H. Indicate whether the given phonological process is possible for each of the words given. Circle "Yes" or "No."

1. clown   weak syllable deletion   Yes   No
2. pup   labial assimilation   Yes   No
3. Jenny   reduplication   Yes   No
4. cry   gliding   Yes   No
5. shot   fronting   Yes   No
6. play   devoicing   Yes   No
7. stove   velar assimilation   Yes   No

8.	ship	stopping	Yes	No
9.	chew	deaffrication	Yes	No
10.	chair	cluster reduction	Yes	No
11.	penny	prevocalic voicing	Yes	No
12.	clay	final consonant deletion	Yes	No

I. Transcribe the following words as spoken by a 5-year-old male child who demonstrates *gliding*.

1. lobster _____
2. nurse _____
3. soldier _____
4. astronaut _____
5. teacher _____
6. truck driver _____
7. dentist _____
8. refrigerator _____
9. telephone _____
10. lamp _____
11. toothbrush _____
12. bathtub _____
13. toilet _____
14. hammer _____
15. alarm clock _____
16. vacuum cleaner _____
17. elephant _____
18. tiger _____
19. squirrel _____
20. spider _____
21. lion _____
22. dolphin _____
23. kangaroo _____
24. octopus _____
25. lawyer _____

J. Transcribe the following words and sentences as spoken by a 7-year-old female child who demonstrates *dentalization* of alveolar fricatives.

1. cherries _____
2. celery _____
3. cheese _____
4. cereal _____
5. grapes _____
6. ice cream _____
7. peas _____
8. pancakes _____
9. eggs _____
10. spider _____
11. octopus _____
12. squirrel _____
13. snake _____
14. skunk _____
15. jeans _____
16. sweater _____
17. pajamas _____
18. sandals _____
19. mittens _____
20. slippers _____

21. We went to Ben Franklin's and looked at the toys.

_____

22. I saw some dolls that I liked.

_____

23. They traveled to Maine from Nebraska.

_____

24. We do spelling and math.

_____

25. Sometimes we play mystery games.

_____

K. Transcribe the following words as spoken by a 7-year-old female child who demonstrates both *vocalization* and *dentalization* of alveolar fricatives.

1. frog	_____		14. lobster	_____
2. zebra	_____		15. rabbit	_____
3. cookies	_____		16. spider	_____
4. hamburger	_____		17. elephant	_____
5. skunk	_____		18. ice cream	_____
6. strawberries	_____		19. butter	_____
7. parakeet	_____		20. cherries	_____
8. carrots	_____		21. squirrel	_____
9. cereal	_____		22. orange	_____
10. hotdog	_____		23. horse	_____
11. pancakes	_____		24. potato	_____
12. celery	_____		25. turtle	_____
13. giraffe	_____			

L. Define each of the following diacritics.

Example:

[n̪]   dentalized production of /n/
    _____

1. [pʰ]

    _____

2. [u̟]

    _____

3. [ɾ̥]

    _____

4. [g̃]

    _____

5. [ƀ]

    _____

6. [ð̃]

    _____

7. [z̩]

    _____

8. [e̥]

    _____

M. Select an English word in which you might find each of the following diacritics. Write the word in IPA using the appropriate transcription.

1. [t¬] _____
2. [m̃] _____
3. [b¬] _____
4. [ɛ̃] _____
5. [t̪̬] _____

6. [n̠] _____
7. [d̪] _____
8. [ɬ] _____
9. [m̥] _____
10. [ʔ] _____

N. Place an "X" next to each item where the diacritic is placed incorrectly. Consonants are represented by the square symbol.

1. ____ ʰ☐
2. ____ ☐˜
3. ____ ☐¬
4. ____ ☐₊

5. ____ ☐⁼
6. ____ ☐̬
7. ____ ☐̠
8. ____ ☐̃

O. Circle the most accurate allophonic transcription for each of the following words.

1. clue	[kʰlu]	[k̥ɬu]	[k¬lu]
2. lymph	[lɪɱf]	[ɬɪmf]	[lɪmp¬f]
3. money	[mʌ̃ni]	[mʌ̃nɪ]	[m̥ʌnɪ]
4. coop	[k¬upʰ]	[kʰupʰ]	[kʰup⁼]
5. trial	[t̪ʰ ɹ̥aɪɬ]	[tʰɾaɪɬ]	[tʰ ɹ̥aɪɬ]
6. skunk	[sk⁼ʌŋkʰ]	[sk¬ʌ̃ŋkʰ]	[sk⁼ ʌ̃ŋkʰ]
7. menthol	[mɛ̃ n̠ θaɬ]	[mɛ̃ n θ a l]	[mɛ̃ n θ̠ a ɬ]
8. sweet	[s̠wit⁼]	[s˜wit¬]	[s˜w̥itʰ]

Study Questions

1. What is clinical phonetics? Outline the steps of the clinical process, as discussed in the text.

2. What is the difference between an articulation disorder and a phonological disorder?

3. Define the terms substitution, distortion, omission, and addition.

4. Which manners of articulation appear first in typically developing children? Which places of articulation appear first?

5. What are the differences between syllable structure processes, assimilatory processes, and substitution processes?

6. Describe the following phonological processes:

   a. stopping
   b. fronting
   c. deaffrication
   d. gliding
   e. vocalization

   f. weak syllable deletion
   g. cluster reduction
   h. final consonant deletion
   i. reduplication
   j. labial assimilation

   k. alveolar assimilation
   l. velar assimilation
   m. prevocalic voicing
   n. devoicing

7. Which of the processes in question 6 disappear by the age of 3;0 in typically developing children?

8. What is an idiosyncratic phonological process? Describe four such processes.

9. What is meant by the terms nasal emission and denasality?

10. Describe two different types of lisps.

11. When do the following stop consonant allophones generally occur in English?

    a. unreleased   b. aspirated   c. unaspirated

12. What is meant by the following terms?

    a. labialization   b. dentalization   c. velarization

13. What is the difference in the use of the symbols front [₊] and back [＿] versus advanced [₊] and retracted [₊]?

14. When would you use the diacritics for voicing and devoicing?

15. What is the extIPA? What is the VoQS? When would these diacritic sets be employed in transcription?

16. Of what importance is being able to perform a systematic allophonic transcription of a speech sample?

17. Describe several strategies you might employ when attempting to transcribe the speech patterns of a disordered client?

18. What would be the advantage of performing a phonological analysis versus an analysis of manner, place, and voicing?

19. What is the difference between an *independent* and a *relational* phonological analysis?

Assignment 7-1
Substitution Processes

Name _____

The productions of the following words all demonstrate one substitution process occurring. Indicate the phonemic alteration, describing the change in terms of place, manner, and/or voicing, and then label the process.

Example:

came → /teɪm/

<u> k → t </u>   <u>voiceless, velar stop → voiceless, alveolar stop</u>   <u> fronting </u>

1. catch → /kæʃ/

_____   _____   _____

2. dish → /dɪs/

_____   _____   _____

3. four → /pɔr/

_____   _____   _____

4. hurt → /hɔt/

_____   _____   _____

5. black→ /blæt/

_____   _____   _____

6. fairy → /fɛwɪ/

_____   _____   _____

7. seas → /tiz/

_____   _____   _____

8. fell → /fɛʊ/

_____   _____   _____

9. case → /teɪs/

_____   _____   _____

10. love → /jʌv/

_____   _____   _____

11. those → /doʊz/

_____   _____   _____

12. jam → /ʒæm/

_____   _____   _____

Assignment 7-2
Assimilation Processes

Name _____

The productions of the following words all demonstrate one assimilation process occurring. Indicate the phonemic alteration, describe the change, and then label the process.

Example:

bag → /bæk/

<u>g → k</u>   voiced, velar stop → voiceless velar stop   <u>devoicing</u>

1. bounce → /daʊns/

_____   _____   _____

2. ship → /pɪp/

_____   _____   _____

3. press → /brɛs/

_____   _____   _____

4. grade → /greɪg/

_____   _____   _____

5. moon→ /nun/

_____   _____   _____

6. crab → /kræp/

_____   _____   _____

7. bean → /bim/

_____   _____   _____

8. pink → /kɪŋk/

_____   _____   _____

9. dad → /dæt/

_____   _____   _____

10. kind → /taɪnd/

_____   _____   _____

11. set → /zɛt/

_____   _____   _____

12. choose → /ʧus/

_____   _____   _____

Assignment 7-3

Name _____

1. Match the transcriptions with the process being demonstrated. Each item has only one correct answer.

a. lake	→ /jeɪk/	a. fronting
b. with	→ /wɪt/	b. stopping
c. very	→ /bɛrɪ/	c. deaffrication
d. camp	→ /tæmp/	d. prevocalic voicing
e. chews	→ /ʃuz/	e. gliding
f. tree	→ /dri/	
g. pitch	→ /pɪʃ/	
h. dish	→ /dɪs/	
i. through	→ /tru/	
j. shop	→ /ʒɑp/	
k. dropped	→ /dwɑpt/	
l. song	→ /sɑn/	

2. Match the transcriptions with the process being demonstrated. Each item has only one correct answer.

____ a. tickle	→ /kɪkl̩/	a. labial assimilation
____ b. feed	→ /fit/	b. alveolar assimilation
____ c. drop	→ /drɑt/	c. velar assimilation
____ d. bath	→ /bæf/	d. prevocalic voicing
____ e. box	→ /gɔks/	e. devoicing
____ f. pad	→ /pæb/	
____ g. case	→ /teɪs/	
____ h. corn	→ /kɔrŋ/	
____ i. was	→ /wʌs/	
____ j. camp	→ /pæmp/	
____ k. bring	→ /grɪŋ/	
____ l. share	→ /ʒɛr/	

3. For each of the following words, apply the phonological process given and transcribe the resulting production.

Example:

lean	final consonant deletion	/li/
a. cost	prevocalic voicing	_____
b. flag	final consonant deletion	_____
c. tacky	velar assimilation	_____
d. park	cluster reduction	_____
e. wish	fronting	_____
f. than	alveolar assimilation	_____
g. glued	gliding	_____
h. cage	devoicing	_____
i. other	stopping	_____

Assignment 7-3 (cont.)

Name _____

j. chocolate   weak syllable deletion   _____

k. badge   deaffrication   _____

l. tough   labial assimilation   _____

4. Circle the transcriptions that could be examples of the process given.

    a. fronting

       leash → /lis/   pack → /pæt/

       door → /tɔr/   juice → /zus/

    b. cluster reduction

       string → /rɪŋ/   lather → /læɾɚ/

       match → /mæs/   from → /rʌm/

    c. labial assimilation

       pig → /bɪg/   drink → /brɪŋk/

       money → /mʌmɪ/   cave → /peɪv/

    d. final consonant deletion

       obey → /ou/   cash → /kæs/

       nest → /nɛs/   both → /boʊt/

    e. velar assimilation

       bingo → /gɪŋgoʊ/   knee → /nik/

       singer → /nɪŋɚ/   class → /glæs/

    f. stopping

       puss → /pʊt/   math → /mæt/

       Vicki →/bɪkɪ/   badge → /bæd/

    g. gliding

       trust → /twʌst/   fly → /fwaɪ/

       turn → /tʊn/   lip → /jɪp/

    h. deaffrication

       Roger → /rɑʒɚ/   catch → /kæʃ/

       sheep → /sip/   measure → /mɛzɚ/

    i. alveolar assimilation

       make → /neɪk/   then → /zɛn/

       bunny → /dʌnɪ/   sand → /tænd/

    j. vocalization

       like → /lɔk/   rain → /weɪn/

       tire → /taɪoʊ/   here → /hɪʊ/

Assignment 7-4

Name _____

Transcribe the following sentences, as spoken by a 7-year-old female child. This child demonstrates both gliding and vocaliation.

1. I put my right shoe on my left foot.

   _____

2. She'll have to wear a raincoat.

   _____

3. There was a hole in the roof.

   _____

4. My Grandma likes roses.

   _____

5. His sandwich fell apart.

   _____

6. I can't decide which I like best.

   _____

7. He pushed us on the merry-go-round.

   _____

8. Shannon was sick of school.

   _____

9. Grandpa fell asleep on the couch.

   _____

10. Jasmine hopes it'll stop raining soon.

    _____

11. My shirt is in the washing machine.

    _____

12. I had a seashell for show 'n' tell.

    _____

Assignment 7-5

Name _____

Transcribe the following utterances, as spoken by a 4-year-old male child. This child demonstrates the idiosyncratic processes of initial consonant deletion and glottal insertion.

1. black _____
2. pink _____
3. red _____
4. yellow _____
5. orange _____
6. white _____
7. blue _____
8. green _____
9. apple _____

10. pear _____
11. green beans _____
12. berries _____
13. icing _____
14. cheese _____
15. hotdog _____
16. cocoon _____
17. magic _____
18. caterpillar _____

19. What is these?
20. big tree and lake
21. See worm eat big leaf.
22. Me see egg right there.
23. Worm no hungry no more.
24. We have that movie.
25. I like long necks . . . him . . . er . . .
    Joshua likes sharp tooths.

26. Do you color dinosaurs with me?

_____
_____
_____
_____
_____
_____
_____
_____
_____

Assignment 7-6

Name _____

1. For each of the following phonemes, provide two allophones. Then transcribe two words in which those allophones may be found.

   Example:

   /p/   i) [pʰ]   push [pʰʊʃ]   ii) [p⁼]   spin [sp⁼ɪn]

   a. /l/   i)   ii)

   b. /t/   i)   ii)

   c. /k/   i)   ii)

   d. /d/   i)   ii)

   e. /r/   i)   ii)

   f. /g/   i)   ii)

   g. /z/   i)   ii)

2. Transcribe each of the following words using the devoicing diacritic [̥].

   a. pew   ____   f. raise   ____

   b. leave   ____   g. fuse   ____

   c. plaque   ____   h. queen   ____

   d. phase   ____   i. live   ____

   e. crazy   ____   j. sweet   ____

3. Transcribe each of the following words using the diacritics for aspirated [ʰ] and for unaspirated [⁼] where necessary.

   a. spank   ____   f. camera   ____

   b. treasure ____   g. table   ____

   c. skewed   ____   h. stared   ____

   d. peeked   ____   i. supposed   ____

   e. clueless ____   j. retain   ____

4. Transcribe the following words using the diacritics for dental [̪] and labiodental [ɱ] articulations, where necessary.

   a. nineteenth ____   f. breadth   ____

   b. emphatic   ____   g. although   ____

   c. enfold   ____   h. emphysema ____

   d. infrared   ____   i. healthier ____

   e. enthused   ____   j. inference ____

Assignment 7-7

Name _____

1. Explain the difference between the following allophones:

   Example:

   ε/ε̃   non-nasalized (oral) /ε/ versus nasalized /ε/

   a. z/z̠
   b. pʰ/p⁼
   c. l/ɫ
   d. ŋ/ŋ̃
   e. d̪/d̠
   f. ɑ/q̣
   g. t/t̬
   h. u/uː
   i. s/s̯
   j. ŋ/m̩
   k. r/r̃

2. Indicate for each of the following whether the diacritic is used correctly by placing an "X" in the proper blank. If the diacritic is incorrect, explain the error.

a. plain	[plẽɪn]	____ correct	____ incorrect
b. licked	[lɪkt]	____ correct	____ incorrect
c. freed	[friːd]	____ correct	____ incorrect
d. spread	[sp⁼rɛd]	____ correct	____ incorrect
e. plaid	[plæd̪]	____ correct	____ incorrect
f. hark	[hɑrkʰ]	____ correct	____ incorrect
g. practice	[præk̚tɪs]	____ correct	____ incorrect
h. swirl	[s̃wɝl]	____ correct	____ incorrect
i. spry	[s̠pry]	____ correct	____ incorrect
j. clasp	[k̠læsp]	____ correct	____ incorrect

8

Dialectal Variation

A s college freshmen, many of you moved away from home for the first time. Once you arrived at college, you immediately found yourself thrust into new surroundings. You became a little fish in a big pond, the pond being comprised of people from various regions of the country. You also had the opportunity to meet people with quite varied social and cultural backgrounds. For the first time in your life, you may have realized the marked variation in the speech and language patterns of people with backgrounds different from your own. The variations in the speech patterns of your new college acquaintances may have been subtle, in the form of a slight "accent." Or perhaps the differences were not so subtle, reflecting a difference in grammatical patterns, vocabulary, and even heavier accents. Prior to this time, the primary speech and language patterns to which you were exposed were probably those of your family and friends and from the newscasters you heard on the radio or saw on TV. You may have been exposed to some stereotypical dialectal patterns only while watching TV, such as a "hick" farmhand or a "fast-talking" person from New York City.

Although you may have never thought about it before, the English spoken in the United States is quite variable in terms of syntax (grammatical rules), vocabulary, and phonology. These variations in speech and language are called **dialects**. Even though you probably do not realize it, everyone speaks with a dialect of some form. The dialect you use in your daily life is the product of the region of the United States in which you grew up, your cultural background, and also the social class to which you belong. Social class in this sense refers to type of occupation (white collar, blue collar, etc.), as well as income level, level of education, and in which part of town you grew up. Factors such as age and gender also play important roles in determining the English patterns you will use on a day-to-day basis. In addition, as a speaker of a language you also possess an individual, idiosyncratic speech pattern, characteristic of your personality. Each person's individual, idiosyncratic speech pattern is referred to as an **idiolect**.

Suppose you grew up in Cleveland and had to travel to Boston on business. You would immediately notice a sizable variation in the pronunciation patterns of the natives of Massachusetts. You would probably consider the native speakers to have an accent. This judgment would be made using your own, learned speaking habits as an internal yardstick or standard. Consider the fact that Boston natives would find your speech to have just as much of an accent as you do theirs. In fact, each of us probably considers our own usage of English as the standard. This raises an interesting question, "Is there a standard form of American English?"

Standard American English (SAE) is a form of English that is relatively devoid of regional characteristics (Wolfram, 1991). In a written form, SAE is the English of dictionaries, grammar books, and most printed matter. In spoken form, the standard is observed most often in the speech of the national network newscasters who, for the most part, have no regional "accents." SAE is the idealized form often adopted when teaching English as a second language to foreign learners. An individual learning English as a second language is considered to be a nonstandard speaker of English because his or her dialect varies from Standard English. Regional and social dialects are sometimes considered to be nonstandard forms of English. In this sense, the term *nonstandard* should not be considered deviant or wrong. It is simply a term used to denote a variation of Standard English.

Is Standard English actually achieved by speakers of American English? This is a difficult question to answer. Virtually every speaker of American English belongs to a dialect group defined by region, culture, or social class. For this reason, it is better to think of American English as having regional standards of pronunciation as opposed to one national standard of pronunciation.

EXERCISE 8.1

Which regional, social, and cultural factors have influenced the particular dialect of English you speak? Do you have any particular idiosyncratic speech patterns that contribute to your idiolect?

Recall that a dialect is a variety of speech or language based on one of several factors, including geographical area or social class. These two factors are typically used in categorizing the various dialects in the United States. Regional dialects are those that are defined by geographical boundaries. Social dialects are defined by membership in a particular social class or cultural group. Both classifications of dialects will be discussed in the following sections. Because this is a phonetics book, the focus will be on the phonological aspects of dialect, commonly referred to as a person's "accent." Differences in dialects related to syntax and vocabulary will not be covered in this text.

As speech and hearing professionals, often you will be evaluating the speech and language capabilities of individuals from various regional, social, and cultural backgrounds. You will need to determine whether these individuals have a handicapping communicative problem, regardless of the particular dialect of English that they have acquired. It is important to realize that dialects of Standard English should *not* be thought of as substandard versions of our language. That is, dialects should not be thought of as "wrong," or in need of remediation. Instead, regional and social dialects should be considered strictly as a variety of Standard English that reflects an individual's social class or the region in which he or she grew up. In fact, dialects should be thought of as a communication difference, as opposed to a communication disorder, the difference being the variation in phonological rules, vocabulary, and syntax of any particular dialect.

In 2003, the American Speech-Language-Hearing Association (ASHA) published a technical report entitled "American English Dialects." This report promotes the idea that "no dialectal variety of American English is a disorder or a pathological form of speech or language" (ASHA, 2003). According to ASHA:

> Each dialect is adequate as a functional and effective variety of American English. Each serves a communication function as well as a social solidarity function. Each dialect maintains the communication network and the social construct of the community of speakers who use it. Furthermore, each is a symbolic representation of the geographic, historical, social, and cultural background of its speakers. (p. 45)

In some instances, speech-language pathologists are asked to assist non-standard English speakers in becoming more easily understood, that is, more intelligible, to the mainstream, Standard English-speaking population. This state of affairs has become increasingly more common with individuals who are learning English as a second language. In this case, speech-language pathologists provide an elective service known as **accent reduction**. The focus of these sessions is simply to help nonstandard speakers of English reduce their accents to be more intelligible. Accent reduction programs are becoming increasingly more common in university settings as the number of foreign instructors in the classroom increases. In fact, in Ohio, state law requires that all university teaching assistants must be proficient in the use of the English language. Therefore, mandatory accent reduction programs are in effect in many of the university speech and hearing clinics for individuals who are limited in their proficiency of English. Keep in mind that the focus of an elective accent reduction program for any nonstandard English speaker "is to assist in the acquisition of the desired competency in the second dialect without jeopardizing the integrity of the individual's first dialect" (ASHA, 2003, p. 46).

Regional Dialects

Several classification schemes have been used by researchers in an attempt to describe and categorize regional dialects in the United States. The regional use of certain vocabulary items have been studied to help define dialectal regions. For instance, in the eastern United States, many people refer to carbonated beverages as "soda," whereas people from the Midwest generally use the term "pop," and some people from the South use the term "coke." Likewise, the terms "pail" and "bucket" and "faucet" and "spigot" are used contrastively, depending on where a person lives. When using vocabulary items to demarcate regional dialects, research has shown conflicting evidence as to the actual number of dialectal regions present in the United States (Carver, 1987; Kurath, 1949). Some research indicates that the United States can be divided into three separate dialectal regions—North, Midland, and South (Kurath, 1949). Another approach divides the United States into two general dialect regions, North and South (Carver, 1987). Each of these regions is further divided into layers, in a hierarchical arrangement. The North dialect region is divided into three layers: Upper North (including New England), Lower North, and the West. The South dialect region has two layers: Upper South and Lower South.

Another approach to defining dialectal regions in the United States is to examine the phonological patterns of English speakers. The linguistics laboratory at the University of Pennsylvania has conducted extensive telephone surveys of over 600 speakers to determine how vowel pronunciation differs across the United States. This investigation, the Telsur Project, systematically examined speakers from 145 urban centers with populations greater than 200,000. These urban centers account for 54 percent of the total United States population (Labov, Ash, & Boberg, 1997). The purpose of this investigation was (1) to identify the major dialectal regions in the U.S. using phonological data instead of vocabulary data, and (2) to determine the specific pronunciation patterns that are found in each of the dialect regions.

Results of the Telsur surveys confirmed the well-known fact that vowel articulation in the United States is not static; the place of articulation of American English vowels is in an active state of change. The changes in place of vowel articulation can be categorized as *chain shifts* and *mergers* (Labov et al., 1997).

A **chain shift** occurs when the place of articulation of one vowel changes, causing the surrounding vowels in the quadrilateral to likewise shift in production. This causes a "chain reaction" in relation to the place of articulation for other vowels. Because chain shifting affects the production of several vowels at the same time, the articulation of a single vowel is not independent of the articulation of other vowels. Instead, vowel articulation is relative; place of articulation of one vowel is determined by the place of production of other vowels. A **vowel merger** occurs when vowels with separate articulations fuse into one similar place of articulation. For example, in many regions in the United States, the vowels /ɑ/ and /ɔ/ have merged so that their production is the same—that is, /ɑ/.

The Telsur project has helped to demarcate three identifiable dialectal regions based on the chain shift and merger phonological data: (1) Inland North, (2) South, and (3) West (Labov, 1991; Labov et al., 1997). Each of these regions will be discussed along with the major pronunciation patterns that help to define that region.

The Inland North

The Inland North is composed of many large urban centers around the Great Lakes as well as in upper New York state (Labov et al., 1997). In cities such as Buffalo, Detroit, Chicago, and Cleveland, people have begun to demonstrate a shift in the place of articulation of the vowel /æ/ so that it is produced higher and more forward in the mouth. This shift causes /ɑ/ to be produced more forward in the mouth (becoming more like /æ/), so that the word "hot" /hɑt/ would be produced as /hæt/. Due to chain shifting, the vowel /ɔ/ is then produced lower in the mouth so that "caught" /kɔt/ would be produced more like /kɑt/.

Chain shifting affects the articulation of the six vowels, /ɔ, ɑ, æ, ɪ, ɛ, and ʌ/, in what is known as the **Northern Cities Shift**. The Northern Cities Shift occurs in western New England, New York state, and the northern parts of Pennsylvania, Ohio, Indiana, Illinois, Michigan, and Wisconsin (Labov, 1991). The shift reflects a forward and/or raised production of the vowels /ɑ and æ/, and a backward and/or lowered production of the vowels /ɔ, ɪ, ɛ, and ʌ/. The shift occurs in a clockwise rotation so that the front-back articulation of /ɑ/ and /ɛ/ becomes quite similar; they both are produced more centrally in the oral cavity. The Northern Cities Shift can be better understood by examining the arrows in the quadrilateral in Figure 8.1.

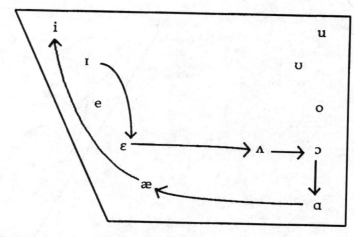

FIGURE 8.1 Vowel quadrilateral of the northern cities shift (after Labov et al., 1997).

EXERCISE 8.2

Transcribe the following words, first in your own dialect, and then as they would be pronounced using the Northern Cities Shift dialect. Use the appropriate diacritics to indicate raising [⊥], lowering [⊤], advancement [₊], or retraction [₊] of the tongue. Refer to Figure 8.1 for your answers.

Examples:

hug	/hʌg/	[hʌg]
red	/rɛd/	[rɛd]

1. lid
2. when
3. rub
4. caught
5. left

The South

The southern dialect region is defined geographically by the Southern, Middle Atlantic, and Southern Mountain states (Labov, 1991). A chain shift known as the **Southern Shift** affects the six vowels /i, ɪ, e, ɛ, u, and o/, and reflects a forward and/or raised production of the vowels /u, o, ɛ, and ɪ/ and a lowered production of the vowels /i and e/. Also, the diphthong /aɪ/ is produced farther forward. The pattern of the Southern Shift is illustrated in Figure 8.2.

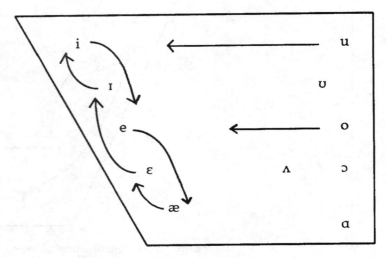

FIGURE 8.2 Vowel quadrilateral of the Southern Shift (after Labov et al., 1997).

EXERCISE 8.3

Use the appropriate diacritical marking for raising, lowering, or fronting to indicate the appropriate transcription as predicted by the Southern Shift. Refer to Figure 8.2 for your answers.

Example:

red   [rɛ̝d]   food   [fʉd]

1. may   _____   _____
2. lick   _____   _____
3. bone   _____   _____
4. like   _____   _____
5. weed   _____   _____

The West

A third and somewhat different pattern of vowel articulation is currently being observed throughout various regions of the United States. This is known as the **Low Back Merger** (Labov, 1991). This change in pronunciation involves the merger of the low, back vowels /ɑ/ and /ɔ/. Speakers who merge these vowels show no phonemic contrast between them during the production of words. For instance, a speaker who merges these vowels would pronounce the names "Dawn" and "Don" the same—that is, /dɑn/. This merger occurs in a large section of the western United States as well as in eastern New England, southern Ohio, Pennsylvania (in the Pittsburgh area), northern Minnesota, and Wisconsin (Labov et al., 1997).

EXERCISE 8.4

Transcribe the following word pairs as you would pronounce them. Do you produce both /ɑ/ and /ɔ/ in your dialect of English? Or do you use the vowels /a/ or /ɒ/ (the rounded version of /ɑ/) in transcription of these words?

1. Lon   _____   lawn   _____
2. clod   _____   Claude   _____
3. caught   _____   cot   _____
4. taught   _____   tot   _____

Traditionally, phonetics books have described three major regional dialects specific to the United States. These regional dialects include: (1) Southern American English, (2) Eastern American English, and (3) General American English (Edwards, 1992; Gray & Wise, 1959; Wise, 1957). Interestingly, these dialectal regions correspond quite closely with the three dialectal regions based on vowel production described in the previous section.

In this text, the discussion on regional dialect will focus primarily on the Southern and Eastern American English dialects. However, a word needs to be said concerning the term *General American English*. General American English traditionally has been used as a term to describe the dialect spoken in areas of the country other than the East or the South. As such, the term General American English is equated with the speech patterns of most of the western United States as well as most of the country east of the Mississippi and north of the Ohio River, not including the East Coast (Hartman, 1985). Because regional dialects do exist in the North and in the western half of the United States, the term General American English is not an accurate term in describing the speaking patterns of so many Americans. The term General American English has also been used to designate a "standard" dialect that lacks any "regional" pronunciation, such as that associated with the South or the East. In this manner, the use of the term is synonymous with the term Standard American English.

In the following discussion on regional dialects, several geographic labels will be adopted to refer to specific regions of the country such as South, South Midland, New England, and Northeast. These labels and the states to which they refer are listed in Table 8.1 (adapted from Cassidy, 1985).

Southern American English

One of the most highly recognized regional dialects in the United States is **Southern American English**. This is the dialect of English spoken primarily in the southern and South Midland states including all or part of Alabama, Arkansas, Delaware, Florida, Georgia, Kentucky, Louisiana, Maryland, Mississippi, Missouri, North Carolina, South Carolina, Tennessee, Texas, Virginia, and West Virginia (see Table 8.1). Although Southern American English varies from Standard English primarily in terms of vowel and diphthong articulation, consonant production is affected as well. Keep in mind that not all speakers from the South speak the same; there are also regional variations of the Southern American English. However, there are some general characteristics of southern speech that are fairly typical across the southern United States. All of these characteristics would

TABLE 8.1   Geographic Labels for Selected Dialectal Areas in the Greater United States

Geographic Label	State Abbreviations
Appalachians	neAL, nGA, eKY, wMD, wNC, cPA, wSC, eTN, wVA, WV
Atlantic	CT, DC, DE, FL, GA, MA, MD, ME, NC, NH, NJ, NY, PA, RI, SC, VA, VT
Great Lakes	nIL, nIN, MI, MN, nwNY, nOH, nwPA
Middle Atlantic	MD, NC, SC, VA
New England	CT, MA, ME, NH, RI, VT
Northeast	New England states, NJ, NY, nPA
Pacific	CA, OR, WA
South Midland	nAL, AR, nGA, sIL, sIN, KY, nLA, nMD, c&sMO, nMS, wNC, sOH, neOK, wSC, wVZ, sWV
South	c&s AL, sDE, FL, c&s GA, c&s LA, e&s MD, c&s MS, c&e NC, c&e SC, eTX, eVA
Southwest	AZ, sCA, NM, OK, TX
West	wND, wSD, wNE, wKS, wOK, wTX, and all points west

Key: e = east; n = north, s = south; w = west, c = central; ne = northeast; nw = northwest
Source: Cassidy, 1985.

not necessarily apply to the same speaker. Likewise, each speaker of Southern American English would vary in the number of words that would demonstrate the dialect. Only some of the more common features of Southern American English are explained below. They are also summarized in Table 8.2.

Front Vowel Production

Variation in Production of /i/ and /ɪ/

- When /ɪ/ occurs before the palatal fricative /ʃ/, it may become tensed, and produced as /i/, as in the words "fish" and "dish." For example:

  fish → /fiʃ/   dish → /diʃ/

  This articulation is seen most often in the South Midland region and also from Delaware and Maryland westward into northwest Missouri (Hartman, 1985).

- In the southern United States, when /i/ precedes /l/, it may become lax and be produced as /ɪ/. For example:

  really → /rɪlɪ/   feel → /fɪl/   meal → /mɪl/

- /ɪ/ tends to occur in unstressed final syllables of words (as opposed to /ə/) as in the words "florist" → /flɔrɪst/ and "pigeon" → /pɪʤɪn/. This use of the vowel /ɪ/ occurs in much of the southern United States (Hartman, 1985.) Other examples include:

TABLE 8.2 Common Features of Southern American English

English Word	Southern English Transcription	Phonological Pattern
fish	/fiʃ/	ɪ → i
really	/rɪlɪ/	i → ɪ
chemist	/kɛmɪst/	use of /ɪ/ in unstressed syllable
pen	/pɪn/	ɛ → ɪ
egg	/eɪg/	ɛ → eɪ
mesh	/meɪʃ/	ɛ → eɪ
Larry	/lærɪ/	ɛ → æ
push	/puʃ/	ʊ → u
result	/rəzʊlt	ʌ → ʊ
two	/tju/	epenthesis of /j/
bought	/bɔt/	use of /ɔ/
Florida	/flɑrɪdə/	ɔ → ɑ
worry	/wʌrɪ/	ɝ → ʌr
terse	/tɜːs/	ɝ → ɜː
fire	/far/	diphthong simplification
winning	/wɪnən/	ŋ → n
here	/hɪə/	r deletion
course	/kɔs, kɔəs, koəs/	r deletion
car	/kɑː/	r deletion

Source: Adapted from Cassidy, 1985; Gray & Wise, 1959; Hartman, 1985; Wise, 1957.

chemist → /kɛmɪst/	waited → /weɪɾɪd/
lettuce → /lɛɾɪs/	granite → /grænɪt/
hopeless → /houplɪs/	forfeit → /fɔrfɪt/

Variation in Production of /ɛ/

- The vowel /ɛ/ may be raised and therefore articulated as /ɪ/ when it precedes the nasal /n/, as in "pen" and "cents." In the context of the nasal /n/, the vowels /ɪ/ and /ɛ/ tend to merge for many speakers, so that the two vowels become indistinguishable in production. Examples include:

pen → /pɪn/	sense → /sɪns/
pin → /pɪn/	since → /sɪns/

- In the South Midland, and in parts of the Southwest, the vowel /ɛ/ is raised to /eɪ/ when it precedes /g/ (Hartman, 1985). Examples include:

egg → /eɪg/	leg → /leɪg/	keg → /keɪg/

- /ɛ/ may be raised to /eɪ/ when it precedes the palatal fricatives /ʃ/ and /ʒ/. Examples include:

mesh → /meɪʃ/	treasure → /treɪʒɚ/

- In words that contain the letter sequence "_arry," /ɛ/ may be lowered to /æ/. Examples include:

  Larry → /lærɪ/   marry → /mærɪ/   carry → /kærɪ/

Back Vowel Production

Variation in Production of /ʊ/ and /u/

- /ʊ/ is sometimes tensed and produced as /u/ when it precedes the fricative /ʃ/. This variation of /ʊ/ occurs in the South Midland states (Hartman, 1985). Examples include:

  push → /puʃ/   bush → /buʃ/

- /j/ is sometimes inserted prior to production of the vowel /u/, when following the alveolar consonants /t/, /d/, or /n/. This epenthesis is evidenced most often from Delaware and Maryland southward into Florida and westward into Arkansas and eastern Texas (Hartman, 1985). For example:

  two → /tju/   new → /nju/   due → /dju/

Variation in Production of / ɔ /

- In the South, it is common for /ɔ/ to be used in pronunciation of words that contain the following allographs: "all," "aul," "aw," "ough," "og," "ong," "on," and "augh" (Hartman, 1985; Wise, 1957).

call	→ /kɔl/	haul	→ /hɔl/
caw	→ /kɔ/	fall	→ /fɔl/
bought	→ /bɔt/	log	→ /lɔg/
long	→ /lɔŋ/	gone	→ /gɔn/
wrong	→ /rɔŋ/	caught	→ /kɔt/

- /ɔ/ may be lowered to /ɑ/ in words with the rhotic diphthong /ɔr/, (represented by the allographs "orr," "or," "ar," and "arr"). Examples include:

Florida → /flɑrɪdə/	warrant → /wɑrɪnt/
forest → /fɑrɪst/	quarrel → /kwɑrl̩/
orange → /ɑrɪnʤ/	quarantine → /kwɑrɪntin/
horrible → /hɑrɪbl̩/	

Central Vowel Production

Variation in Production of /ʌ/ and /ɝ/

- In stressed syllables containing the grapheme sequence "ul," /ʊ/ is often produced. This articulation is most common in the South Midland states (Hartman, 1985). For example:

  result → /rɪzʊlt/   bulk → /bʊlk/

- /ʌ/ (plus consonantal /r/) is sometimes produced instead of /ɝ/ in words spelled "orr" or "urr," such as:

  worry → /wʌrɪ/   furry → /fʌrɪ/   hurry → /hʌrɪ/

- The central vowel /ɜ/ may be produced among southern speakers who delete postvocalic /r/ from their speech. This vowel is the nonrhotacized partner of the vowel /ɝ/. /ɜ/ is produced similarly to /ɝ/ in terms of place of articulation. The main difference in production is the lack of rhotacization, which results in the vowel being produced as an "r-less" vowel. To produce /ɜ/, try saying the word "girl" without the "r," that is, producing the /ɝ/ vowel without an "r" quality. When /ɜ/ is produced, it tends to be lengthened. Examples include:

  terse → [tɜːs]   word → [wɜːd]   earth → [ɜːθ]

Diphthong Production

Diphthong Simplification

- In the South Midland states, the diphthong /aɪ/ often is produced as the low central monophthong /a/, as in the words "fire," "tire," "child," and "mild" (Hartman, 1985). For example,

  fire   → /far/   tire   → /tar/
  child → /tʃald/   mild → /mald/

- The diphthong /ɔɪ/ also becomes a monophthong in parts of the South, so that it is produced as /ɔ/ (before /l/), as in the words "boil" and "oil." Note that the production of the vowel /ɔ/ also becomes lengthened.

  foil → [fɔːl]   oil → [ɔːl]

Consonant Production

Variation in Production of /ŋ/

- In words ending with "ing," /ŋ/ is sometimes fronted and produced as the alveolar nasal /n/, as in:

  "winning" → /wɪnɪn/   "skipping" → /skɪpən/

Variation in Production of /r/

One of the most common speech traits of many southern speakers is the varied use of the consonant /r/ and the rhotic vowels /ɝ/ and /ɚ/. In word-final and postvocalic positions, /r/ (or /ɚ/) are often deleted, especially in parts of Virginia and in coastal South Carolina and Georgia (Hartman, 1985). One example of the deleted /r/ is the use of the non-retroflexed vowel /ɜ/ already discussed.

- In words that contain the r-colored vowels, /ɪr/, /ɛr/, and /ʊr/, /r/ may become de-rhotacized and produced as schwa. For example:

  beer → /bɪə/   hair → /hɛə/   sure → /ʃʊə/

The r-colored vowel /ɔr/ has variable regional pronunciations in southern speech (Hartman, 1985; Wise, 1957). For instance the word "Ford" may be pronounced as /fɔd/, /fɔəd/, or /foəd/. Both /fɔəd/ or /foəd/ are produced as diphthongs. Other examples include:

course → /kɔs/, /kɔəs/, /koəs/
more → /mɔ/, /mɔə/, /moə/
door → /dɔ/, /dɔə/, /doə/

In syllables containing /ɑr/, the /r/ is deleted and the vowel /ɑ/ is lengthened. /ə/ is not produced, as with the other r-colored vowels. For instance:

car   → [kɑ:] (note the lengthened vowel)
farmer → [fɑ:mə]
marlin → [mɑ:lɪn]
armor → [ɑ:mə]

- /ə/ is often produced at the end of unstressed syllables, as in the words "later" → /leɪɾə/ and "rumor" → /rumə/. Other examples include:

other → /ʌðə/	razor → /reɪzə/	martyr → /mɑ:ɾə/
tire → /taɪə/	flour → /flaʊə/	

EXERCISE 8.5

Determine the phonological pattern for each of Southern American English pronunciations given below. Write your answer in the blank.

Example:

running	/rʌnɪn/	ŋ → n
1. curry	/kʌrɪ/	
2. Warren	/wɑrɪn/	
3. tear (noun)	/tɪə/	
4. bar	/bɑ:/	
5. trial	/tral/	
6. spoiled	/spɔ:ld/	
7. concern	/kənsɜ:n/	
8. cushion	/kuʃɪn/	
9. precious	/preɪʃɪs/	
10. floor	/flɔə/	

Eastern American English

What is commonly recognized as **Eastern American English** is spoken predominantly by individuals in the New England states and by people from parts of New York, New Jersey, and Pennsylvania. The dialectal patterns that will be introduced in the following section are speech patterns observed among several of the Eastern regional dialects. For instance, individuals in Boston may exhibit quite distinct articulation patterns when compared to individuals from other cities in Massachusetts and from other cities in New England. Similarly, some individuals in New York City often have a distinct dialectal pattern. Due to the varied nature of "Eastern" regional dialects, only the more commonly shared dialectal patterns will be discussed below. Keep in mind that any one speaker of Eastern American English dialect will not demonstrate all of the examples given. A summary of the major characteristics of Eastern American dialect is displayed in Table 8.3.

Front Vowel Production

Variation in Production of /ɛ/

- The front vowel /æ/ may sometimes (but not always) be produced in words with allographs of the phoneme sequence /ɛr/, that is, "air," "ar," "arr," and "ear." Examples include:

bear	→ /bɛr/ or /bær/	carry	→ /kɛrɪ/ or /kærɪ/
flair	→ /flɛr/ or /flær/	sparrow	→/spɛroʊ/ or /spæroʊ/
parents	→ /pɛrənts/ or /pærənts/		

TABLE 8.3 Features of Eastern American Dialect

English Word	Eastern English Transcription	Phonological Pattern
sparrow	/spæroʊ/	ɛ → æ
half	/haf/	æ → ɑ
stop	/stɒp/	ɑ → ɒ
Florida	/flɑrɪdə/ or /flɒrɪdə/	ɔ → ɑ or ɒ
taught	/tɔt/ or /tɒt/ (or /tɑt/)	ɑ → ɔ or ɒ
new	/nju/	epenthesis of /j/
room	/rʊm/	u → ʊ
hurry	/hʌrɪ/	ɝ → ʌr
third	/θɜːd/	ɝ → ɜː
here	/hɪə/	/r/ deletion
chord	/kɔd/, /kɔəd/, /koəd/	/r/ deletion
car	/kɑː/	/r/ deletion
Linda	/lɪndɚ/	epenthesis of /r/

Source: Adapted from Gray & Wise, 1959; Hartman, 1985; Wise, 1957.

Variation in Production of /æ/

- In New England and on the Atlantic Coast, some speakers may produce the back vowel /ɑ/ before the fricatives /f, v, s, θ, and ð/ and before the nasal phoneme /n/ (Wise, 1957). Examples include:

half → /hæf/ or /hɑf/	rather → /ræðə/ or /rɑðə/
dance → /dæns/ or /dɑns/	path → /pæθ/ or /pɑθ/
aunt → /ænt/ or /ɑnt/	pass → /pæs/ or /pɑs/

- The low central vowel /a/ is used by some speakers in the New England states in the same phonetic contexts presented directly above, that is:

half → /haf/	rather → /raðə/
dance → /dans/	path → /paθ/
aunt → /ant/	pass → /pas/

Back Vowel Production

Variation in Production of /u/

- When /u/ follows the alveolar consonants /t/, /d/, or /n/, /j/ is sometimes added prior to the vowel (as seen in some Southern American English dialects). In addition, this articulation is seen in speakers from San Francisco and Hawaii (Hartman, 1985). For example:

two → /tju/	new → /nju/	due → /dju/

- In the Northeast, and to a lesser extent in the Great Lakes region, either of the high, back vowels /u/ or /ʊ/ may be produced in the phonetic context represented by /u/ (Hartman, 1985). For example:

room → /rum/ or /rʊm/	roof → /ruf/ or /rʊf/
hoof → /huf/ or /hʊf/	

Variation in Production of /ɑ/

- In eastern New England as well as in western Pennsylvania and parts of Ohio, words pronounced with the phoneme /ɑ/ also may be pronounced with the rounded back phoneme /ɒ/ (Hartman, 1985). To produce this phoneme, prolong a production of /ɑ/ (its unrounded counterpart). As you produce the phoneme, round your lips. You now should be producing /ɒ/. Examples include:

stop → /stɑp/ or /stɒp/	trot → /trɑt/ or /trɒt/
father → /fɑðə/ or /fɒðə/	bottle → /bɑɾl̩/ or /bɒɾl̩/

Variation in Production of /ɔ/

- In the East, it is common for /ɔ/ to be used in pronunciation of words that contain the following allographs: "all," "aul," "aw," "ough," "og," "ong," "on," and "augh" (Hartman, 1985; Wise, 1957).

call	→ /kɔl/	haul	→ /hɔl/
caw	→ /kɔ/	fall	→ /fɔl/
bought	→ /bɔt/	slaughter	→ /slɔrə/
long	→ /lɔŋ/	gone	→ /gɔn/

- Some speakers in the East will use the vowels /ɑ/ or /ɒ/ in production of words that contain the phoneme sequence /ɔr/ or /wɔr/ plus a vowel (Wise, 1957). Examples include:

Florida → /flɔrɪdə/ or /flɑrɪdə/ or /flɒrɪdə/
orange → /ɔrɪndʒ/ or /ɑrɪndʒ/ or /ɒrɪndʒ/
warrant → /wɔrɪnt/ or /warənt/ or /wɒrɪnt/
quarry → /kwɔrɪ/ or /kwarɪ/ or /kwɒrɪ/

Central Vowel Production

Variation in Production of /ɝ/

- Stressed schwar /ɝ/ may be produced as /ʌ/ (plus /r/) in words in which /ɝ/ is followed by another vowel. Examples include "hurry" /hɝɪ/ → /hʌrɪ/ or "burrow" /bɝou/ → /bʌrou/. The words "hurry" and "burrow" may also be pronounced by some Eastern speakers as /hɜrɪ/ or /bɜrou/ (Wise, 1957). Additional examples include:

blurring → /blʌrɪŋ/ or /blɜrɪŋ/
thorough → /θʌrou/ or /θɜrou/
whirring → /wʌrɪŋ/ or /wɜrɪŋ/

Consonant Production

Variation in Production of /r/

- Postvocalic /r/ is deleted by speakers in eastern New England and in the New York City metropolitan area (Hartman, 1985). The loss of /r/ in the eastern United States follows a pattern quite like that seen in Southern American English dialect. For instance the nonrhotacized vowel /ɜ/ is produced in words such as "herd" /hɜːd/ and "wordy" /wɜːdɪ/. Similarly, /ə/ will often occur at the ends of words, in unstressed syllables, as in "faster" → /fastə/ and "better" → /bɛɾə/. Schwa /ə/ also occurs in the r-colored vowels /ɔr/, /ɪr/, /ɛr/, /ʊr/. Examples include:

cord → /kɔə/		chair → /tʃɛə/	
here → /hɪə/		lure → /lʊə/	

As in Southern American English, the r-colored vowel /ɔr/ has variable pronunciations in Eastern American dialect. For example, the word "sword" may be pronounced as /sɔd/, /sɔəd/, or /soəd/. In syllables containing /ɑr/ or /ar/, the /r/ is silent and the vowel /ɑ/ (or /a/) is lengthened accordingly. /ə/ is not pronounced as with the other r-colored vowels. For instance:

barn → [bɑːn] or [baːn]
harder → [hɑːdə] or [haːdə]
marlin → [mɑːlɪn] or [maːlɪn]
barter → [bɑːɾə] or [baːɾə]

- An interesting characteristic of some Northeastern speakers is the addition of the phoneme /ɚ/ in connected speech (rhotacization). This occurs when a word that ends with /ə/ is followed by a word beginning with a vowel. For example, "Cuba and America" would be pronounced as /kjubɚ n̩ əmɛrɪkə/. In addition, /ɚ/ may be found to occur in words normally ending in /ə/ or /ɔ/, as in "Linda" /lɪndɚ/, "soda" /soʊdɚ/, "idea" /aɪdiɚ/, and "saw" /sɔɚ/.

EXERCISE 8.6

Determine the phonological pattern for each of the Eastern American English pronunciations given below. Write your answer in the blank.

Example:

hair	/hɛə/	r → ə
1. slot	/slɒt/	
2. laugh	/lɑf/	
3. third	/θɜːd/	
4. ward	/wɔd/	
5. can't	/kɑnt/	
6. marry	/mærɪ/	
7. Maria	/mərɪɚ/	
8. choir	/kwaɪə/	
9. stirring	/stʌrɪŋ/	
10. darker	/dɑːkə/	

Social Dialects

In addition to the various regional dialects observed across the United States, American English also has several dialects based upon social class and cultural background. The predominant dialects in this category include African American Vernacular English (AAVE), Spanish-Influenced English, and Asian/Pacific-Influenced English. The development of AAVE, a dialect spoken by many African Americans in the United States, is directly related to the history of their migratory patterns from Africa to the southern United States, beginning in the 1600s. The development of Spanish- and Asian/Pacific-Influenced English is somewhat different. These dialects are a result of Spanish and Asian/Pacific individuals speaking English as a second language. Because Spanish, Asian, and Pacific languages often are comprised of phonemes vastly different from the phoneme set found in English, it is not surprising that speakers of other languages will markedly vary in their pronunciation of the English language.

African American Vernacular English

African American Vernacular English (AAVE) is a common dialect of English spoken in the United States. Not all African American people speak this dialect, nor is this dialect limited solely to African Americans. The term AAVE is the most recent term used to label this dialectal form of English. Previous labels applied by linguists and, speech-language pathologists for this dialect have included *ebonics* (ASHA, 1983), *Black English* (Owens, 1991; Terrell & Terrell, 1993), *Vernacular Black English* (Wolfram, 1991; Wolfram & Fasold, 1974), and *Black English Vernacular* (Iglesias & Anderson, 1993).

AAVE has quite an interesting history. Its origins took root when Europeans traveled to Africa for reasons of business and commerce. A **pidgin** language developed between these two groups of people. A pidgin language develops when two different groups of people, with two distinct languages, attempt to communicate. The resulting pidgin language is typically characterized as having both a reduced vocabulary and grammar. The pidgin language that led to the development of AAVE shared characteristics of both African and European languages. When slaves arrived in the United States, both the slaves' overseers as well as the owners of the plantations introduced new vocabulary items and grammatical structures to the pidgin. Children born to the slaves were taught this more fully developed pidgin language as their native language. Once a pidgin language is passed on to a new generation of users, the language is considered to be what is known as a *creole* language. AAVE has evolved from this creole and is characteristic of a rich history of grammar and vocabulary from both African and European languages.

AAVE, as it is known today, has several regional variations. The form of AAVE spoken in a northern city, such as Cleveland, differs from the version of AAVE spoken in the South. Although AAVE is characterized by several lexical, grammatical, and phonological features, we will focus only on the more noted phonological features common to AAVE.

Consonant Characteristics

AAVE can be characterized by several phonological patterns that may affect phoneme production. These patterns include (1) the omission or substitution of the medial or final consonant in a word, (2) the omission of unstressed initial phonemes or syllables, and (3) the reduction of word-final consonant clusters (Terrell & Terrell, 1993). Using this classification, a summary of the major phonological traits associated with AAVE are presented in the next section and are also summarized in Table 8.4.

Omission or Substitution of the Medial or Final Consonant in a Word

- *final stop deletion*

   Final /t/ or /d/ may be deleted in some cases.

   Examples:
   hat → /hæ/   bad → /bæ/

   The phoneme /d/ also may be deleted when it is followed by the morpheme /s/.

   Examples:
   kids → /kɪz/   needs → /niz/   feeds → /fiz/

- *final nasal deletion*

   Final nasals are sometimes deleted from a word. The preceding vowel is then nasalized.

TABLE 8.4   Examples of AAVE Phonology

English Word	AAVE Transcription	Phonological Pattern
hat	/hæ/	final stop deletion
pin	/pɪː/	final nasal deletion
through	/θu/	/r/ deletion
wolf	/wʊf/	/l/ deletion
Ruth	/ruf/	θ → f (place change)
bid	/bɪːt/	devoicing of final stop
bid	/bɪʔ/	glottal stop replacement
winning	/wɪnən/	ŋ → n (place change)
isn't	/ɪdn̩t/	stopping
these	/diz/	stopping
about	/baʊt/	deletion of unstressed initial syllable
haste	/heɪs/	word-final cluster reduction
pen	/pɪn/	ɛ → ɪ (vowel raising)
tire	/tar/	diphthong simplification

Source: Adapted from Terrell & Terrell, 1993; Wolfram, 1994; Wolfram & Fasold, 1974.

Examples:
pin → /pɪ̃/   home → /hõʊ̃/

- *liquid deletion*

  /r/ may be deleted both in the prevocalic and postvocalic positions of words.

  Examples:

  through → /θu/   secretary → /sɛkətɛrɪ/
  throw   → /θoʊ/   professor → /pəfɛsɚ/
  more   → /moʊ/   story   → /stoʊɪ/
  sure   → /ʃoʊ/   Harold   → /hɛʊld/

  Postvocalic /l/ may also be deleted as in:

  wolf → /wʊf/   help → /hɛp/
  told → /toʊd/   bolt → /boʊt/

- *place of articulation change for /θ/ and /ð/*

  The fricatives /θ/ and /ð/ are sometimes produced as /f/ and /v/, respectively, both in the medial and final positions of words.

  Examples:
  Ruth → /ruf/   breathe → /briv/   bathe → /beɪv/
  both → /boʊf/   birthday → /bɝfdeɪ/   brother → /brʌvə/

- *devoicing of final stops*

  Final voiced stop consonants are sometimes devoiced. The longer vowel length normally associated with voiced stops is maintained (Wolfram, 1994).

Examples:
bid → /bɪːt/   bad → /bæːt/   rag → /ræːk/

- *glottal stop replacement*

  In some instances, a final stop may be produced as a glottal stop. Examples include:

  bid → /bɪʔ/   dad → /dæʔ/   bag → /bæʔ/

- *place of articulation change for /ŋ/*

  /n/ sometimes replaces /ŋ/ in words containing "ing." For example:

  winning → /wɪnɪn/ or /wɪnən/
  hanging → /hæŋɪn/ or /hæŋən/
  baking → /beɪkɪn/ or /beɪkən/

- *stopping*

  When a voiced fricative precedes a nasal consonant, it may be articulated as a voiced stop (Wolfram, 1994).

  Examples:
  isn't → /ɪdn̩t/   seven→ /sɛbm̩/
  wasn't → /wʌdn̩t/   even → /ibm̩/

  In some instances, word-initial /ð/ or /θ/ are stopped, resulting in production of /d/ or /t/, respectively.

  Examples:
  these → /diz/   them →/dɛm/   nothing → /nʌtn̩/

Omission of Unstressed Initial Phonemes and Unstressed Initial Syllables

The unstressed, initial syllable of a word may be elided. Sometimes this elision involves only one phoneme, as in the word "about."

Examples:
about   → /baʊt/   around→ /raʊnd/
because → /kʌz/   tomato → /meɪɾoʊ/

Reduction of Word-Final Consonant Clusters

Consonant clusters at the ends of words are often reduced when the final consonant is a stop. This simplification occurs when both consonants in the cluster share the same voicing pattern, that is, both voiced or both voiceless (Wolfram, 1994).

Examples:
haste   → /heɪs/   desk → /dɛs/
begged → /bɛg/   rind → /raɪn/
wished → /wɪʃ/   ghost → /goʊs/
changed → /ʧeɪnʤ/   list   → /lɪs/

Words with a final cluster comprised of the fricative /s/ followed by a stop (e.g., ghost) will have an AAVE plural form comprised of /əz/ (Wolfram, 1994). The plural form /əz/ is typical of Standard English words ending in /s/, for example, "lace" /leɪs/ → "laces" /leɪsəz/.

Examples:

ghosts → /goʊsəz/   desks → /dɛsəz/

lists   → /lɪsəz/   artists → /ɑrɾɪsəz/

Vowel Characteristics

In addition to the consonant characteristics presented above, there are several vowel productions associated with AAVE. These include vowel raising and diphthong simplification.

- *vowel raising*

  Similar to Southern American dialect, the vowel /ɛ/ may be raised and produced as /ɪ/ when it is followed by the nasal consonant /n/. This occurrence makes the vowels /ɪ/ and /ɛ/ indistinguishable from one another. That is the words "ten" and "tin" would both be pronounced as /tɪn/. Other examples include:

  any   → /ɪnɪ/   Ben, been → /bɪn/

  many, Minnie → /mɪnɪ/   pen, pin → /pɪn/

- *diphthong simplification*

  Diphthongs are sometimes simplified to a monophthong. Recall that this is a characteristic also observed in southern speech patterns.

  Examples:

  tire   → /tar/   oil → /ɔːl/   hour → /ar/

  dime → /dam/   toil → /tɔːl/   flour → /flar/

EXERCISE 8.7

Examine each of the words below. Then look at the AAVE phonological pattern that should be applied to each word. Provide the appropriate transcription in the blank at the right.

Example:

east   final cluster reduction   /is/

1. ran   final nasal deletion   _____
2. with   θ → f place change   _____
3. character   liquid deletion   _____
4. weeds   stop deletion   _____
5. hasn't   fricative stopping   _____
6. yelling   ŋ → place change   _____
7. blast   final cluster reduction   _____
8. behind   deletion of unstressed initial syllable   _____
9. Denny   ɛ → ɪ (vowel raising)   _____
10. cat   /ʔ/ replacement   _____

Learning English as a Second Language

The demographic profile of the population of the United States has changed markedly over the last three decades. There has been a steady increase in the number of immigrants coming to the United States from other countries. It is estimated that 28.4 million residents of the United States were foreign-born in 2000. The foreign-born population accounts for 10.4 percent of the total U.S. population (Schmidley, 2001). (Foreign-born individuals are those who are not currently U.S. citizens or those who have become citizens through naturalization.) This reflects an increase from 19.8 million in 1990. According to U.S. census figures, individuals from Mexico, China, the Philippines, India, Cuba, Vietnam, El Salvador, the Dominican Republic and the former Soviet Union account for the vast increase in the foreign-born population (Schmidley, 2001). The largest number of foreign-born residents come from Latin America (51 percent), with 27.6 percent of the foreign born coming from Mexico. Individuals from Asia account for 25.5 percent of the foreign-born population, whereas individuals from Europe account for 15.3 percent.

Fourteen percent of the U.S. population (age 5 or older) speaks a non-English language at home. This reflects a 4 percent rise in speakers of a second language since 1990 (U.S. Census Bureau, 2003). Approximately 39 percent of the residents of California, 37 percent of the residents of New Mexico, and 31 percent of the residents of Texas speak a non-English language. In addition, Arizona, Florida, Hawaii, New York, and New Jersey each report that more than 20 percent of their residents speak a second language. Close to one-half of all U.S. residents who speak a second language live in California, Texas, or New York (U.S. Census Bureau, 2003).

Children born to immigrant families will often be first-generation learners of English. These children will learn English while using their native language as a template for the proper use of English grammatical rules, vocabulary, and pronunciation. The phonological problems a bilingual child may have in production of English speech patterns may be due to the *interference* of the phonological system of the child's first language. Because of interference, a child will begin to develop a dialect of spoken English based on a set of phonemes and phonological rules from the first language.

In addition to the phonology of the child's first language, several other factors contribute to the dialect spoken by second-language learners of English. The dialect of the family's first language also will have an impact on the dialect of English spoken in the home. As an example, the English dialect spoken by someone originally from Mexico City would be different from the English dialect of someone originally from Chihuahua, because the dialects of Spanish spoken in these two Mexican cities vary. Also, a second-language learner's dialect will reflect regional variations of English depending on where the family has settled in the United States.

As practicing clinicians, you need to have a heightened awareness of the dialects and language practices of second-language learners, especially when working in the schools. In many cases, when bilingual children begin school, they may have little familiarity with English. These children are considered to be **limited English proficient** (LEP) speakers. They initially will use their first language as their primary mode of communication. Most typically developing LEP children will develop English due to interaction with other English-speaking individuals and will, in time, become fluent in both languages (Paul, 1995). As English develops, the LEP child may display a dialectal variation of English due to factors associated with the child's environment and to familial language practice. If the child's language and speech performance are related to dialectal variation and not a communication disorder, therapeutic treatment is not necessarily indicated. However, it is not uncommon for LEP children to have other communication deficits associated with hearing loss, cleft palate, fluency disorders, language disorders, or phonological disorders (not due to interference). In any of these instances, treatment might be indicated.

Adult second-language learners also have problems with learning the intricacies of English pronunciation. This group of adults may elect to receive treatment for accent reduction in order to improve overall speech intelligibility. This is especially important if an individual wishes to be more easily understood in the work place, especially in fields such as education and business.

Spanish-Influenced English

According to the March 2002 *Current Population Reports,* the Hispanic population in the United States numbered 37.4 million, or 13.3 percent of the total population. This makes the Hispanic population the largest minority group in the United States (Ramirez & de la Cruz, 2003).

The term *Hispanic* is used to refer to an individual with a Spanish background from any race, regardless of whether Spanish is spoken in the home (Kayser, 1993). A little over two-thirds of the Hispanic population in the United States comes from Mexico (66.9 percent), followed by Central and South America (14.3 percent), Puerto Rico (8.6 percent), Cuba (3.7 percent), and "Other" (6.5 percent), which includes other individuals of Spanish descent (Ramirez & de la Cruz, 2003). Spanish is spoken in nearly 60 percent of the homes in the United States in which a second language is spoken. In addition, almost half of all Spanish speakers live in either Texas or California (U.S. Census Bureau, 2003).

Most Hispanic children in the United States are born into families in which Spanish is the primary language spoken, both by parents and by other family members (Perez, 1994). The extent to which a Hispanic child becomes masterful in the use of the English language depends on (1) the age when the child was first exposed to English, (2) the degree of acceptance of English by the immediate family members, (3) the degree of exposure to English in the child's daily environment, and (4) whether the child's family is monolingual or bilingual (Perez, 1994; Reed, 1994).

In relation to bilingualism, the family members may be fluent in both Spanish and English. However, not all bilingual individuals are proficient in both languages. Some bilingual individuals are more fluent in one language than the other. In some cases, there may be limited proficiency in both languages. It is possible then for Hispanic children to be fluent in both languages, have limited English proficiency, or have limited proficiency in either language.

Phonological Characteristics of Spanish-Influenced English

Because some Hispanic children may be considered LEP when they enter school, speech-language pathologists should understand how Spanish may influence the further development of English. Otherwise, it would not be possible to tell whether a child's particular speech patterns were consistent with Spanish-influenced english (SIE) or the result of a speech disorder.

The phonemic system of Spanish varies from that of English, both in terms of vowels and consonants. In English, the vowel system is represented by approximately 14 phonemes. Spanish, on the other hand, has only five vowels: /i, e, a, o, and u/ (Iglesias & Goldstein, 1998; Perez, 1994). Therefore, a Spanish individual speaking English will often experience difficulty with vowel production, due to interference. Vowel production in SIE often involves articulation of vowels that are adjacent to the intended vowel in the quadrilateral (Perez, 1994). Some of the more common vowel articulations consistent with SIE are described below and are summarized in Table 8.5.

Due to interference, the word "pick" would be pronounced in SIE as /pik/, because /ɪ/ is not typical of Spanish. Some other SIE vowel productions due to interference include:

eɪ → e	bake → /bek/ (the vowel will sound similar to /ɛ/)
æ → ɑ	tack → /tɑk/
ʊ → u	good → /gud/
oʊ → o	hope → /hop/ (the vowel will sound similar to /ɔ/)

Also, several vowel confusions in SIE are not always predictable from an interference view of speech production. For instance, the production of "fit" for the word "feet" (i → ɪ), is not predictable from interference, because /ɪ/ does not exist in Spanish. Other vowel patterns sometimes seen in SIE that are not explained by interference include the following (from Perez, 1994):

eɪ → ɛ	date → /dɛt/
ɛ → æ	men → /mæn/
æ → ɛ	tack → /tɛk/
u → ʊ	room → /rʊm/
ʌ → ɑ or a	some → /sɑm/ or /sam/
ɝ → ɛr	girl → /gɛrl/

There are several consonants that are shared by both Spanish and English. Spanish includes the stops /p, t, k, b, d, and g/, the nasals /m/ and /n/, the fricatives /f/ and /s/, the affricate /ʧ/, and the approximants /w, l, and j/ (Iglesias & Goldstein, 1998). Even though these consonants are common to both languages, there are some allophonic variants in production of these consonants when comparing the two languages. For example, in Spanish, the voiceless stops /p, t, and k/ are not aspirated as they are in English.

Several English consonants also occur in Spanish only as allophones. For example, the fricative /ð/ occurs in Spanish as an allophone of the voiced, stop /d/, and /ŋ/ occurs as an allophone of /n/ (Bleile & Goldstein, 1996). In addition, Spanish has several phonemes that are not part of English. These include the voiceless, velar fricative /x/, the palatal nasal /ɲ/, and the trilled /r/ (Bleile & Goldstein, 1996). (Recall that the English approximant /r/ is not trilled and is officially represented by the IPA symbol /ɹ/.)

Due to the various differences in the consonantal systems of English and Spanish, it is not surprising that a Spanish-speaking individual often will have difficulty producing unfamiliar English phonemes. Some of these problems are due to interference, others are not. Some examples of consonant articulations common to SIE are described below and are also displayed in Table 8.5.

TABLE 8.5 Common Spanish-Influenced English Vowel and Consonant Productions

English Word	Spanish-Influenced English Transcription	Phonological Pattern
	Vowel Articulations	
lid	/lid/	ɪ → i
need	/nɪd/	i → ɪ
mate	/met/ (will sound similar to /ɛ/	eɪ → e
late	/lɛt/	eɪ → ɛ
tennis	/teɪnɪs/	ɛ → eɪ
dead	/dæd/	ɛ → æ
bag	/bɑg/ or /bɛg/	æ → ɑ or ɛ
look	/luk/	ʊ → u
pool	/pʊl/	u → ʊ
boat	/bot/ (will sound similar to /ɔ/)	oʊ → o
bug	/bɑg/ or /bag/	ʌ → ɑ or a
word	/wɛrd/	ɚ → ɛr
	Consonant Articulations	
think	/tɪŋk/	θ → t stopping
them	/dɛm/	ð → d stopping
vase	/bes/	v → b stopping
you	/ʤu/	j → ʤ affrication of a glide
sheep	/ʧip/	ʃ → ʧ affrication of a fricative
choose	/ʃuz/	ʧ → ʃ deaffrication
just	/jʌst/	ʤ → j deaffrication
zoo	/su/	consonant devoicing
was	/wʌs/	consonant devoicing
spot	/əspat/ or /ɛspat/	epenthesis of /ə/
leaks	/lik/	reduction of word-final consonant clusters

Source: Adapted from Penfield & Ornstein-Galicia, 1985; Perez, 1994; Wise, 1957.

Some of the common consonant patterns observed in SIE (with examples) include:

- *stopping*
  with → /wɪt/   those → /doʊz/   vine → /baɪn/

- *affrication of fricatives and glides*
  shoe → /ʧu/   yes → /ʤɛs/

- *deaffrication*

  chase → /ʃes/   just → /jʌst/

- *devoicing of consonants (prevocalic and postvocalic)*

  zoo → /su/   leave → /lif/   ridge → /rɪtʃ/

- *reduction of word-final consonant clusters*

  rest → /rɛs/   won't → /wɔn/

  worked → /wɝk/   wound → /wun/

- *epenthesis of /ə/ preceding initial /s/ + stop clusters*

Although the consonant clusters /sk/, /st/, and /sp/ are commonly found at the beginning of English words, they do not occur at the beginning of Spanish words. In SIE, a vowel (/ə/ or /ɛ/) is added prior to one of these word-initial clusters, splitting the components of the cluster (Wolfram, 1994).

In this manner, each element of the cluster will appear in two separate syllables. The result is a new first syllable comprised of the added vowel + /s/. The next syllable begins with the stop consonant from the cluster. For example:

spot → /əspat/ or /ɛspat/   school → /əskul/ or /ɛskul/
stand → /əstand/ or /ɛstand/

EXERCISE 8.8

Determine the phonological pattern being demonstrated in each of the following SIE pronunciations. Write your answer in the blank.

Example:

need	/nɪd/	i → ɪ

1. eyes	/aɪs/	_____
2. much	/matʃ/	_____
3. squirrel	/skwɛrl̩/	_____
4. yes	/dʒɛs/	_____
5. spoiled	/əspɔɪld/	_____
6. clasp	/klɑsp/	_____
7. winner	/winɚ/	_____
8. voice	/bɔɪs/	_____
9. should	/ʃud/	_____
10. badge	/bætʃ/	_____

Asian/Pacific-Influenced English

The March 2002 U.S. *Current Population Reports* indicates that 12.5 million residents of the United States are members of the Asian and Pacific Islander (API) population. The API population currently comprises approximately 4.4 percent of the total U.S. population (Reeves & Bennett, 2003). Almost 7 million people living in the United States speak an Asian or Pacific Island language. This is an increase of 2.5 million since 1990. Approximately 40 percent of these individuals live in California. The most common Asian languages spoken in the United States include Chinese (over 2 million speakers), Pilipino (1.2 million speakers), Vietnamese (1 million speakers), Korean (894,000 speakers), and Japanese (478,000 speakers). Forty percent of all Chinese speakers live in California (Reeves & Bennett, 2003).

The languages spoken in Asia and the Pacific Islands are quite diverse. There are over 1,200 languages spoken by the 5 million residents of the Pacific Islands alone (Cheng, 1994). In reference to structure, Asian languages differ markedly from one another, both in terms of grammatical rules and phonology. Similarly, Asian languages vary greatly from the grammatical rules and phonology of English. For instance, in Chinese, each printed character is only one syllable in length. Therefore, when a Chinese person is learning English, there is a tendency to pronounce multisyllabic words syllable by syllable, in a telegraphic, or staccato, manner.

In addition, several Asian languages, such as Chinese and Vietnamese, are *tone languages*. In a tone language, a word's meaning may differ when pronounced with a varying tone or intonation pattern. For instance, in Mandarin, one of the major Chinese dialects spoken in the United States, the syllable /ba/ may mean "eight," "to pull," "handle," "to give up," or "okay," depending on the intonation produced as the word is articulated (Cheng, 1994). In a tone language, intonation is considered to be phonemic because each tone will convey a different meaning to the listener. As you know, in English, tone is not phonemic. Instead, tone generally indicates the speaker's mood or intent or signals whether the utterance is a statement or a question.

Children whose parents immigrated to the United States from Asia or one of the Pacific Islands may have initial difficulty learning English as a second language. The same variables related to bilingualism and second language learning previously discussed with Hispanic children also apply to children from Asia or the Pacific Islands. The articulation patterns that Asian speakers produce in speaking English are, at least in part, due to interference of the speaker's native language. For instance in Chinese and Vietnamese, consonant clusters do not exist. In Korean, consonant clusters do not exist in initial or final positions of words (Cheng, 1987b). Therefore, when an Asian speaker produces an English word containing a cluster, there is a tendency to simplify the cluster.

It is also quite common in English for words to end with a consonant. In fact, all of the following English phonemes are commonly found at the ends of words: /p, t, k, b, d, g, m, n, ŋ, r, l, ʃ, s, θ, f, ʒ, z, ð, v, ʧ, and ʤ/. In Asian languages, such as Chinese, Vietnamese, and Japanese, the number of consonants that end a word is quite small compared to English. In Japanese, the only final consonant is /n/ (Cheng, 1987b). In Mandarin, there are only two final consonants, /n/ and /ŋ/, and in Cantonese (the other major Chinese dialect spoken in the United States), there are only seven final consonants, /m, n, ŋ, p, t, k, and ʔ/ (Cheng, 1987b). Therefore, Asian speakers of English often will delete the final consonants of English words because it is not common for words to end with consonants in their native languages.

When examining the phonemic inventories of several of the Asian languages, it becomes immediately apparent that the number of consonant and vowel phonemes vary when compared to English. In addition, there are English consonants not typical of Asian languages, and phonemes in Asian languages not typical of English. For this reason, articulation difficulties arise when an Asian speaker is learning to speak English. Table 8.6 displays some of the consonant productions characteristic of Asian/Pacific-influenced English (APIE). This table highlights English consonant production by speakers of Cantonese, Mandarin, Vietnamese, Korean, Japanese, and Pilipino. Although in APIE some consonant productions involve allophonic variants—that is, [p]/[pʰ]—Table 8.6 only highlights phonemic articulations. Some of the more common vowel interference problems seen in APIE are also summarized in Table 8.7.

TABLE 8.6 Common Consonant Productions for English Phonemes, as spoken by Chinese, Vietnamese, Korean, Japanese, and Pilipino speakers (Mandarin and Cantonese dialects of Chinese are shown separately)

Intended Phoneme		Cantonese	Mandarin	Vietnamese	Korean	Japanese	Pilipino
Fricatives	θ	s, f	s, f	s		s, z	t
	ð	d	z, d		ʤ	z, j	d
	ʃ	s		s, t	s		s
	ʒ					ʤ, ʃ	d, ds
	f	~		p		h	p
	v	f, w	f, w		b, p	b	b
	z	s		s	s	dz, ʤ, s	s
Affricates	ʧ		ʃ	s, t, ʃ	t		ts
	ʤ	z			ʒ		ds
Liquids	r	l	l	z	l		
	l		r	n		r	r

Source: Adapted from Baker, 1982; Cheng, 1987a, 1987b, 1994; and Shen, 1962.

TABLE 8.7 Some Common Vowel Productions in APIE

Chinese	• æ → e or ɛ; ɛ → e; ɪ → i; ɔ → o; ʊ → u; ʌ → ɑ
	• /ə/ is added to consonant clusters
Vietnamese	• ɪ → i; æ → ʌ; ʊ → u
Korean	• problems with the production of /i, ɪ, u and ɔ/
Japanese	• epenthesis of the vowels /ə/ or /u/ to the ends of syllables and words. (Most Japanese words end in an open syllable.)
	• ɪ → i; æ, a or ə → ɑ; ɚ → ɑ; ʊ → u; ʌ → æ; eɪ → e; æ → ɛ
Pilipino	• tensing of lax vowels, i.e., ɪ → i; ʊ → u; ɔ → o

Source: Adapted from Baker, 1982; Cheng, 1987a, 1987b, 1994.

EXERCISE 8.9

Apply the given phonological pattern to each transcription in order to produce an Asian/Pacific-influenced English (APIE) pronunciation of each word. Provide both the APIE transcription and the orthography.

SAE Transcription	Phonological Pattern	APIE Transcription	Orthography
Example:			
/raɪs/	r → l	/laɪs/	rice
Chinese			
1. /θɪŋk/	θ → s	_____	_____
2. /ʃuz/	ʃ → s	_____	_____
3. /vaɪn/	v → w	_____	_____
4. /bɑt/	ɑ → ʌ	_____	_____
Japanese			
5. /ðɪs/	ð → z	_____	_____
6. /fri/	f → h	_____	_____
7. /ʃɪp/	ɪ → i	_____	_____
Pilipino			
8. /faɪn/	f → p	_____	_____
9. /tʃɛk/	tʃ → ts	_____	_____
10. /fɪt/	ɪ → i	_____	_____

Phonological Interference: Russian and Arabic Speakers

Due to the large influx of individuals from Europe and other Asian countries to the United States, it might be instructive to look at some other examples of phonological interference from two vastly different languages, Arabic and Russian. Both Arabic and Russian have very different phonemic systems when compared to English. Each language will be examined separately to help clarify why it is difficult for native speakers of Arabic and Russian to learn American English.

Russian-Influenced English

Russian has only five vowels, /i, ε, a, u, and o/, and only one true diphthong, /aʊ/ (Berger, 1952). For this reason, Russian speakers learning English have much difficulty with vowel production. The Russian consonant system varies greatly when compared to English as well. For example, all stop consonants in Russian are unaspirated. Therefore, English words that begin with a voiceless stop may be unaspirated when spoken by a Russian individual learning English. An unaspirated voiceless stop at the beginning of a word will tend to sound voiced. For example, "tame" will sound like "dame." Likewise, "pig" will have a tendency to sound like "big." In Russian, voiced stops do not occur in final word positions (Baker, 1982; Berger, 1952). Some examples include "lag" → /lak/ and "range" → /rentʃ/. Russian voiced stops and fricatives cannot appear together in the final position of a word. Therefore, the word "rags" would be pronounced as /rɛks/ (both the /g/ and /z/ being produced as their voiceless cognates /k/ and /s/).

In Russian, voiceless and voiced phonemes cannot occur together at word boundaries (Berger, 1952). For example, "hit the ball," would be produced as /hɪdðəbɔl/. Note that the /t/ in "hit" becomes voiced. This is an example of regressive assimilation; the /ð/ in "the" causes the /t/ in "hit" to be produced as /d/. A similar example would be "nice boy" being pronounced as /naɪzbɔɪ/.

There are several consonants in English that do not exist in Russian, causing interference problems for Russian speakers. These include /ð, θ, w, and ŋ /. The phoneme /h/ is also problematic for some Russian speakers; it is sometimes produced as the voiceless velar fricative /x/ (Berger, 1952). This phoneme is found in the name of the German composer "Bach." Production of /v/ can also be difficult, sometimes being produced as the voiced bilabial fricative /β/, sometimes as /w/, and sometimes as /vw/ (Berger, 1952). For example, "vodka" could be produced as /βɔdkə/, /wɔdkə/, or /vwɔdkə/. See Table 8.8 for a summary of Russian-influenced English pronunciation.

TABLE 8.8 Common Russian-Influenced English Vowel and Consonant Productions

English Word	Russian-Influenced English Transcription	Phonological Pattern
Vowel Articulations		
sit	/sit/	ɪ → i
book	/buk/	ʊ → u
hat	/hɛt/	æ → ɛ
caught	/kot/	ɔ → o
come	/kam/	ʌ → a
Consonant Articulations		
tone	/don/	t → d
rag	/rɛk/	g → k
rags	/rɛks/	gz → ks
this	/dɪs/	ð → d
thin	/tin/	θ → t
sink	/sink/	ŋ → n
quota	/kvotə/	w → v
vodka	/wɔdkə/	v → w
vote	/vwot/	v → vw
hate	/xɛt/	h → x

Source: Adapted from Baker, 1982; Berger, 1952; Power, 2003a.

Arabic-Influenced English

Arabic has only three vowels, /i/, /a/, and /u/, which occur in both short and long forms. The only diphthongs in Arabic are /eɪ/ and /aʊ/. Also, several English consonants do not exist in Arabic. These include the stops /p/ and /g/, the fricatives /v/ and /ʒ/, and the nasal /ŋ/ (Altaha, 1995; *Handbook of the International Phonetic Association*, 1999). However, some of these phonemes exist in some dialects of Arabic. In Arabic, it is not possible to have a cluster of two or three consonants at the beginning of a word. For this reason, vowels are inserted in production of clusters, as in /sikrim/ for "scream" and /sitrit/ for "street" (Altaha, 1995).

Arabic speakers learning English will sometimes pronounce silent letters, since Arabic's alphabet is phonemic—for example, "knot" → /knɔt/, "could" → /kuld/, and "lamb" → /læmb/. Other difficulties that arise from English spelling intrusions include problems pronouncing words with the letter "c"— for example, "city" → /kɪtɪ/ and "soccer" → /sɔsɚ/. As can be seen "c" is sometimes pronounced as /k/ when it should be pronounced as /s/, and vice versa. In a similar manner, since the letter "g" can be pronounced as either /dʒ/ or /g/, Arabic speakers may produce "gear" as /dʒir/ and "origin" as /ɔrigin/. Also, the spelling "dg" may be pronounced as two separate phonemes, as in /bʌdgit/

TABLE 8.9 Common Arabic-Influenced English Vowel and Consonant Productions

English Word	Arabic-Influenced English Transcription	Phonological Pattern
Vowel Articulations		
brought	/bot/	ɔ → o
bit	/bet/	ɪ → e
because	/bikuz/	ʌ → u
cup	/kæp/	ʌ → æ
set	/sæt/	ɛ → æ
bread	/brid/	ɛ → i
note	/nat/	o → a
Consonant Articulations		
party	/bɑrtɪ/	p → b
very	/fɛrɪ/	v → f
thin	/sɪn/	θ → s
lesion	/liʃən/	ʒ → ʃ
witch	/wɪʃ/	tʃ → ʃ
Jim	/ʃɪm/	dʒ → ʃ
bathe	/bez/	ð → z
think	/θɪnk/	ŋ → n
scream	/sikrim/	epenthesis of i

Source: Adapted from Altaha, 1995; Baker, 1982; Power, 2003b.

for "budget" (Altaha, 1995). Refer to Table 8.9 for a summary of the pronunciation difficulties associated with Arabic-Influenced English.

EXERCISE 8.10

For the following, indicate (with an "X"), the productions that are consistent with the phonological patterns associated with Russian-Influenced English. For these words, fill in the blank with the correct description of the pattern.

Example:

_X_	look	/lʊk/	ʊ → u
_____	1. pack	/bæk/	_____
_____	2. very	/wɛrɪ/	_____
_____	3. patch	/pæʃ/	_____
_____	4. think	/θɪnk/	_____
_____	5. candy	/kɛndɪ/	_____
_____	6. written	/rɪtn̩/	_____
_____	7. meant	/mʌnt/	_____
_____	8. them	/dɛm/	_____

EXERCISE 8.11

For the following, indicate (with an "X"), the productions that are consistent with the phonological patterns associated with Arabic-Influenced English.

Example:

_X_	vest	/væst/
_____	1. pink	/pɪnk/
_____	2. Paul	/bɔl/
_____	3. thought	/dɔt/
_____	4. check	/ʃæk/
_____	5. reed	/ræd/
_____	6. vine	/faɪn/
_____	7. lucky	/loʊkɪ/

Review Exercises

A. Transcribe each of the following words as if they were pronounced by a Southern American English speaker. All of these words involve some form of deleted /r/.

Example:

  shirt   /ʃɜːt/

1. writer   _____
2. Clark   _____
3. aware   _____
4. score   _____
5. curtains   _____
6. appear   _____
7. danger   _____
8. murder   _____
9. charter   _____
10. bourbon   _____

B. Provide English orthography for each of the following Southern American English pronunciations.

1. /lɪmɪn/   _____   9. /rɪzʊlt/   _____
2. /ɑrɪnʤ/   _____   10. /flʌrɪ/   _____
3. /preɪʃɪs/   _____   11. /wɜːðɪ/   _____
4. /kuʃɪn/   _____   12. /ʧɛə/   _____
5. /stju/   _____   13. /sɪstə/   _____
6. /veɪrɪəs/   _____   14. /pjʊə/   _____
7. /wɔʧ/   _____   15. /kɑːt/   _____
8. /rɪl/   _____   16. /spoət/   _____

C. Transcribe each of the following words as if they were pronounced by an Eastern American English speaker. All of these words involve some form of deleted /r/.

1. beware   _____   6. store   _____
2. start   _____   7. squirt   _____
3. hanger   _____   8. glare   _____
4. severe   _____   9. doctor   _____
5. clergy   _____   10. carbon   _____

D. Provide English orthography for each of the following Eastern American English pronunciations.

1. /klɒgd/   _____   9. /kɔfɪ/   _____
2. /tjuzdeɪ/   _____   10. /pærət/   _____
3. /kɑnt/   _____   11. /sɒrɪ/   _____
4. /brʊm/   _____   12. /ɛksploə/   _____
5. /mæroʊ/   _____   13. /ʧɑːrə/   _____
6. /blʌrɪŋ/   _____   14. /laʤəst/   _____
7. /fɔn/   _____   15. /dɪmɑnd/   _____
8. /baθ/   _____   16. /kənspaɪə/   _____

E. Examine each of the words below. Then read the description describing an AAVE phonological pattern that should be applied to each word. Provide the appropriate transcription in the blank at the right.

Example:

east	final cluster reduction	/is/

1. moth   θ → f place change   _____
2. beneath   deletion of unstressed initial syllable   _____
3. then   ɛ → ɪ place change   _____
4. can   final nasal deletion   _____
5. protection   /r/ deletion   _____
6. them   stopping of fricative   _____
7. behind   diphthong reduction   _____
8. wastes   plural of /s/ + stop   _____
9. eleven   stopping   _____
10. driving   ŋ → n place change   _____

F. For the following, indicate (with an "X") the productions that are consistent with the phonological patterns associated with AAVE. For those words, write the phonological pattern in the blank.

Example:

X	east	/is/	final cluster reduction

____	1. bread	/brɛ/	_____
____	2. broom	/brʊm/	_____
____	3. suppose	/poʊz/	_____
____	4. shake	/seɪk/	_____
____	5. raced	/reɪs/	_____
____	6. chalk	/ʃɑk/	_____
____	7. when	/wɪn/	_____
____	8. light	/lat/	_____
____	9. hold	/hoʊd/	_____
____	10. has	/hæs/	_____
____	11. cola	/koʊlɚ/	_____
____	12. washing	/wɑʃən/	_____
____	13. could	/kʊʔ/	_____
____	14. landed	/jændəd/	_____
____	15. corn	/koʊn/	_____

G. For the following, indicate (with an "X") the productions that are consistent with the phonological patterns associated with SIE. For those words, write the description of the phonological pattern in the blank.

Example:

X	need	/nɪd/	i → ɪ

	1. bath	/bæt/	_____
	2. been	/bin/	_____
	3. writer	/raɪɾə/	_____
	4. oven	/avən/	_____
	5. bold	/boʊd/	_____
	6. Jimmy	/jɪmɪ/	_____
	7. bird	/bɜːd/	_____
	8. cushion	/kuʃən/	_____
	9. class	/klɑs/	_____
	10. shallow	/ʧæloʊ/	_____
	11. vine	/baɪn/	_____
	12. them	/ðɪm/	_____
	13. stood	/əstʊd/	_____
	14. zebra	/sibrə/	_____
	15. can't	/kant/	_____

H. Examine the phonological pattern in the APIE pronunciation of each of the following words. From Table 8.7, determine the Asian language(s) in which the pattern may occur. Write your answers in the blanks.

Example:

them	/dɛm/	Pilipino, Mandarin, and Cantonese

1. like	/naɪk/	_____
2. very	/wɛrɪ/	_____
3. vine	/baɪn/	_____
4. shine	/saɪn/	_____
5. joke	/zoʊk/	_____
6. raise	/leɪz/	_____
7. thank	/sæŋk/	_____
8. chant	/tsænt/	_____
9. zoo	/dzu/	_____
10. them	/zɛm/	_____

I. Using Tables 8.7 and 8.8, determine whether the phonological pattern given is indicative of either Arabic-Influenced or Russian-Influenced English (or both). Mark the appropriate blank with an "X".

Example:

	Russian	*Arabic*	*Both*
ʒ → ʃ	____	X	____
1. p → b	____	____	____
2. v → w	____	____	____
3. ð → d	____	____	____
4. ɔ → o	____	____	____
5. ʌ → u	____	____	____
6. dʒ → ʃ	____	____	____
7. θ → t	____	____	____
8. ŋ → n	____	____	____
9. æ → ɛ	____	____	____
10. θ → s	____	____	____

J. Eastern American English Transcription Practice.
Transcribe each of the following sentences as spoken by a female from New York City.

1. Ma, I gotta go to the store with Paul today.

   _____

2. What are you talking about? Forget about it already.

   _____

3. Carly, why do you have to ruin everything?

   _____

4. I have a dentist appointment at 6:30.

   _____

5. Robert needs to go to the barber, his hair is too long.

   _____

6. I walked over to the mall yesterday afternoon to get a new pair of shoes.

   _____

7. My dog likes to run all around the yard and bark.

   _____

8. When I was playing basketball, I ran all over the court.

   _____

9. I gotta go food shopping. I need watermelon, corn, and soda.

   _____

10. My friend Mary is a weirdo. She don't want to leave me alone.

   _____

K. Eastern American English Transcription Practice.

Transcribe each of the following sentences as spoken by a female from Massachusetts.

1. Park the car in the garage.

   _____

2. I am going to the market in Boston.

   _____

3. I love to shop Harvard Square.

   _____

4. Have you guys been to the Cape or Martha's Vineyard for the summer?

   _____

5. Don't forget to bring your pocketbook.

   _____

6. Donna loves to drink tonic.

   _____

7. Can you wear your dungarees and sneakers?

   _____

8. Get a fork for that huge helping of pasta and gravy.

   _____

9. Go ahead and give mommy some jimmies for her banana split.

   _____

10. John Miller is a decent human being.

   _____

L. Southern American English Transcription Practice.

Transcribe each of the following sentences as spoken by a female from Tennessee.

1. She's driving to Louisiana tomorrow morning.

   _____

2. I'm going to boil a dozen eggs for Easter.

   _____

3. Last night, I was talking to my friend Mary Lynn.

   _____

4. I am fixing to have to buy some tires for my car.

   _____

5. I am looking for my blue ballpoint pen.

   _____

6. You better cover that broiling pan with aluminum foil.

   _____

7. Wait a minute, Larry. I need another minute to make up my mind.

———————————————————————————

8. I left the chicken out on the counter and it spoiled.

———————————————————————————

9. The University of Tennessee is in Knoxville.

———————————————————————————

10. Hurricanes and tornadoes are both large damaging wind storms.

———————————————————————————

M. African American Vernacular English Transcription Practice.

Transcribe each of the following sentences as spoken by a female from Ohio.

1. The boy needs more money.

———————————————————————————

2. We fixin to go to the store.

———————————————————————————

3. He be playing ball at the park.

———————————————————————————

4. There four new kids in my class.

———————————————————————————

5. My sister and brother was at that concert.

———————————————————————————

6. My family go to church every Sunday.

———————————————————————————

7. Your momma car in the middle of the street.

———————————————————————————

8. She found five quarters in her purse.

———————————————————————————

9. Kwanzaa got her hair done.

———————————————————————————

10. The students helped themselves to breakfast.

———————————————————————————

N. Spanish-Influenced English Transcription Practice.

Transcribe each of the following sentences as spoken by a female from Spain.

1. Please put the flowers in the vase.

———————————————————————————

2. It was a very special occasion.

———————————————————————————

3. You should quit yelling at your mother.

4. I was not sure I would be able to help.

5. My favorite teacher's name is Mister Jones.

6. Don't let your dog play in my yard.

7. Why don't you put these clothes in the garage?

8. Yesterday, I went to the zoo with Doug.

9. Shelley put the potato chips on the lower shelf.

10. I was very excited about winning the football game.

O. Asian-Influenced English Transcription Practice.

Transcribe each of the following sentences as spoken by a female from Japan.

1. I have one younger brother in my family.

2. I would like a grilled cheese sandwich for lunch, please.

3. It is supposed to rain heavily for much of the week.

4. The river is heavily polluted.

5. My sister Kyoko will be 23 years old next Thursday.

6. Would you like to go shopping with me after I get off work?

7. Would your other brother help me lift this? It's heavy.

8. Thank you very much for the beautiful flowers.

9. I have a hard time distinguishing between the singular and plural forms.

10. The only connecting flight is through Portland, Oregon.

P. Asian-Influenced English Transcription Practice.

Transcribe each of the following sentences as spoken by a male from Hong Kong. This male speaks the Cantonese dialect of Chinese.

1. Typing email helps me think in English.

   _____

2. I went to the zoo to see the new panda bears.

   _____

3. What do you think of the new television show?

   _____

4. I have two or three friends who are going to the soccer game.

   _____

5. Usually, she is not so forgetful.

   _____

6. I bet you that I will win the race.

   _____

7. My girlfriend sent me flowers last week for my birthday.

   _____

8. There are several people I need to get to know.

   _____

9. The layout of this city is not very convenient.

   _____

10. I plan to go to Purdue for my master's degree.

   _____

Q. Russian-Influenced English Transcription Practice.

Transcribe each of the following sentences as spoken by a male from Russia.

1. I would like a vodka and tonic, please.

   _____

2. Put the books over there on the table.

   _____

3. It was difficult for me to learn the correct pronunciation.

   _____

4. I have been living in the United States since last August.

   _____

5. He has many problems with his vocabulary.

   _____

6. The Russian economy depends on the current price of oil.

   _____

7. My younger brother Alexander is studying metallurgy at Moscow State University.

8. The author of the book was a famous writer.

9. I had several visitors from Virginia last month.

10. How many other people needed to take the class?

R. Arabic-Influenced English Transcription Practice.

Transcribe each of the following sentences as spoken by a male from Saudi Arabia.

1. Please use that word in a sentence.

2. I need sugar substitute for my coffee.

3. Dr. Cooper told me to make a copy of my homework assignment.

4. Their friend Robin got married to Victor, my next door neighbor.

5. I was depressed because we have had so much bad weather.

6. Pete got a prison sentence because he hit the policeman.

7. My favorite cotton shirt shrunk in the laundry.

8. Penny visited her fiancé on Friday.

9. I need to study English phonology to improve my pronunciation.

10. I grew a beard so that I would appear older.

Complete Assignment 8-1.

Study Questions

1. What is a dialect? What is the difference between a regional dialect and a social dialect?

2. What is meant by the term Standard American English?

3. What is chain shifting? How is chain shifting affecting English vowel production?

4. Describe several features of Southern American and Eastern American dialects that are different in terms of vowel production. Describe several features that are the same.

5. How does /r/ deletion affect pronunciation in eastern and southern speech patterns?

6. What is AAVE? Describe its origin and how it has developed into the dialect that is currently spoken in the United States.

7. Describe several vowel and consonant features of AAVE that differ from Standard American English.

8. What is the basic difference between the dialect associated with AAVE and the dialects associated with Spanish- and Asian/Pacific-influenced English?

9. What is meant by the term interference? How does interference affect phoneme acquisition by an individual learning English as a second language?

10. Describe several consonant and vowel characteristics typical of Spanish-influenced English.

11. Describe some of the phonological characteristics typical of Asian/Pacific-influenced English.

12. Describe some general characteristics of Asian languages that add to the difficulty of learning English as a second language.

13. How does the Russian phonological system differ from English?

14. How does the Arabic phonological system differ from English?

15. Should individuals who speak with a dialect receive treatment in order to reduce their "accents"?

Assignment 8-1   Name _____

"The Grandfather Passage" (Darley, Aronson, & Brown, 1975) will be spoken by several individuals who demonstrate different regional and cultural dialects of American English. Transcribe the passage carefully for each speaker, using systematic phonemic transcription. In some instances, it may be necessary to use systematic narrow transcription. In addition to the phonological patterns produced by these speakers, pay attention to the suprasegmental patterns displayed.

You wish to know all about my grandfather. Well, he is nearly 93 years old, yet he still thinks as swiftly as ever. He dresses himself in an old black frock coat, usually several buttons missing. A long beard clings to his chin, giving those who observe him a pronounced feeling of the utmost respect. When he speaks, his voice is just a bit cracked and quivers a bit. Twice each day he plays skillfully and with zest upon a small organ. Except in the winter when the snow or ice prevents, he slowly takes a short walk in the open air each day. We have often urged him to walk more and smoke less, but he always answers, "Banana oil!" Grandfather likes to be modern in his language.

1. African American Vernacular English (Ohio)

   _____
   _____
   _____
   _____
   _____
   _____
   _____
   _____
   _____
   _____

2. Eastern American English (Massachusetts)

   _____
   _____
   _____
   _____
   _____
   _____
   _____
   _____
   _____
   _____

Assignment 8-1 (cont.)   Name _____

3. Asian/Pacific-influenced English (China–Cantonese)

_____

_____

_____

_____

_____

_____

_____

4. Spanish-Influenced English (Spain)

_____

_____

_____

_____

_____

_____

_____

_____

5. Southern American English (Tennessee)

_____

_____

_____

_____

_____

_____

_____

_____

Assignment 8-1 (cont.)   Name _____

6. Asian/Pacific-influenced English (Japan)

_____

_____

_____

_____

_____

_____

_____

_____

7. Eastern American English (New York City)

_____

_____

_____

_____

_____

_____

_____

_____

8. Russian-Influenced English

_____

_____

_____

_____

_____

_____

_____

_____

Assignment 8-1 (cont.)

Name _____

9. Arabic-Influenced English

_____

_____

_____

_____

_____

_____

_____

_____

_____

References

Altaha, F. M. (1995). Pronunciation errors made by Saudi University students learning English: Analysis and remedy. *I.T.L Review of Applied Linguistics, 109–110,* 110–123.

American Speech-Language-Hearing Association (ASHA). (1983). Social dialects. *ASHA, 25*(9), 23–27.

American Speech-Language-Hearing Association (ASHA). (2003). *Technical report: American English dialects.* (ASHA Supplement 23), 45–46.

Baker, A. (1982). *Introducing English pronunciation: A teacher's guide to tree or three? and ship or sheep?* Cambridge, UK: Cambridge University Press.

Ball, M., Esling, J., & Dickson, J. (1995). The VoQS system for the transcription of voice quality. *Journal of the International Phonetics Association, 25*(2), 71–80.

Berger, M. D. (1952). *The American English pronunciation of Russian immigrants.* Unpublished doctoral dissertation, Columbia University, New York.

Bleile, K., & Goldstein, B. (1996). Dialect. In K. Bleile, *Articulation and phonological disorders: A book of exercises* (pp. 73–82). San Diego: Singular Publishing Group.

Boone, D., & McFarlane, S. (1994). *The voice and voice therapy* (5th ed.). Boston: Allyn and Bacon.

Borden, G., Harris, K., & Raphael, L. (1994). *Speech science primer* (3rd ed.). Baltimore: Williams and Wilkins.

Calvert, D. (1986). *Descriptive phonetics.* New York: Thieme.

Carrell, J., & Tiffany, W. (1960). *Phonetics: Theory and application to speech improvement.* New York: McGraw-Hill.

Carver, C. (1987). *American regional dialects: A word geography.* Ann Arbor: University of Michigan Press.

Cassidy, F. (Ed.). (1985). *Dictionary of American regional English: Volume I. Introduction and A-C.* Cambridge, MA: The Belknap Press of Harvard University Press.

Cheng, L. (1987a). Cross-cultural and linguistic considerations in working with Asian populations, *ASHA, 29*(6), 33–38.

Cheng, L. (1987b). *Assessing Asian language performance*. Rockville, MD: Aspen.

Cheng, L. (1994). Asian/Pacific students and the learning of English. In J. Bernthal & N. Bankson (Eds.), *Child phonology: Characteristics, assessment and intervention with special populations* (pp. 255–274). New York: Thieme.

Chomsky, N., & Halle, M. (1968). *The sound pattern of English*. Cambridge, MA: MIT Press.

Cruttenden, A. (2001). *Gimson's pronunciation of English* (6th ed.). London: Edward Arnold.

Crystal, D. (1987). *The Cambridge encyclopedia of language*. Cambridge, UK: Cambridge University Press.

Daniloff, R., Schuckers, G., & Feth, L. (1980). *The physiology of speech and hearing*. Englewood Cliffs, NJ: Prentice-Hall.

Darley, F., Aronson, F., & Brown, J. (1975). *Motor speech disorders*. Philadelphia: W.B. Saunders, Co.

Duckworth, M., Allen, G., Hardcastle, W., & Ball, M. (1990). Extensions to the International Phonetic Alphabet for the transcription of atypical speech. *Clinical Linguistics and Phonetics, 4*(4), 273–280.

Edwards, H. (1992). *Applied phonetics*. San Diego, CA: Singular Publishing Group.

Elbert, M., & Gierut, J. (1986). *Handbook of clinical phonology: Approaches to assessment and treatment*. San Diego: College-Hill Press.

Erber, N. (1983). Speech perception and speech development in hearing-impaired children. In I. Hochberg, H. Levitt, & M. Osberger (Eds.), *Speech of the hearing impaired: Research, training and personnel preparation* (pp. 131–145). Baltimore: University Park Press.

Fudge, E. (1984). *English word-stress*. London: George Allen & Unwin Publishers.

Gray, G., & Wise, C. (1959). *The bases of speech* (3rd ed.). New York: Harper and Row.

Grunwell, P. (1987). *Clinical phonology* (2nd ed.). Baltimore: Williams and Wilkins.

Handbook of the International Phonetic Association. (1999). Cambridge, UK: Cambridge University Press.

Hartman, J. (1985). Guide to pronunciation. In F. Cassidy (Ed.), *Dictionary of American regional English: Volume I, Introduction and A-C* (pp. xli–lx). Cambridge, MA: The Belknap Press of Harvard University Press.

Hodson, B. W., & Paden, E. P. (1991). *Targeting intelligible speech: A phonological approach to remediation* (2nd ed.). Austin, TX: Pro-Ed.

Iglesias, A., & Anderson, N. (1993). Dialectal variation. In J. Bernthal & N. Bankson (Eds.), *Articulation and phonological disorders* (3rd ed., pp. 147–161). Englewood Cliffs, NJ: Prentice-Hall.

Iglesias, A., & Goldstein, B. (1998). Language and dialectal variations. In J. Bernthal & N. Bankson (Eds.), *Articulation and phonological disorders* (4th ed., pp. 148–171). Boston: Allyn and Bacon.

Ingram, D. (1976). *Phonological disability in children*. London: Edward Arnold.

Jakobson, R., Fant, G., & Halle, M. (1952). *Preliminaries to speech analysis: The distinctive features and their correlates*. Cambridge, MA: MIT Press.

Jones, D. (1963). *The pronunciation of English*. Cambridge, UK: Cambridge University Press.

Jones, D. (1967). *An outline of English phonetics*. Cambridge, UK: W. Heffner and Sons.

Kayser, H. (1993). Hispanic cultures. In D. Battle (Ed.), *Communication disorders in multicultural populations* (pp. 114–157). Boston: Andover Medical Publishers.

Kent, R. (1997). *The speech sciences.* San Diego: Singular Publishing Group.

Kurath, H. (1949). *Word geography of the eastern United States.* Ann Arbor: University of Michigan Press.

Labov, W. (1991). The three dialects of English. In P. Eckert (Ed.), *New ways of analyzing sound change* (pp. 1–44). San Diego: Academic Press.

Labov, W., Ash, S., & Boberg, C. (n.d.). *Telsur Project at the Linguistics Laboratory, University of Pennsylvania Web Site.* Retrieved September 15, 2003, from http://www.ling.upenn.edu/phono_atlas/maps/Map8.html

Labov, W., Ash, S., & Boberg, C. (1997). *A national map of the regional dialects of American English.* Retrieved September 15, 2003, from the University of Pennsylvania Telsur Project Web site: http://www.ling.upenn.edu/phono_atlas/NationalMap/NationalMap.html

Ladefoged, P. (2001). *A course in phonetics* (4th ed.). Fort Worth, TX: Harcourt Brace.

Lehiste, I. (1970). *Suprasegmentals.* Cambridge: MIT Press.

Lowe, R. (1996). *Workbook for the identification of phonological processes.* Austin, Texas: Pro-Ed.

MacKay, I. (1987). *Phonetics: The science of speech production* (2nd ed.). Boston: College-Hill Press.

Ohde, R., & Sharf, D. (1992). Phonetic analysis of normal and abnormal speech. New York: Merrill.

Owens, R. (1991). *Language disorders: A functional approach to assessment and intervention* (2nd ed.). Boston: Allyn and Bacon.

Paul, R. (1995). *Language disorders from infancy through adolescence: Assessment and intervention.* St. Louis: Mosby.

Penfield, J., & Ornstein-Galicia, J. (1985). *Chicano English: An ethnic contact dialect.* Philadelphia: John Benjamins Publishing.

Perez, E. (1994). Phonological differences among speakers of Spanish-influenced English. In J. Bernthal & N. Bankson (Eds.), *Child phonology: Characteristics, assessment and intervention with special populations* (pp. 245–254). New York: Thieme.

Pike, K. L. (1945). *The intonation of American English.* Ann Arbor: University of Michigan Press.

Poole, I. (1934). Genetic development of articulation of consonant sounds in speech. *Elementary English Review, 11,* 159–161.

Power, T. (2003a). *Practice for Russian language backgrounds.* Retrieved September 15, 2003, from http://www.btinternet.com/~ted.power/l1russian.html

Power, T. (2003b). *Practice for Arabic language backgrounds.* Retrieved September 15, 2003, from http://www.btinternet.com/~ted.power/l1arabic.html

Prather, E. D., Hedrick, D. L., & Kern, C. A. (1975). Articulation development in children aged two to four years. *Journal of Speech and Hearing Disorders, 40,* 179–191.

Ramirez, R. R., & de la Cruz, G. P. (2003). *The Hispanic population in the United States: March 2002.* (U.S. Census Bureau, Current Population Reports, Series P20-545). Washington, DC: U.S. Government Printing Office.

Reed, V. (1994). *An introduction to children with language disorders* (2nd ed.). New York: Merrill.

Reeves, T., & Bennett, C. (2003). *The Asian and Pacific Islander population in the United States: March 2002.* (U.S. Census Bureau, Current Population Reports, Series P20-540). Washington, DC: U.S. Government Printing Office.

Sander, E. (1972). When are speech sounds learned? *Journal of Speech and Hearing Disorders, 37,* 55–63.

Schmidley, A. D. (2001). *Profile of the foreign-born population in the United States 2000.* (U.S. Census Bureau, Current Population Reports, Series P23-206). Washington, DC: U.S. Government Printing Office.

Shen, Y. (1962). *English phonetics.* Ann Arbor: University of Michigan Press.

Shriberg, L., & Kent, R. (2003). *Clinical phonetics* (3rd ed.). Boston: Allyn and Bacon.

Smit, A., Hand, L., Freilinger, J., Bernthal, J., & Bird, A. (1990). The Iowa articulation norms project and its Nebraska replication. *Journal of Speech and Hearing Disorders, 55,* 779–798.

Stampe, D. (1969). *The acquisition of phonetic representation.* Paper presented at the Fifth Regional Meeting of the Chicago Linguistic Society.

Stevick, R. D. (1968). *English and its history.* Boston: Allyn and Bacon.

Stoel-Gammon, C. (1996). Phonological assessment using a hierarchical framework. In K. N. Cole, P. S. Dale, & D. J. Thal (Eds.), *Communication and language intervention series: Vol. 6. Assessment of communication and language* (pp. 77–95). Baltimore: Brookes.

Stoel-Gammon, C., & Dunn, C. (1985). *Normal and disordered phonology in children.* Austin, TX: Pro-Ed.

Templin, M. C. (1957). *Certain language skills in children.* Minneapolis: The University of Minnesota Press.

Terrell, S., & Terrell, F. (1993). African American cultures. In D. Battle (Ed.), *Communication disorders in multicultural populations* (pp. 3–37). Boston: Andover Medical Publishers.

U.S. Census Bureau. (2003). *Table 5. Detailed list of languages spoken at home for the population 5 years and over by state: 2000.* Retrieved September 15, 2003, from http://www.census.gov/population/cen2000/phc-t20/tab05.pdf

Velleman, S. L. (1998). *Making phonology functional: What do I do first?* Boston: Butterworth-Heinemann.

Wellman, B., Case, M., Mengert, E., & Bradbury, D. (1931). *Speech sounds of young children.* (University of Iowa studies in Child Welfare, 5.) Iowa City: University of Iowa Press.

Wise, C. (1957). *Applied phonetics.* Englewood Cliffs, NJ: Prentice-Hall.

Wolfram, W. (1991). *Dialects and American English.* Englewood Cliffs, NJ: Prentice-Hall.

Wolfram, W. (1994). The phonology of a sociocultural variety: The case of African American Vernacular English. In J. Bernthal & N. Bankson (Eds.), *Child phonology: Characteristics, assessment and intervention with special populations* (pp. 227–244). New York: Thieme.

Wolfram, W., & Fasold, R. W. (1974). *The study of social dialects in American English.* Englewood Cliffs, NJ: Prentice-Hall.

Answers to Questions

Chapter 2

Chapter Exercises

2.1

4	lazy	4	smooth	3	cough		
5	spilled	6	driven	1	oh		
3	comb	2	why	5	raisin		

2.2

	shoe	X	mea<u>s</u>ure		o<u>ce</u>an		suffi<u>c</u>ient
	<u>ch</u>ord		liquor		bis<u>c</u>uit	X	rag
	m<u>oo</u>n		thr<u>ou</u>gh	X	th<u>ou</u>gh		s<u>ui</u>t
X	w<u>oo</u>d		d<u>o</u>ne		fl<u>oo</u>d		r<u>u</u>b
	i<u>c</u>e	X	wa<u>s</u>		pre<u>ss</u>		<u>s</u>cissors

2.3 Possible answers include:

1. deduct	4. scrutinize	7. dishonest	10. magnetize
2. protection	5. laborious	8. indecent	
3. potential	6. greatly	9. later	

2.4

1	caution	2	running	2	lived	3	relistened
2	warmly	1	finger	2	talker	1	kangaroo
3	prorated	2	clarinetist	2	sharply	2	swarming

2.5

1. lend	ɛ
2. man	æ
3. flick	ɪ
4. should	ʊ
5. rude	u
6. week	i

2.6 1. ram   _ɛ_
    2. laugh   _f_
    3. wish   _ʃ_
    4. sung   _ŋ_
    5. bath   _θ_
    6. leave   _v_

2.7 Sample minimal pairs include:

1. lame, came	6. harm, hard
2. rate, sate	7. toad, toes
3. doll, hall	8. well, wedge
4. wood, hood	9. cheat, cheese
5. coil, toil	10. rug, rush

2.8 1. /m, n, ŋ /
    2. /k, g, ŋ /
    3. /v/
    4. voice
    5. voiced

2.10 _1, 3, 5_ phonemic

     _2, 4, 5_ allophonic

      _2, 4_ impressionistic

2.11

ouch	**crab**	**hoe**	oats	elm	**your**
re act	**car go**	**be ware**	a **tone**	**cour** age	eat ing

2.12

shrine	scold	plea	produce	schism	**away**
elope	selfish	**auto**	biceps	flight	truce

2.13

through	spa	**rough**	bough	row	spray
law **ful**	**fun** ny	cre **ate**	**in verse**	**can** dy	re ply

2.14

O	pliant	C	comply	O	coerced	C	minutes
O	decree	C	encase	C	flatly	O	preface

2.15

C	pliant	O	comply	C	coerced	C	minutes
O	decree	C	encase	O	flatly	C	preface

2.16

propose	**contest**	**protest**	congress	**research**
project	consume	**compress**	reasoned	**confines**

2.17

decoy	**mirage**	**pastel**	puzzle	**regret**	**platoon**
stipend	thesis	**undo**	reason	falter	**Maureen**
timid	planted	**derail**	virtue	**restricts**	peon
transcend	**parade**	circus	**suspend**	movie	shoulder
lucid	**cajole**	**devoid**	**cassette**	**provide**	merchant

2.18	**pondering**	**edited**	**consequent**	**misery**	**calendar**	**ebony**
	plentiful	**asterisk**	pharyngeal	persona	distinctive	example
	surrounded	December	**caribou**	**underling**	Barbados	lasagna
	terrified	hydrangea	**telephoned**	contended	perfected	**India**
	musical	**skeletal**	courageous	umbrella	**Philistine**	perusal

2.19	**stupendous**	pliable	**creative**	carefully	elevate	magical
	corporal	answering	spectacle	**presumption**	**placenta**	**bananas**
	plantation	clarinet	murderer	predisposed	**decorum**	horribly
	heroic	violin	integer	**discover**	clavicle	**majestic**
	daffodil	**subscription**	expertise	**immoral**	muscular	**Hawaii**

Review Exercises

A.
1.	bread	4	5.	**plot**	4	9.	**fat**	3
2.	coughs	4	6.	stroke	5	10.	tomb	3
3.	throw	3	7.	**fluid**	5	11.	walked	4
4.	news	3	8.	**spew**	4	12.	**last**	4

B.
1.	clueless	2	6.	rewrite	2
2.	tomato	1	7.	winterized	3
3.	pumpkin	1	8.	edits	2
4.	likable	2	9.	thoughtlessness	3
5.	cheddar	1	10.	coexisting	3

C.
1.	box	flack	**puss**	6.	through	chow	**flew**
2.	buzz	**dogs**	fits	7.	tomb	**limb**	bob
3.	flag	lounge	**league**	8.	fleas	**wheeze**	mice
4.	cooked	**pant**	nagged	9.	laugh	**giraffe**	bough
5.	throw	cow	**beau**	10.	path	bathe	**cloth**

D.
1.	net	ten	6.	main	name
2.	sell	less	7.	pin	nip
3.	pots	stop	8.	ban	nab
4.	gnat	tan	9.	tack	cat
5.	need	dean	10.	tune	newt

E.
1.	church	**chef**	chop
2.	see	cent	**cut**
3.	**think**	this	these
4.	knee	**came**	nut
5.	phone	**please**	frost
6.	**song**	sure	sheep
7.	**gnat**	grim	groan
8.	cup	choir	**chore**
9.	gerbil	**goat**	George
10.	**their**	thanks	thing

F. Possible answers include:

1. sp<u>i</u>t	slit		6. f<u>a</u>n	fun	
2. <u>h</u>and	band		7. <u>th</u>ink	rink	
3. <u>p</u>ink	sink		8. ha<u>d</u>	hid	
4. <u>s</u>in	win		9. <u>t</u>ook	cook	
5. pai<u>l</u>	paid		10. r<u>o</u>b	rib	

G.
1. **maybe, baby**   6. **bribe, tribe**
2. plaid, prod   7. smart, dart
3. **looks, lacks**   8. dinner, runner
4. mail, snail   9. window, minnow
5. **prance, prince**   10. **lumpy, bumpy**

H.
1. mar<u>b</u>le	C		6. a<u>w</u>esome	O	
2. <u>pr</u>evious	O		7. mis<u>t</u>ake	C	
3. pa<u>tr</u>on	C		8. luck<u>y</u>	O	
4. <u>tr</u>ifle	O		9. prof<u>it</u>	C	
5. <u>so</u>dium	O		10. <u>s</u>ystem	C	

I.

	Onset Yes	No	Coda Yes	No
1. mentions	X		X	
2. icon		X		X
3. camper	X		X	
4. instinct		X	X	
5. able		X		X
6. lotion	X			X
7. charming	X		X	
8. asterisk		X	X	
9. Japan	X			X
10. aloof		X		X

J.
1	1. loser	2	6. provoke	1	11. plastic
2	2. unsure	1	7. stagnant	2	12. divorce
1	3. anxious	2	8. beside	1	13. western
2	4. disturb	2	9. germane	1	14. language
1	5. Grecian	2	10. gourmet	2	15. defer

K.   __2__   1. provincial   __1__   6. hypocrite   __3__   11. picturesque

       __1__   2. sorceress   __3__   7. indisposed   __1__   12. relegate

       __1__   3. indigent   __2__   8. uncertain   __2__   13. foundation

       __2__   4. commander   __2__   9. magenta   __2__   14. contagious

       __3__   5. arabesque   __1__   10. platypus   __1__   15. constable

L.   __3__   1. problematic   __3__   6. correlation   __3__   11. protozoan

       __1__   2. mercenary   __1__   7. catamaran   __3__   12. contradiction

       __2__   3. statistical   __2__   8. continuant   __1__   13. protoplasm

       __1__   4. ecosystem   __1__   9. allegory   __3__   14. Argentina

       __2__   5. gregarious   __2__   10. carnivorous   __2__   15. obstructionist

Chapter 3

Chapter Exercises

3.1 Possible answers include:

voiced   /r/, /l/, /d/

voiceless   /p/, /t/, /h/

3.2 The phoneme /p/ is produced by closing the lips.
The phoneme /w/ is produced by rounding the lips; the lips do not close.

3.3 The phoneme in the word <u>th</u>ink is voiceless: /θ/
The phoneme in the word <u>th</u>at is voiced: /ð/

Review Exercises

A.   velar   soft palate or velum

     alveolar   alveolar ridge

     lingual   tongue

     labial   lips

     palatal   hard palate

     glottal   glottis

     dental   teeth

B. 1. b
   2. c
   3. d
   4. a

C. 1. fundamental frequency   6. subglottal
   2. mandible   7. habitual
   3. in front of   8. eustachian tubes
   4. below   9. blade, apex
   5. diaphragm   10. front, back

Chapter 4

Preliminary Exercise 1

U	1. lean	R	6. throw
R	2. hook	U	7. back
R	3. road	U	8. then
U	4. mint	U	9. wait
R	5. chew	R	10. should

Preliminary Exercise 2

T	1. seek	L	3. singe	T	5. hot	L	7. map
L	2. push	L	4. head	T	6. hoot	T	8. clerk

Chapter Exercises

4.1—The Vowel /i/

A.
paper	train	**Cleveland**	**seaside**
please	picture	trip	trail
tribal	**machine**	labor	**trees**
settle	**screen**	**Toledo**	lip
nice	foreign	**Levi**	**jeans**

B.
/ist/	/flip/	/**min**/	/**hid**/
/**iv**/	/hig/	/lim/	/wins/
/rift/	/if/	/**trit**/	/**lik**/

C.
/lip/	leap	/it/	eat	/brizd/	breezed
/pip/	peep	/hip/	heap	/spik/	speak
/mit/	meat, meet	/sip/	seep	/klin/	clean
/rid/	reed, read	/did/	deed	/krist/	creased

D.
___	dream	drip	X	east	eaves
X	seek	wheel	___	chief	vein
___	same	land	___	base	lease
X	creek	steam	___	need	pain
X	bean	heed	X	creed	cream

4.2—The Vowel /ɪ/

B.
peace	friend	enthrall	**bitter**
mythical	**silver**	woman	**tryst**
click	**ingest**	**build**	**fear**
thread	**pink**	**bowling**	tried
pride	**clear**	**sporty**	**synchronize**

C. /vɪl/   /**sɪst**/   /**fɪld**/   /**wɪns**/
    /**izɪ**/   /klip/   /**spid**/   /hik/
    /**hɪr**/   /ɪl/   /sɪg/   /**pɪgɪ**/

D. /stip/   steep   /pɪk/   pick

    /pliz/   please   /kɪst/   kissed

    /mɪt/   mitt   /bik/   beak

    /dɪd/   did   /pɪp/   pip

    /fɪr/   fear   /mɪstɪ/   misty

    /rilɪ/   really   /ɪndid/   indeed

E. X   feel   teach   X   win   king

      ___   lip   thread   X   mint   inch

      X   been   drink   X   deed   flea

      ___   vent   list   X   dish   ill

      ___   tied   pig   X   kick   mill

F. 1. ___ flirt   5. X smeared   9. ___ stirred

    2. X peerless   6. ___ worried   10. ___ stared

    3. ___ bird   7. X steered   11. X earring

    4. ___ shrill   8. ___ harder   12. ___ cursor

4.3—The Vowel /e/ - /eɪ/

B. **trail**   **rage**   wheel   **palatial**
    vice   **razor**   manage   green
    transit   machine   **whale**   **potato**
    lazy   bread   football   temperate
    dale   tackle   **daily**   bright

C. /**freɪd**/   /deɪs/   /dɪnt/   /**deɪlɪ**/
    /**kreɪt**/   /**biz**/   /**spid**/   /**deɪm**/
    /**neɪp**/   /trips/   /**treɪ**/   /fril/
    /pɪln/   /**blid**/   /feɪlm/   /streɪp/

D. /bleɪz/   blaze   /pleɪket/   placate

    /pleɪd/   played   /rimeɪn/   remain

    /beɪn/   bane   /ɪnmeɪt/   inmate

    /iveɪd/   evade   /ribet/   rebate

    /krɪmp/   crimp   /steɪnd/   stained

    /rikt/   reeked   /deɪzɪ/   daisy

E. <u>O</u> crayon   <u>C</u> unmade

    <u>O</u> prepay   <u>O</u> stay

    <u>C</u> baking   <u>O</u> tailor

    <u>O</u> masonry   <u>C</u> betrayed

F. <u>   </u> braid hid   <u>X</u> state rain

    <u>   </u> feed hate   <u>   </u> fist flea

    <u>X</u> lane aim   <u>X</u> cringe hid

    <u>X</u> fill kissed   <u>   </u> deal will

    <u>   </u> treat sling   <u>X</u> wheel meat

4.4—The Vowel /ɛ/

B.
pimple	trip	**ensure**	tryst
syrup	**caring**	women	**contend**
pencil	butter	build	**pretzel**
thing	**thread**	**prepare**	tried
jeep	pistol	**unscented**	**remember**

C.
/**mɛrɪ**/	/hint/	/split/	/istɛr/
/**slɛpt**/	/fɛr/	/ɪrk/	/**meɪd**/
/**sɪsɪ**/	/kleɪ/	/wɛl/	/**krɪp**/

D.
/reɪk/	rake	/stɛr/	stare
/fɪz/	fizz	/treɪl/	trail
/smɛl/	smell	/prɪtɛnd/	pretend
/sid/	seed	/hɛvɪ/	heavy
/kreɪn/	crane	/friz/	freeze
/breɪzd/	braised	/blɛst/	blessed

E. <u>X</u> fill fear   <u>X</u> step edge

    <u>X</u> made cage   <u>   </u> bread breathe

    <u>   </u> wind best   <u>   </u> flit red

    <u>   </u> trade peel   <u>X</u> sill kit

    <u>X</u> rid sing   <u>X</u> care meant

F. <u>C</u> 1. trail   <u>O</u> 6. spree

    <u>O</u> 2. repay   <u>C</u> 7. arouse

    <u>C</u> 3. strike   <u>C</u> 8. rough

    <u>O</u> 4. plea   <u>O</u> 9. undo

    <u>C</u> 5. late   <u>O</u> 10. chow

G. 1. <u>X</u> share   6. <u>X</u> careful

2. ___ early   7. <u>X</u> sparrow

3. ___ dearly   8. ___ third

4. <u>X</u> compare   9. ___ corridor

5. ___ fluoride   10. ___ certain

4.5—The Vowel /æ/

B. **straddle**   **practice**   **lapse**   **revamp**
    pale   **panther**   **repast**   straight
    Lester   pacific   **pacify**   farmer
    baseball   **hanged**   **chances**   cards
    jazz   pistol   tamed   **bombastic**

C. /**klæd**/   /prid/   /strɪv/   /wæd/
    /**slæpt**/   /**bɪrd**/   /bæz/   /**trækt**/
    /web/   /steɪp/   /**sprɪg**/   /læzɪ/

D. /klæn/   <u>clan</u>   /spɪr/   <u>spear</u>

/sprɪnt/ <u>sprint</u>   /hɛrɪ/   <u>hairy, Harry</u>

/rɛk/   <u>wreck</u>   /pækt/   <u>packed</u>

/teɪstɪ/ <u>tasty</u>   /dræg/   <u>drag</u>

/præns/ <u>prance</u>   /bɛrɪ/   <u>berry</u>

/læft/   <u>laughed</u>   /tinz/   <u>teens</u>

E. ___   badge   rage   <u>X</u>   hair   bend

___   seed   shade   <u>X</u>   lick   beer

___   cab   blonde   ___   beak   bless

<u>X</u>   tray   whale   ___   trap   bake

<u>X</u>   crank   shag   <u>X</u>   lapse crag

4.6—The Vowel /u/

A. **ghoul**   oboe   **crew**   plural
    butter   stuck   **Lucifer**   must
    should   luck   lusty   shook
    fuchsia look   molding   **stupor**
    loosely **glue** blouse   **choose**

B. /ust/   /**krud**/   /prus/   /**tul**/
    /suv/   /tug/   /pus/   /**wund**/
    /**pul**/   /rup/   /**lus**/   /slug/

C. /spun/   spoon   /sup/   soup
    /tun/   tune   /lud/   lewd
    /rut/   root   /stru/   strew
    /mud/   mood   /flu/   flew, flue, flu
    /klu/   clue   /grum/   groom
    /ruf/   roof   /snut/   snoot

D. ___ 1. could   showed   ___ 6. brood   hood
    _X_ 2. suit   loon   _X_ 7. stood   could
    ___ 3. lute   book   ___ 8. hoops   poor
    _X_ 4. crew   scoot   _X_ 9. feud   moose
    _X_ 5. push   foot   ___ 10. muse   cook

E. ___ 1. oozing   _X_ 6. fuming
    _X_ 2. cute   ___ 7. Pluto
    _X_ 3. huge   _X_ 8. useful
    ___ 4. ruined   _X_ 9. viewing
    ___ 5. sloop   ___ 10. spooky

4.7—The Vowel /ʊ/

B. hole   **wooden**   snooze   stunned
    shut   punched   luscious   spook
    hood   **couldn't**   **pulled** **shook**
    flushed   **mistook**   beauty   person
    rudely   **cooker**   brood   **stood**

C. /**buk**/   /stʊ/   /**rul**/   /sul/
    /lʊv/   /**lum**/   /rʊk/   /**frut**/
    /**trups**/   /stʊr/   /**buts**/   /slʊg/

D. /pʊs/   puss   /tʊr/   tour
    /tru/   true   /hʊk/   hook
    /stʊd/   stood   /lum/   loom
    /dum/   doom   /fluk/   fluke
    /gru/   grew   /prun/   prune
    /good/   good   /krʊk/   crook

E. ___ 1. loot   foot   ___ 6. what   look
    _X_ 2. tune   mute   _X_ 7. nook   stood
    _X_ 3. coupe   soon   ___ 8. rust   rook
    ___ 4. flood   cute   _X_ 9. goof   cruise
    _X_ 5. would   soot   ___ 10. mutt   look

4.8—The Vowel /o/ - /ou/

B.

mope	aloof	root	**toll**
noose	**slowed**	pond	push
soda	lost	**loaded**	**lasso**
nosy	book	sugar	**remote**
dole	**spoke**	doily	**wholly**

C.

/tou/	/boʊn/	/stʊp/	/prʊb/
/bʊt/	/floʊd/	/boʊd/	/krud/
/stub/	/stud/	/flʊk/	/woʊnt/

D.

/moʊld/	mold	/tupeɪ/	toupee
/kupt/	cooped	/bruzd/	bruised
/boʊnɪ/	bony	/bændeɪd/	Band-Aid
/ivoʊk/	evoke	/kʊkɪ/	cookie
/stoʊd/	stowed	/koʊɛd/	coed
/doʊpɪ/	dopey	/rizum/	resume

E.

o	Romania	ou	snowman
ou	corroded	o	location
ou	stolen	ou	jello
ou	magnolia	o	coagulate

4.9—The Vowel /ɔ/

A.

/bɔt/	/drʊm/	/stɔn/	/brɔn/
/koʊt/	/grɔn/	/tɔk/	/pʊl/
/lups/	/fɔrt/	/flum/	/ɔrn/

B.

/spɔrt/	sport	/sprɔl/	sprawl
/kʊd/	could	/stʊd/	stood
/proʊb/	probe	/frɔt/	fraught
/pruv/	prove	/kɔrps/	corpse
/stɔrd/	stored	/hʊkt/	hooked
/ɔfʊl/	awful	/doʊnet/	donate

C.

1. ___	farm	4. X	storm	7. ___	lured		
2. ___	third	5. ___	worm	8. ___	worth		
3. X	horrid	6. X	thorn	9. ___	spar		

4.10—The Vowel /ɑ/

B.

/wond/	/tɔb/	**/hɑrm/**	**/blɑb/**
/koʊd/	/sɔt/	/blɑd/	**/ɑrmɪ/**
/frɔd/	/pʊnt/	**/ɑd/**	**/kɑd/**

C. /frɑst/ frost   /zɑr/ czar

/lʊkt/ looked   /prund/ pruned

/bɔrd/ board, bored   /blɔnd/ blonde

/kroʊm/ chrome   /ɑnsɛt/ onset

/wɑnt/ want   /krɔdæd/ crawdad

/stɑrvd/ starved   /ɑrdvɑrk/ aardvark

D.
1. ___ war   7. ___ orchard
2. ___ cleared   8. X March
3. ___ quartz   9. ___ poorly
4. ___ flare   10. X smarter
5. X starred   11. X carbon
6. ___ dirt   12. ___ spore

4.11—The Vowel /ə/

A. rowing **decision** **control** **untamed** laundry
lasagna injure glamour **opera** **petunia**
wooded poorly **motion** puppy cockroach
Laverne ruled holding **fuchsia** **lotion**

B. /sətɪn/ /zəbrɑ/ **/əbeɪt/** **/əluf/**
/drɑmə/ /ləpʊr/ **/bəlun/** /rədæn/
/səpoʊz/ /rəpik/ **/brəzɪl/** **/əndu/**

C. /pinət/ peanut   /kəntein/ contain

/əkrɑs/ across   /lɛmən/ lemon

/vəlɔr/ velour   /bətɑn/ baton

/səpɔrt/ support   /əwɔrd/ award

/kɔfɪn/ coffin   /eɪprəl/ April

/plətun/ platoon   /kəsɛt/ cassette

4.12—The Vowel /ʌ/

B. awful **blunder** laundry Hoover
custard laborious **Sunday** lawyer
pushy cushion **hundred** **trumpet**
cologne **abundant** plural shouldn't
charades mundane wander conducive

C. 1. hooked   /hʌkt/   X
    2. bond   /bʊnd/   X
    3. bluff   /blʌf/   ___
    4. hood   /hʊd/   X
    5. cluck   /klʌk/   ___
    6. rookie   /rʌkɪ/   X
    7. mistook   /mɪstʊk/   ___
    8. lucky   /lʌkɪ/   ___
    9. rubbing   /rʊbɪŋ/   X
    10. crooked   /krɔkəd/   X

D. /klʊstɪ/   /əpʌft/   /dʊkɪ/   /sʌntæn/
    /**rizən**/   /krɑmd/   /**pʊlɪ**/   /vɪstʌ/
    /**mʌstɪ**/   /əndʌn/   /**plʌmət**/ /**plæzə**/

E. /pɛrəs/   Paris   /robʌst/   robust
    /hʌnɪ/   honey   /sʌdən/   sudden
    /əlɑt/   allot; a lot   /kəbus/   caboose
    /kənvɪns/ convince   /tʌndrə/   tundra
    /gɑrdəd/   guarded   /kəlæps/   collapse
    /flʌbd/   flubbed   /bəfun/   buffoon

F. lumber   /ʌ/ /ə/   suspend /ʌ/ /ə/
    abort   /ʌ/ /ə/   suppose /ʌ/ /ə/
    shaken   /ʌ/ /ə/   induct   /ʌ/ /ə/
    contain /ʌ/ /ə/   serpent /ʌ/ /ə/
    thunder /ʌ/ /ə/   rusty   /ʌ/ /ə/

G. ___ 1. nuts   could   ___ 6. crook fund
    ___ 2. foot   stoop   X   7. blood crust
    X   3. done   rubbed   X   8. runs   floods
    X   4. crumb rust   X   9. loom   food
    X   5. cook   should   ___ 10. rush   look

4.13—The Vowel /ɚ/

B. **clover**   rebel   barley   dearly
    fearless   endear   **perjure**   **fester**
    carbon   torment   **harbor**   electric
    tremor   written   poorly   breezy
    laundered   **perhaps**   torpedo   **surprise**

C. /kɑnvɚt/　　/pəteɪn/　　/pɚsɛnt/　　/lɛpəd/
　 /rɑbɚ/　　　/tɚoʊd/　　/drɪmɚ/　　/fɚəst/
　 /sɚvɛs/　　　/ɚɛdɪ/　　　/ʌnfɛr/　　/hɪndɚ/

D. /drɛsɚ/　　　dresser _____　　/kəntɔrt/　　contort _____
　 /kæmrə/　　　camera _____　　/pɚɑnə/　　piranha _____
　 /rʌbɚ/　　　rubber _____　　/pɚu/　　　Peru _____
　 /mɑrbəl/　　marble _____　　/sɪmɚ/　　simmer _____
　 /tɚeɪn/　　　terrain _____　　/kɛrosin/　　kerosene _____
　 /flʌstɚd/　　flustered _____　　/əweɪtəd/　　awaited _____

4.14—The Vowel /ɝ/

B. forward　　muster　　warship　　steered　　morale
　 disturbed　pretend　**wordy**　　distort　　persistent
　 terrible　　**turban**　January　　**conserve**　choir
　 conversion　arid　　**stirrup**　barren　　fearless

C. /kʌstɚd/　　/lɝdɪ/　　/kɚrɪr/　　/vɝsəz/
　 /pɝsən/　　　/hɝdəd/　　/fɝmɚ/　　/dɝsənt/
　 /plædʒɚ/　　/fɔrən/　　/ɝbɔrt/　　/kɝsɚ/

D. /smɝkt/　　　smirked _____　　/kənvɚt/　　convert _____
　 /ovɝt/　　　overt _____　　　/wɪspɚ/　　whisper _____
　 /kɛrət/　　　carrot _____　　　/bɝbən/　　bourbon _____
　 /sʌbɚb/　　　suburb _____　　　/skwɝəl/　　squirrel _____
　 /supɝb/　　　superb _____　　　/səhɛrə/　　Sahara _____

E. erasure　　/ɝ/ /ɚ/　　　ermine　/ɝ/ /ɚ/
　 surprise　　/ɝ/ /ɚ/　　　color　　/ɝ/ /ɚ/
　 furnace　　/ɝ/ /ɚ/　　　infer　　/ɝ/ /ɚ/
　 curtail　　/ɝ/ /ɚ/　　　terror　　/ɝ/ /ɚ/
　 immerse　　/ɝ/ /ɚ/　　　duster　/ɝ/ /ɚ/

F. ___ 1. herd　cheered　　　___ 6. hair　queer
　 ___ 2. cord　word　　　　 X 7. birch　lurk
　 ___ 3. lured　stored　　　 X 8. hoard　lord
　 X 4. ark　smart　　　　___ 9. pear　heard
　 X 5. fears　cheer　　　___ 10. term　peered

G.   ɝ   1. myrth   ɪr   11. appearance
     ɛr   2. flared   ɛr   12. Carol
     ɪr   3. cirrus   ɝ   13. furtive
     ɛr   4. serenade   ɛr   14. larynx
     ɝ   5. Merlin   ɪr   15. experience
     ɛr   6. cherub   ɝ   16. disturbing
     ɔr   7. portion   ɪr   17. clearance
     ɑr   8. farming   ɝ   18. nervous
     ɛr   9. sparrow   ɝ,ʊr   19. furious
     ɝ   10. nervous   ɛr   20. clairvoyant

4.15—The Diphthong /aɪ/

B. power   spacious   machine   replaced
   slice   delicious   **formica**   traded
   contrite **spider**   maybe   **piped**
   lever   **Cairo**   **cider**   **supplied**
   rivalry razor   piano   spigot

C. /**fraɪdeɪ**/   /braɪmɚ/   /taɪfraɪn/   /rəvaɪz/
   /məbaɪ/   /**naɪlɔn**/   /prədaɪt/   /**traɪdɛnt**/
   /**traɪd**/   /laɪɚ/   /**haɪəst**/   /**straɪpt**/

D. /sɚpraɪz/   surprise ___   /klaɪmaks/   climax ___
   /kəlaɪd/   collide ___   /preɪlin/   praline ___
   /treɪlɚ/   trailer ___   /baɪsɛps/   biceps ___
   /praɪmeɪt/ primate ___   /waɪɚd/   wired ___
   /vaɪrəs/   virus ___   /taɪred/   tirade ___
   /deɪlaɪt/   daylight ___   /daɪmənd/   diamond ___

4.16—The Diphthong /ɔɪ/

B. repay   **hoisted**   **voiceless** reward
   loiter crowded   fiery   tiled
   straight   feisty   **coy**   **cloying**
   crime   **broiler**   stoic   **destroy**
   goiter razor   **avoid**   supplied

C. /**kwaɪət**/   /sprɔɪdɪn/   /dɔɪɚz/   /**plɔɪdənt**/
   /**mɝdɚ**/   /**blaɪndlɪ**/ /ənstraɪt/   /**taɪpsɛt**/
   /**pɔɪzən**/   /**vɔɪdəd**/   /rikɔɪld/   /taɪwɑn/

D. /ɔɪlɪ/ oily   /ændrɔɪd/ android

  /maɪstroʊ/ maestro   /laɪvlɪ/ lively

  /taɪfɔɪd/ typhoid   /ɪnvɔɪs/ invoice

  /parbɔɪl/ parboil   /ɔɪstɚ/ oyster

  /haɪndsaɪt/ hindsight   /haɪɔɪd/ hyoid

  /baɪaʊt/ buyout   /deɪlaɪt/ daylight

4.17—The Diphthong /aʊ/

B. toilet   **dowdy**   **frown**   **bounty**
  mousy   **allowed**   loaded   probate
  beauty   explode   soils   **proud**
  astound   toil   **chowder**   crowbar
  hello   toad   chastise   scrolled

C. /taɪɚd/   /laʊzɪ/   /aɪvrɪ/   /hoʊmbɔɪ/
  /rɪbaʊ/   /blaʊkɚ/   /rɔɪdɪ/   /kaʊtaʊ/
  /waʊntɪd/   /roʊgbɪ/   /paʊzɚ/   /aʊɚlɪ/

D. /bɔɪfrɛnd/ boyfriend   /roʊboʊt/ rowboat

  /klɑndaɪk/ Klondike   /pispaɪp/ peace pipe

  /daʊntaʊn/ downtown   /sɚaʊnd/ surround

  /sloʊɚ/ slower   /doʊnʌt/ doughnut

  /faʊndəd/ founded   /klaɪənt/ client

  /vaɪzɚ/ visor   /braʊzɚ/ browser

Review Exercises

A.

ʊ	high	back	yes	lax
ɝ	mid	central	yes	tense
ə	mid	central	no	lax
o	high-mid	back	yes	tense
u	high	back	yes	tense
ɛ	low-mid	front	no	lax
ɚ	mid	central	yes	lax
ʌ	low-mid	back-central	no	lax
e	high-mid	front	no	tense
ɪ	high	front	no	lax
ɑ	low	back	no	tense
ɔ	low-mid	back	yes	tense
æ	low	front	no	lax

B. 1. æ, bad
    2. ʌ, sun
    3. ɛ, slept
    4. u, soup
    5. ɔ, cord
    6. ʊ, foot
    7. ɪ, fizz
    8. ɑ, park
    9. ɝ, word
    10. oʊ, crows

C. 1. Sunday   L   T
    2. bashful   L   L
    3. laundry   T   L
    4. confused   L   T
    5. fender   L   L
    6. concern   L   T
    7. regroup   T   T
    8. obese   T   T
    9. layette   T   L
    10. abrupt   L   L

D. 1. foolish   R   U
    2. curfew   R   R
    3. decade   U   U
    4. collate   R   U
    5. football   R   U
    6. Pluto   R   R
    7. person   R   U
    8. pursuit   R   R
    9. rugby   U   U
    10. lower   R   U

E. /eɪ/   1. straight
    /i/   2. bees
    /ɛ/   3. bread
    /æ/   4. can
    /ɪ/   5. filled
    /ɪ/   6. bring
    /æ/   7. lapse
    /æ/   8. sang
    /ɛ/   9. fair
    /i/   10. mean
    /ɛ/   /ɪ/   11. empty
    /eɪ/   /ɪ/   12. rabies
    /ɪ/   /ɛ/   13. instead
    /æ/   /i/   14. stampede
    /eɪ/   /e/   15. vacate
    /i/   /ɪ/   16. pleasing
    /æ/   /ɪ/   17. transit
    /ɪ/   /æ/   18. beer can
    /ɪ/   /æ/   19. implant
    /ɛr/   /ɪ/   20. barely

F. /oʊ/   1. moat
    /ʊ/   2. push
    /ɑ/   3. laud
    /ɑ/   4. locks
    /u/   5. crude
    /oʊ/   6. chose
    /ɑ/   7. raw
    /ʊ/   8. lure
    /ɔr/   9. sword
    /ɑr/   10. card
    /ɑ/   /ʊ/   11. awful
    /ɔr/   /ɑ/   12. Clorox
    /oʊ/   /oʊ/   13. loco
    /oʊ/   /oʊ/   14. oboe
    /ɑ/   /oʊ/   15. taco
    /ɑ/   /ɑr/   16. monarch
    /ɑ/   /ɔr/   17. popcorn
    /u/   /ʊ/   18. truthful
    /ɑ/   /u/   19. costume
    /u/   /ɑ/   20. crouton

G. /ɝ/ /ə/   1. certain   /ɝ/   /ə/   11. purpose

    /ʌ/ /ə/   2. rusted   /ʌ/   /ə/   12. sudden

    /ɚ/ /ɝ/   3. perturb   /ʌ/   /ɚ/   13. luster

    /ə/ /ɝ/   4. assert   /ɝ/   /ə/   14. purchase

    /ʌ/ /ɚ/   5. upper   /ɝ/   /ə/   15. sherbet

    /ɝ/ /ɚ/   6. merger   /ʌ/   /ɚ/   16. mother

    /ʌ/ /ə/   7. clutter   /ə/   /ɝ/   17. converge

    /ɝ/ /ə/   8. verbal   /ɝ/   /ɚ/   18. herder

    /ə/ /ɝ/   9. traverse   /ɝ/   /ə/   19. worded

    /ɝ/ /ə/ 10. learner   /ʌ/   /ɚ/   20. mustard

H. 1. word   /wɝd/   16. maestro   /maɪstroʊ/
    2. lard   /lɔrd/   /ɑr/   17. flour   /floʊɚ/   /aʊ/
    3. carp   /kɝp/   /ɑr/   18. pouring   /pɔrɪŋ/
    4. war   /wɑr/   /ɔr/   19. liar   /laɪɚ/
    5. mere   /mɪr/   20. appear   /əpɛr/   /ɪr/
    6. wide   /weɪd/   /aɪ/   21. tighter   /taɪtɝ/   /ɚ/
    7. curd   /kʊrd/   /ɝ/   22. parrot   /pɝət/   /ɛr/
    8. stay   /steɪ/   23. corner   /kɔrnɚ/
    9. pray   /praɪ/   /eɪ/   24. oyster   /ɔɪstɛr/   /ɚ/
   10. crow   /kraʊ/   /oʊ/   25. squarely /skwɛrlɪ/
   11. coin   /kɔɪn/   26. silence   /sɪləns/   /aɪ/
   12. pride   /praɪd/   27. smarter   /smɔrtɚ/   /ɑr/
   13. firm   /fɪrm/   /ɝ/   28. avoid   /əvaɪd/   /ɔɪ/
   14. tour   /tʊr/   29. prowess   /prowəs/   /aʊ/
   15. fair   /fɛr/   30. license   /leɪsəns/   /aɪ/

I. 1. p____   pier (peer), pour (poor), pore , par, pear (pair), purr
    2. r____   rear, roar, rare
    3. d____t   dart, dirt
    4. w____d   weird, ward, word
    5. k____d   cord, card, cared, curd

J. 1. ____d   id, aid, Ed, add, oohed, owed, odd
    2. ____n   in, an, own, on, urn (earn)
    3. l____st   least, list, laced, lest, last, lost, lust
    4. sk____n   skin, skein, scan, scone
    5. st____d   steed, stayed (staid), stead, stewed, stood, stowed, stirred, stud
    6. b____rd   beard, bared, board (bored), bard, bird
    7. t____nt   tint, taint, tent, taunt
    8. s____t   seat, sit, sate, set, sat, suit, soot, saught, sot
    9. r____t   writ, rate, rat, root, rote, rot, rut
   10. r____bd   ribbed, robed, robbed, rubbed
   11. sp____t   spit, spate, spat, spot, spurt
   12. w____d   weed, wade, wed, wooed, wood (would), wad, word

K.
1. customs
2. abound
3. toward
4. slender
5. carefree
6. vacant
7. bunted
8. cloudy
9. stapler
10. contort
11. sirens
12. cloistered
13. Ohio
14. radio
15. corrosive
16. platonic
17. resonate
18. digress
19. siphoned
20. Arkansas
21. wonderful
22. calendar
23. remorseful
24. stupendous
25. laxative
26. sincerely
27. colander
28. Raisinettes
29. baritone
30. December
31. Mexico
32. quagmire
33. orderly
34. herbicide
35. repulsive
36. character
37. sassafras
38. xylophone
39. quarterback
40. embarrassed

L.

/ɛ/	/ɪ/	1. epic	/ɪ/	/ɪ/	21. inkling
/æ/	/ɚ/	2. faster	/ɛr/	/æ/	22. Fairbanks
/ʌ/	/ɚ/	3. wonder	/ɑr/	/u/	23. car pool
/ɑ/	/ɛ/	4. octet	/ə/	/i/	24. machine
/ʊ/	/ə/	5. woolen	/æ/	/ə/	25. Athens
/i/	/oʊ/	6. depot	/ɑ/	/ə/	26. autumn
/oʊ/	/ɚ/	7. soldier	/i/	/ə/	27. rebus
/ɪ/	/ɪ/	8. itchy	/ɔr/	/ɛ/	28. torment
/ɝ/	/ɪ/	9. worship	/ʌ/	/ɚ/	29. utter
/æ/	/ə/	10. palace	/ʊ/	/ə/	30. bushel
/ɛr/	/ɪ/	11. barely	/ɔr/	/ɚ/	31. corner
/eɪ/	/ə/	12. nation	/ɑ/	/ɪ/	32. quandary
/i/	/ə/	13. genius	/æ/	/ɚ/	33. aster
/ʌ/	/ɚ/	14. cupboard	/oʊ/	/u/	34. phone booth
/ɑr/	/u/	15. cartoon	/ɝ/	/ə/	35. turban
/æ/	/ɪ/	16. nasty	/i/	/eɪ/	36. key case
/ɪr/	/ə/	17. fearless	/ɔr/	/ɚ/	37. boarder
/ʌ/	/ɚ/	18. number	/ɛr/	/ɪ/	38. blaring
/æ/	/ə/	19. sanction	/æ/	/ə/	39. strangle
/oʊ/	/ə/	20. ocean	/ɔ/	/ə/	40. awesome

M. /ɔɪ/ /ɚ/   1. broiler   /ɛ/   /ɚ/   16. gender

/aʊ/ /æ/   2. mousetrap   /aɪ/ /ə/   17. China

/ɔr/ /ɑ/   3. boardwalk   /ɔ/   /ɪ/   18. jaundiced

/oʊ/ /ɚ/   4. closure   /ɝ/   /ɔɪ/ 19. turquoise

/aɪ/ /ɑ/   5. nylons   /i/   /ɔɪ/ 20. invoice

/ɛr/ /ɔɪ/ 6. steroid   /aɪ/ /æ/   21. financed

/ɑr/ /ʌ/   7. starstruck   /ɝ/   /ə/   22. merchant

/ə/   /i/   8. regime   /o/   /eɪ/ 23. proclaim

/æ/   /ʊ/   9. bashful   /oʊ/ /e/   24. probate

/ɝ/   /ɚ/   10. perjure   /ə/   /aɪ/ 25. July

/ɪr/ /ɪ/   11. spearmint   /ɑr/ /ə/   26. martian

/aɪ/ /ʌ/   12. lightbulb   /u/   /ɚ/   27. future

/i/   /ɔɪ/ 13. destroy   /ɑ/   /ɛ/   28. prospect

/æ/   /ə/   14. banquet   /ɑ/   /ə/   29. product

/aɪ/ /ɔr/ 15. eyesore   /o/   /u/   30. tofu

Chapter 5

Preliminary Exercise 1

a 1. s̲eem   b 6. oil̲y

c 2. tra̲de   a 7. hot̲dog

b 3. a̲w̲ay   b 8. ha̲s̲ten

a 4. c̲ruise   b 9. o̲pen

c 5. oa̲f   c 10. foot̲ball

Preliminary Exercise 2

f 1. /r/

a 2. /d/

e 3. /w/

b 4. /f/

d 5. /n/

c 6. /tʃ/

Preliminary Exercise 3

___	1.	me, we	___	6.	shoot, suit
X	2.	seal, zeal	___	7.	flame, blame
___	3.	plan, clan	X	8.	dram, tram
___	4.	lice, rice	___	9.	yes, chess
X	5.	grain, crane	X	10.	vender, fender

Chapter Exercises

5.1—The Stop Consonants

A.

___	1.	wish	___	6.	runs	___	11.	church	X	16.	think
X	2.	spring	X	7.	whisper	X	12.	tomb	___	17.	rummage
___	3.	loom	X	8.	question	X	13.	logical	___	18.	realm
X	4.	brush	X	9.	system	___	14.	jeans	X	19.	guess
X	5.	window	___	10.	phase	X	15.	Stephen	X	20.	fox

B.
1. *Contains a high front vowel* — perky, green
2. *Contains a voiceless alveolar stop* — about
3. *Contains no stops* — man
4. *Contains a velar stop* — perky, could, plaque, green
5. *Contains a central vowel* — about, perky
6. *Ends with a voiceless sound* — about, plaque
7. *Begins with a voiced sound* — man, about, green
8. *Contains a back vowel and a voiced stop* — could
9. *Begins with a voiceless sound* — perky, could, plaque
10. *Contains a front vowel and a voiceless stop* — perky, plaque

C.

___	1.	table	___	6.	uncle	___	11.	pushin'	___	16.	talkin'
T	2.	better	G	7.	written	T	12.	splatter	G	17.	bitten
___	3.	errand	G	8.	beaten	T	13.	rotted	T	18.	wedded
___	4.	listen	___	9.	walked	G	14.	sweatin'	G	19.	rotten
G	5.	quittin'	___	10.	Lincoln	T	15.	bottle	T	20.	fodder

D.

t	1.	wished	t	6.	danced	d	11.	sailed	d	16.	crabbed
d	2.	loaded	t	7.	wrapped	t	12.	leased	t	17.	placed
t	3.	endorsed	d	8.	hanged	t	13.	reached	t	18.	meshed
d	4.	dangered	t	9.	hoped	d	14.	toted	d	19.	burned
d	5.	robbed	d	10.	traded	t	15.	wrecked	d	20.	carved

E. 1. /kipɚt/
   2. /təkɪd/
   3. /ədɛbt/
   4. /pauɾɚ/

   5. /pɝkt/
   6. /pækət/
   7. /tɛpɪd/
   8. /taɪɾɚ/

   9. /pɝpət/
   10. /pɪkɪ/
   11. /ətæk/
   12. /tɔrkot/

   13. /tʊkɪ/
   14. /gækət/
   15. /dɛrbɪ/
   16. /pipʔd/

F. 1. pottery
   2. puckered
   3. potato
   4. doctor
   5. target
   6. puppet

   7. guppy
   8. packing
   9. diapered
   10. paperboy
   11. daiquiri
   12. dieted

G. 1. direct   no error
   2. tighter   no error
   3. petted   /pɛɾəd/
   4. corker   no error
   5. Carter   /kɑrɾɚ/

   6. partake   /pɑrteɪk/
   7. repeat   /ripit/ or /rəpit/
   8. poet   no error
   9. oboe   no error
   10. paper   /peɪpɚ/

H. 1. /kɪd/   kid
   2. /igɚ/   eager
   3. /tɛpɪd/   tepid
   4. /əbʌt/   abut
   5. /dɑkt/   docked
   6. /gɔdɪ/   gaudy

I. 1. /keɪp/
   2. /pɛrd/
   3. /dɔg/ or /dɑg/
   4. /taɪd/
   5. /kɛpt/
   6. /dɛt/
   7. /beɪk/
   8. /pɔr/
   9. /bɔrd/
   10. /pɔrk/
   11. /pit/
   12. /toʊp/
   13. /tʊk/
   14. /pʌt/
   15. /koʊt/
   16. /əpɑrt/
   17. /gɑrdəd/
   18. /boʊɾɚ/
   19. /babɪ/
   20. /bɑrɾɚ/

   21. /bɪgɚ/
   22. /bikɚ/
   23. /tubɚ/
   24. /kæbɪ/
   25. /pɪrd/
   26. /bækt/
   27. /pɝkɪ/
   28. /gɪrd/
   29. /dægɚ/
   30. /gɪdɪ/
   31. /kɑrpət/
   32. /dɑktɚ/
   33. /tɪkət/
   34. /dɛkt/
   35. /taɪɚd/
   36. /bɪgɚ/
   37. /dəbeɪt/ or /dibeɪt/
   38. /tɔrɪd/
   39. /pɛrət/
   40. /dɝɾɪ/

5.2—The Nasal Consonants

A.
X	1. ring	X	6. jasmine	X	11. moan	X	16. ripen
X	2. bomb	___	7. crease	X	12. spanking	X	17. unfair
___	3. pet	X	8. inside	___	13. possible	X	18. monkey
___	4. stop	___	9. trait	X	14. trench	___	19. lure
X	5. tomb	X	10. loaner	X	15. lung	___	20. failure

B.
X	1. **angle**	___	8. singe	X	15. banging
___	2. angel	___	9. ginger	X	16. manx
X	3. brink	___	10. danger	___	17. ingest
X	4. **mango**	X	11. blinker	X	18. singer
___	5. Angie	X	12. **hanger**	X	19. **hunger**
X	6. **single**	X	13. ringing	X	20. **jangle**
___	7. conjure	X	14. **mingle**	___	21. congeal

C. See exercise B directly above (**bold words**).

D.
___	1. hinge	___	7. ring	X	13. tango
X	2. bangle	___	8. drank	___	14. flange
___	3. wings	___	9. onyx	___	15. engine
X	4. single	X	10. tingle	X	16. English
___	5. wrong	___	11. bungee	___	17. tongue
X	6. mangle	X	12. kangaroo	___	18. dangerous

E.
___	1. pharynx	X	7. engine	X	13. ginger
X	2. England	___	8. flank	___	14. blanket
X	3. bungee	___	9. tingle	___	15. tongue
___	4. length	X	10. lunge	X	16. danger
___	5. lungs	___	11. strength	X	17. vengeance
___	6. jungle	___	12. tango	X	18. ranges

F. 1. *Contains an initial labial sound*   mutton, bank
    2. *Contains a voiced initial sound*   good, mutton, bank, napped
    3. *Ends with a stop*   good, bank, napped, code
    4. *Contains a central vowel*   mutton, curving, taken, carton
    5. *Ends with a voiceless sound*   bank, napped
    6. *Contains a velar nasal*   curving, bank
    7. *Contains a syllabic consonant*   mutton, carton
    8. *Contains no nasals*   good, code
    9. *Contains a low front vowel and a labial consonant*   bank, napped
    10. *Contains a velar consonant and a back vowel*   good, carton, code

G. 1. /kæmp/   4. /pɪnt/   7. /kræŋkɪ/   10. /bʌmpɪ/
    2. /neɪm/   5. /tɪŋgə/   8. /kɔrn/   11. /pɪntoʊ/
    3. /mɛlɪ/   6. /nɪŋgɪd/   9. /dænk/   12. /pɑrmɔɪ/

H. 1. nab   7. candy
    2. conned   8. appoint
    3. amass   9. cooking
    4. anger   10. tumor
    5. morning   11. tighten
    6. bending   12. minded

I. 1. camper   no error   6. pecking   /pɛkɪŋ/
    2. adorn   no error   7. Dayton   /deɪ ʔn̩/
    3. duffer   /dʌfɚ/   8. batter   /bæɾɚ/
    4. bunting   no error   9. baking   /beɪkɪŋ/
    5. bingo   /bɪŋgoʊ/   10. doorknob   /dɔrnɑb/

J. 1. /kænd/   canned
    2. /mʌnɪ/   money
    3. /əteɪn/   attain
    4. /kɑŋgoʊ/   congo
    5. /bɝpt/   burped

K.
1. /mɪŋk/		21. /ʌndɚ/	
2. /pɝt/		22. /tæŋkəd/	
3. /tæn/		23. /pinʌt/	
4. /kɪŋ/		24. /dændɪ/	
5. /dʌn/		25. /parteɪk/	
6. /nid/		26. /mʌndeɪ/	
7. /bæŋ/		27. /noʊmæd/	
8. /noʊm/		28. /baŋgoʊ/	
9. /mʌŋk/		29. /mædəm/	
10. /kɔɪn/		30. /gændɚ/	
11. /ɝn/		31. /omɪt/	
12. /nut/		32. /nəgeɪt/	
13. /taʊn/		33. /tunɪk/	
14. /mud/		34. /daŋkɪ/	
15. /naɪt/		35. /kəmænd/	
16. /dʌm/		36. /mɪrɚ/	
17. /kʊd/		37. /kaʊnˀn̩/ or /kaʊntɪn/	
18. /tɔrn/		38. /dɛrɪŋ/	
19. /tʌŋ/		39. /ɛmpaɪɚ/	
20. /gɔn/		40. /kaʊɚd/	

5.3—The Fricative Consonants

A.
X 1. push	X 6. brazen	___ 11. Montana	___ 16. hombre
X 2. thesis	X 7. cares	X 12. pleasure	X 17. leaks
___ 3. loom	___ 8. burlap	X 13. leather	X 18. worthy
X 4. happy	X 9. croissant	___ 14. marrow	___ 19. crouton
X 5. caution	X 10. vender	X 15. other	X 20. rajah

B.
___ 1. mishap	___ 8. badge	ʃ 15. Sean	
ʒ 2. usually	ʒ 9. lesion	ʃ 16. passion	
ʒ 3. decision	ʃ 10. lotion	ʃ 17. ricochet	
___ 4. cheese	ʒ 11. corsage	___ 18. college	
___ 5. largest	___ 12. changed	ʒ 19. allusion	
___ 6. reason	ʃ 13. friction	___ 20. inject	
ʃ 7. election	___ 14. juice	ʒ 21. Persia	

C.
ð 1. smoothly	θ 7. wrath	θ 13. thimble	
θ 2. method	ð 8. writhe	θ 14. booth	
ð 3. other	ð 9. lathe	θ 15. oath	
ð 4. those	θ 10. thought	ð 16. scathing	
θ 5. moth	ð 11. clothes	ð 17. another	
ð 6. gather	ð 12. weather	θ 18. anything	

D. 1. /mu____/   v, s, z   move, moose, moos

2. /wɪ____/   f, θ or ð, z, ʃ   whiff, with (θ or ð), whiz, wish

3. /ʌ____ɚ/   ð, ʃ   other, usher

4. /lɛ____ɚ/   v, ð, s, ʒ   lever, leather, lesser, leisure

5. /____ɛrɪ/   f, v, ʃ, h   fairy (ferry), very, sherry, hairy

6. /ru____/   f, θ, z, ʒ   roof, Ruth, ruse, rouge

7. /____aɪ/   f, v, θ, ð, s, ʃ, h fie, vie, thigh thy, sigh, shy, high (hi)

8. /____ɪr/   f, v, s, ʃ, h   fear, veer, seer (sear), shear, here (hear)

E. 1. *Begins with a voiceless fricative*   hug, soon

2. *Begins with a voiced obstruent*   them, beige, vend

3. *Ends with a voiceless obstruent*   wreath, tape, cash

4. *Contains a front vowel and a voiceless fricative* wreath, cash

5. *Contains an alveolar sound*   tape, soon, vend

6. *Contains all voiced phonemes*   them, beige, vend

7. *Constrains a stop and a fricative*   beige, hug, cash, vend

8. *Contains a nasal and a fricative*   them, soon, vend

9. *Contains a fricative and a central vowel*   hug

10. *Contains no fricatives*   tape

F.   z 1. babes   z 7. bananas   z 13. dramas

s 2. chafes   s 8. drinks   s 14. croaks

z 3. cars   z 9. passes   s 15. meats

s 4. books   z 10. throws   z 16. affairs

s 5. carpets   z 11. loaves   s 17. loafs

z 6. pushes   s 12. roasts   z 18. birds

G. 1. /ʃʊk/   5. /vɛrɪ/   9. /pɝs/   13. /feɪvɚ/
2. /ʒɪŋ/   6. /ðaɪ/   10. /ʃɑrk/   14. /kreɪzd/
3. /zɔrt/   7. /θrʊ/   11. /ɪrðu/   15. /bɪʒɚ/
4. /θɝd/   8. /vɔɪnz/   12. /ʃæku/   16. /hoʊðɚ/

H. 1. Asian   9. serviced
2. vortex   10. others
3. varnish   11. frozen
4. bother   12. shivered
5. spared   13. fatten
6. thanks   14. horror
7. hearsay   15. gazebo
8. urban   16. birthdays

I. 1. bijou   /biʒu/
    2. neither   /niðɚ/
    3. verify   /vɛrɪfaɪ/
    4. hosed   /hoʊzd/
    5. Hoosier   no error
    6. amnesia   no error
    7. assure   no error, (or /əʃɝ/)
    8. favored   /feɪvɚd/
    9. shining   /ʃaɪnɪŋ/
   10. earthy   /ɝθɪ/

J. 1. /gɑrθ/   21. /θʌndɚ/
    2. /fɛns/   22. /hɛðɚ/
    3. /ʃɝ/ or /ʃɔr/   23. /sæʔn̩/
    4. /doʊzd/   24. /ʃipɪʃ/
    5. /sɔrd/   25. /sɚaʊndz/
    6. /haɪvz/   26. /hɔrʔn̩/
    7. /ʃaʊt/   27. /θɝɾɪ/
    8. /θɔrnz/   28. /vɪʒən/
    9. /ðoʊz/   29. /fɛrɪŋks/
   10. /heɪst/   30. /θɝd beɪs/
   11. /pɚhæps/   31. /gɔɪɾɚ/
   12. /ʃɔrtɚ/, /ʃɔrɾɚ/ 32. /tɛrɚ/
   13. /pɚuzd/   33. /θaʊzənd/
   14. /ənvɝst/   34. /kɑ(ɔ)ntɔ(ʊ)r/
   15. /mʌðɚ/   35. /ʃɔrtkek/
   16. /kənsumd/   36. /vɛrid/
   17. /mɚaʒ/ or /mɚɑʒ/ 37. /də(i)faɪz/
   18. /poʊʃənz/   38. /dɪ(ə)skʌst/
   19. /ovɝt/   39. /ʃɔrthænd/
   20. /tɑrzæn/   40. /mʌɾɚd/

5.4—The Affricate Consonants

A. ___ bon voyage   ___ fantasia   ʤ   cabbage
    ___ barrage   ʧ   touches   ___ exertion
    ʤ   arrange   ʧ   pasture   ___ sabotage
    ʧ   charming   ʤ   nitrogen   ʤ   gender
    ʧ   vulture   ʧ   riches   ___ glacier
    ___ mushroom   ___ charade   ʤ   eject
    ʤ   gerbil   ʤ   rigid   ʧ   unchained

B. 1. /____ɛr/   f, ð, ʃ, h, ʧ   fair, there, share, hair, chair

2. /____æt/   f, v, ð, s, h, ʧ   fat, vat, that, sat, hat, chat

3. /____oʊ/   f, ð, s, ʃ, h, ʤ   foe, though, sew (so), show, hoe, Joe

4. /____ɑrm/   f, h, ʧ   farm, harm, charm

5. /____ɪn/   f, θ, s, ʃ, ʧ, ʤ   fin, thin, sin, shin, chin, gin

6. /ri____/   f, θ, ʧ   reef, wreath, reach

7. /bæ____/   θ, s, ʃ, ʧ, ʤ   bath, bass, bash, batch, badge

8. /bi____/   f, z, ʧ   beef, bees, beach

C. 1. *Contains an initial voiced phoneme*   other, none, jeans, measure

2. *Contains a fricative*   other, shrunk, jeans, hedge, measure

3. *Contains affricate and front vowel*   jeans, hedge

4. *Contains an affricate and a nasal*   jeans, churned

5. *Contains a palatal obstruent*   shrunk, jeans, hedge, churned, measure

6. *Contains an obstruent and a central vowel*   other, shrunk, churned, measure

7. *Contains a stop, nasal and affricate*   churned

8. *Contains all voiced sounds*   other, none, jeans, measure

D. 1. /skrʌnʧ/   5. /muʒd/   9. /oʊðən/   13. /fæʃtɚ/
2. /puʤɪ/   6. /kɪʧən/   10. /ʤeɪd/   14. /gaʊʧt/
3. /ʧɔrz/   7. /moʊʧ/   11. /hʌʤ/   15. /ʤʌmpɪ/
4. /hɑrʃɚ/   8. /ʃɑrm/   12. /ʧɜn/   16. /pɑrʧt/

E. 1. chirped   9. surely
2. junk   10. jersey
3. chit chat   11. purchase
4. wishbone   12. chocolate
5. adjoined   13. mature
6. macho   14. chummy
7. garage   15. agitate
8. pasture   16. jezebel

F. 1. major   /meɪʤɚ/   6. usher   no error
2. March   no error   7. sergeant   /sɑrʤənt/
3. jumped   no error   8. massage   no error
4. Wichita   no error   9. gorge   /gɔrʤ/
5. wedged   /wɛʤd/   10. manger   /meɪnʤɚ/

G.
1. /ʃɑkt/
2. /steɪʃən/
3. /bʊtʃɚ/
4. /nɪkɚz/
5. /ɛkstrə/
6. /tændʒənt/
7. /sʌðən/
8. /nɛktaɪ/
9. /kɔrsaʒ/
10. /spɪrɪ(ə)ts/
11. /vɪvɪ(ə)d/
12. /ʃʌɾɚ/
13. /ə(ɛ)ksaɪt/
14. /æksan/
15. /skaʊɚd/
16. /kɑrvd/
17. /aʊtʃaɪn/
18. /dʒɛndɚ/
19. /kɛrləs/
20. /nɝtʃɚ/

21. /kæʒmɪr/
22. /tʃapɪŋ/
23. /kæʃbɑks/
24. /dʒɛndɚz/
25. /tʃɑrmɪŋ/
26. /ʃɑrpənd/
27. /kæʃɪr/
28. /gɑrbədʒ/
29. /ɔrkə(ɪ)dz/
30. /stræŋ(k)θən/
31. /ɛ(ə)gzɪsts/
32. /dʒɪndʒɚ/
33. /θɔrnɪ/
34. /idʒɪ(ə)pt/
35. /tʃaʊmeɪn/
36. /pɚvɝs/
37. /dʌtʃə(ɪ)s/
38. /æŋkʃə(ɪ)s/
39. /mɪstʃə(ɪ)f/
40. /kæp(t)ʃɚ/

5.5—The Approximant Consonants

A.

w	awkward	r	reasoned	w	suede	w,l	jonquil
l	bellow	__	towered	j	fewer	r	screaming
w	quick	__	Jupiter	r,l	peril	r,l	barley
__	today	l	lazy	w	swiped	j	puny
r	torpedo	r	repaid	j	yawned	__	fired

B.

__	tune	__	hood	__	choosy
__	jealous	__	piano	X	compute
X	putrid	__	maybe	X	usual
__	loop	__	jar	X	yours
X	skew	__	adjourn	__	daisy
__	keynote	X	Cupid	__	boysenberry

C.

__	awesome	X	why	X	warrior
X	well	__	awry	X	swept
X	stalwart	__	wrath	X	quirk
__	how	__	rowboat	__	borrowed
__	showed	X	reward	__	wrist
__	lower	__	Howard	X	wayward

D.

___	lurk	___	surround	___	purchase
X	barter	X	rewritten	___	perfected
___	burgundy	___	tires	X	scorpion
X	unreal	X	fourth	___	flirtatious
X	guarded	X	spirited	X	grandiose
X	grasp	___	curvature	___	divert

E.
1. /ʤelou/
2. /blaɪð/
3. /rɪljə/
4. /roulɚ/
5. /ʤɑr/
6. /sɝklz̩/
7. /fjɜt/
8. /kwɔrl̩d/
9. /wulṇ/
10. /pjaɪd/
11. /spjud/
12. /walʃat/
13. /swɪlz/
14. /riwɝd/
15. /pouləs/
16. /fjunts/

F.
1. yellow
2. robust
3. warrior
4. yearned
5. beetles
6. grouched
7. repute
8. guava
9. liquid
10. tiled
11. curtailed
12. quarrel
13. luckily
14. Latin
15. buckwheat
16. question

G.
1. bowling — no error
2. wrongful — /raŋfʊl/
3. warbled — no error
4. pewter — /pjuɾɚ/
5. quandary — /kwɑndrɪ/
6. regional — no error
7. lawyer — no error, or /lɔɪɚ/
8. flurries — /flɝɪz/
9. fuming — no error
10. baloney — /bəlounɪ/

H.
1. /kwɪksænd/
2. /slauʧt/
3. /ʤɝɪ/ or /ʤʊrɪ/
4. /əkweɪnt/
5. /ʃouldɚ/
6. /slɪðɚ/
7. /sarʤənt/
8. /skjuɚ/
9. /kɔrʤəl/
10. /jusfʊl/
11. /wɪθdru/
12. /wɝʃɪp/
13. /ɛ(ə)nʃraɪnd/
14. /fjumd/
15. /lʌn(t)ʃən/
16. /ʤunjɚ/
17. /ənskeɪðd/
18. /ʃrɪvl̩/
19. /jæŋkiz/
20. /kwɔrɾɚ/
21. /bjugl̩/
22. /ʧɪzl̩/
23. /junə(ɪ)k/
24. /ʧarl̩z/
25. /bəlaŋ(g)ɪŋ/
26. /rubrɪ(ə)k/
27. /junik/
28. /bi(ə)kwɪðd(θt)/
29. /kaɪæk/
30. /bɪljɚdz/
31. /aɪwɑ(ɔ)ʃ/
32. /lɪŋwəl/
33. /kwɔrl̩d/
34. /æŋgwɪ(ə)ʃt/
35. /autwɚd/
36. /rʌp(t)ʃɚ/
37. /ʃu wæks/
38. /kwouʃənt/
39. /straŋglɚ/
40. /əlʊr/

Review Exercises

A.
?	1. writin'	?	6. certain
ɾ	2. rudder	ɾ	7. crater
___	3. about	___	8. winter
ɾ	4. nutty	?	9. Martin
n̩	5. harden	n̩	10. sudden

B.
___	1. wheel	___	6. pull
X	2. written	___	7. contagious
X	3. regal	X	8. that'll
X	4. Seton Hall	X	9. grab 'em by the neck
X	5. candles	___	10. hold 'er by the tail

C.

/k/	stop	velar	voiceless
/r/	liquid	palatal	voiced
/θ/	fricative	interdental	voiceless
/ŋ/	nasal	velar	voiced
/dʒ/	affricate	palatal	voiced
/b/	stop	bilabial	voiced
/ʃ/	fricative	palatal	voiceless
/j/	glide	palatal	voiced
/f/	fricative	labiodental	voiceless
/n/	nasal	alveolar	voiced

D. Possible answers include:
1. deed, need
2. cone, cove
3. hum, thumb
4. hip, ship
5. rag, lag, nag

E. 1. sin-sing   place
    2. jaw-raw   manner
    3. sue-shoe   place
    4. tin-tip   voice, manner, place
    5. clue-crew   place
    6. cop-mop   voice, manner, place
    7. choke-joke   voice
    8. pet-met   voice, manner
    9. done-gun   place
    10. even-Eden   manner, place
    11. Yale-rail   manner
    12. late-lake   place
    13. fame-shame   place
    14. cat-cad   voice
    15. pass-pad   voice, manner

F. 1. jester   /ʤ/   voiced   prevocalic
    2. version
    3. itchy   /ʧ/   voiceless   intervocalic
    4. cash
    5. switched   /ʧ/   voiceless   postvocalic
    6. January   /ʤ/   voiced   prevocalic
    7. regime
    8. mashing
    9. crush
    10. urgent   /ʤ/   voiced   intervocalic

G. 1. celery   /s/   voiceless   alveolar   fricative
    2. breech   /ʧ/   voiceless   palatal   affricate
    3. phase   /f/   voiceless   labiodental   fricative
    4. wreck   /r/   voiced   palatal   liquid
    5. call   /l/   voiced   alveolar   liquid
    6. method   /θ/   voiceless   interdental   fricative
    7. yes   /j/   voiced   palatal   glide
    8. crude   /d/   voiced   alveolar   stop
    9. chasm   /k/   voiceless   velar   stop
    10. edge   /ʤ/   voiced   palatal   affricate
    11. walk   /w/   voiced   labiovelar   glide
    12. cohesion   /ʒ/   voiced   palatal   fricative

H.
1. /bɝθ marks/
2. /kandʒɚɪŋ/
3. /bɪtʃkomɚ/
4. /ʌðɚwaɪz/
5. /dʒɔrdʒ buʃ/
6. /væɾɪkən/
7. /zɪŋk aksaɪd/
8. /hæŋkɚtʃɪf/
9. /ɛkspədaɪt/
10. /faʊndeɪʃən/
11. /ædmɪɾəd/
12. /ðɛræftɚ/
13. /ɪndʒʌŋkʃən/
14. /kənvɝdʒəns/
15. /sæbətɑʒ/
16. /fəzɪʃən/
17. /bʌʔn̩ hol/
18. /dɪskɝədʒd/
19. /ivalvd/
20. /ɪndɪdʒənt/

21. /kɑzmos/
22. /tʃɪmpænziz/
23. /dɪskardəd/
24. /prɛstɪdʒəs/
25. /tʃarmɪŋ/
26. /tɝkɪʃ bæθ/
27. /bɑðɚsəm/
28. /dʒæk naɪf/
29. /ɛnzaɪm/
30. /tuθ fɛɾɪ/
31. /tʃɛɾɪ paɪ/
32. /koɑθɚ/
33. /haɪəsɪnθ/
34. /ɛndʒɔɪmənt/
35. /farməsɪst/
36. /ənwɝðɪ/
37. /wən hʌndɾətθ/
38. /pæstʃɚaɪzd/
39. /fɪdʒəɾi/
40. /fɑðɚz deɪ/

I.
1. /eɔrɾə/
2. /ɛrlaɪnɚ/
3. /kəndʒild/
4. /kaɔkeɪʒən/
5. /vokeɪʃən/
6. /fjunəl̩/
7. /rɛdʒɪstɚd/
8. /jɛstɚdeɪ/
9. /novɛmbɚ/
10. /trʌbl̩səm/
11. /əphoʊlstɚd/
12. /ɪmpjudɪnt/
13. /tɔrɛntʃəl/
14. /dɪstrɪbjut/
15. /daɪəfræm/
16. /æpətaɪt/
17. /pɚsəvɪr/
18. /kɚeɪdʒəs/
19. /mʌskjulɚ/
20. /pəpaɪrəs/

21. /sikwɛnʃəl/
22. /pɔrtreɪl/
23. /θæŋksgɪvɪŋ/
24. /zaɪləfon/
25. /arɾɪtʃok/
26. /pɪdʒənhol/
27. /wɪljəmzbɚg/
28. /ʌndɚgroθ/
29. /hjuməɚs/
30. /wɪrɪnəs/
31. /junəvɚs/
32. /əngæðɚd/
33. /mænjuskrɪpt/
34. /əbskjɝli/
35. /nuklɪəs/
36. /kwɑdræŋɡl̩/
37. /harmənaɪz/
38. /rɛdʒɪstrar/
39. /par bɔɪld/
40. /strʌkʃəl̩/

Chapter 6

Chapter Exercises

6.1   1. /θ/   5. /t/
       2. /d/   6. /h/
       3. /t/   7. /v/
       4. /d/   8. /h/

6.2   1. noon   /nuən/   X
       2. pants   /pænts/   ___
       3. choose   /tʃjuz/   X
       4. friends   /frɛndz/   ___
       5. lamb   /læm/   ___
       6. straw   /strɔr/   X
       7. rinse   /rɪns/   ___
       8. milk   /mɛlk/   ___
       9. clam   /kəlæm/   X
      10. Wednesday   /wænzdeɪ/   ___

6.3   1. [mɪrəkl̩]   3. [ɑ(ɔ)θəˈaɪz]   5. [məkænɪkl̩]
          [məˈækjələs]   [əθɔrɛɾi]   [mɛkənɪstɪk]
       2. [əkjuz]   4. [dəmɑləʃ]
          [ækjəzeɪʃn̩]   [dɛməlɪʃan]

6.4   1. your mother   /jɔr mʌðɚ/   /jəmʌðɚ/
       2. right and left   /raɪt ænd lɛft/   /raɪtn̩lɛft/
       3. food for thought   /fud fɔr θɑt/   /fudfəθɑt/
       4. What will they do?   /wʌt wɪl ðeɪ du/   /wətl̩ðeɪdu/
       5. Thank him.   /θeɪŋk hɪm/   /θeɪŋkəm/
       6. as big as   /æz bɪg æz/   /æzbɪgəz/
       7. of mice and men   /ʌv maɪs ænd mɛn/   /əvmaɪsn̩mɛn/
       8. What is her name?   /wʌt ɪz hɚ neɪm/   /wʌtsəneɪm/

6.5   1. /aɪ bɛt ju aɪ kæn hɛlp ðɛm gɛt aut əv ðæt mɛs ‖/
          /aɪbɛtʃuaɪkənhɛlpm̩gɛtaurəðætmɛs ‖/

       2. /aɪ kat ju tʃiriŋ an ðæt tɛst ‖ aɪ æm gouɪŋ tu tɛl ðə titʃɚ ‖/
          /aɪkatʃutʃɪriŋanðæt tɛst ‖ əmgunətɛlðətitʃɚ ‖/

       3. /wʌt ɪz hɪz rizn̩ fɔr nat biiŋ eɪbl̩ tu kʌm tu ðə pɑrti ‖/
          /wətsɪzrizn̩fənatbiəneɪbl̩təkəmtəðəpɑrti ‖/

       4. /wʌts ðə mæɾə wɪθ θɛlmə ‖ lɛt mi si ɪf aɪ kæn tʃɪr hɚ ʌp ‖/
          /wətsðəmæɾəwɪθ θɛlmə ‖ lɛmɪsiəfaɪkəntʃɪrəəp ‖/

       5. /wʌt dɪd ju du tu jɚ kɑr ‖ aɪ ʃud bi eɪbl̩ tu gɛt ɪt gouɪŋ ‖/
          /wədʒəduɾəjɚkɑr ‖ aɪʃədbieɪbl̩təgɛtɪtgoən ‖/

6.6 1. ˌinˈtense
    2. ˈfalse ˌhood
    3. ˈLu ˌcite
    4. ˌroˈsette
    5. ˈtea ˌbag
    6. ˈfrostˌbite
    7. ˌoˈbese
    8. ˈen ˌtree
    9. ˌeˈrode
    10. ˈhand ˌshake
    11. ˌreˈact
    12. ˈhouse ˌhold

6.7 1. ˈleopard
    2. ˈsweater
    3. ˈrhythm
    4. conˈtend
    5. ˈmurky
    6. aˈnoint
    7. ˈmagnet
    8. beˈlief
    9. ˈscary
    10. ˈnaked
    11. exˈtreme
    12. paˈrade

6.8 1. ˈmeasuring
    2. staˈtistics
    3. laˈryngeal
    4. ˈwarranted
    5. couˈrageous
    6. ˈGermany
    7. unˈbearable
    8. Caˈnadian
    9. soˈrority
    10. fraˈternity
    11. ˈAlbuquerque
    12. dysˈphonia

6.9 1. ˌmyˈopic
    2. ˈcyber ˌspace
    3. ˈarchi ˌtect
    4. ˌiˈdea
    5. ˌciˈtation
    6. ˈcircum ˌstance
    7. ˌbacˈteria
    8. ˌefferˈvescent
    9. ˈali ˌmony
    10. comˈmuni ˌcate
    11. ˈele ˌvator
    12. ˌIndiˈana

6.10 The underlined words should be:
    1. matinee
    2. East
    3. Flo
    4. uncle
    5. Mr.

6.11 1. The girl's name was <u>Chris</u>.
        Her name wasn't Pat.

    2. Jared only forgot to get the <u>toothpaste</u> at the store.
        Jared remembered to get everything else.

    3. Why did they <u>walk</u> to the playground?
        Why didn't they drive?

    4. Why did they walk to the <u>playground</u>?
        Why didn't they walk to the zoo?

    5. <u>Mark</u> got a new blue bike for his birthday.
        Louise didn't get a new bike.

    6. Mark got a new blue <u>bike</u> for his birthday.
        He did not get a blue baseball cap.

    7. Mark got a new <u>blue</u> bike for his birthday.
        The bike wasn't green.

6.12   The answers are in bold.

Waitress:	Would you like something to **drink**?
Customer:	**Lemonade**, please. I would also like to **order**.
Waitress:	Would you like an **appetizer**?
Customer:	**No, thank you.**
Waitress:	Would you like to hear about our **specials**?
Customer:	**Please.**
Waitress:	We have **grilled salmon** and **fettuccine alfredo**.
Customer:	I'll have the **fettuccine**.
Waitress:	Would you like our **house dressing** on your **salad**? It's **Italian**.
Customer:	I would like to have **blue cheese**, please.
Waitress:	I'll also bring out some **fresh rolls**.
Customer:	**Thank you.**
Waitress:	**You're welcome.**

6.13   1. a. ˌSteve's ˈroommate is from ˌMinneapolis.
         b. ˌSteve's ˌroommate is from Minneˈapolis.

       2. a. ˌTim went ˌskydiving on ˈSaturday.
         b. ˈTim went ˌskydiving on ˌSaturday.

       3. a. The ˈanswer on the ˌexam was ˌ"false."
         b. The ˌanswer on the ˌexam was ˈ"false."

       4. a. ˌMary's ˌbirthday is next ˈTuesday.
         b. ˌMary's ˈbirthday is next ˌTuesday.

       5. a. ˈI'd like a ˌsteak for ˌdinner.
         b. ˌI'd like a ˈsteak for ˌdinner.

       6. a. ˌI went to New York ˈCity to see some ˌplays.
         b. ˌI went to ˌNew York City to see some ˈplays.

       7. a. ˌMy ˈprofessor ˌshaved his ˈmustache.
         b. ˌMy ˈprofessor ˌshaved his ˌmustache.

       8. a. ˌI need poˈtatoes from the ˌstore.
         b. ˈI need ˌpotatoes from the ˌstore.

6.14   The answers are in bold.

1. When will you leave?	Rising	**Falling**
2. Is your brother home?	**Rising**	Falling
3. I need to go the library.	Rising	**Falling**
4. What's your favorite season?	Rising	**Falling**
5. Did you get paid yet?	**Rising**	Falling
6. The dog ran away.	Rising	**Falling**
7. Sophie is my oldest friend.	Rising	**Falling**
8. How did you know about that?	Rising	**Falling**
9. Honest?!?	**Rising**	Falling
10. I'm sure!!!	Rising	**Falling**

6.15   1. [piːz]   4. [spɑː]
       2. [liːv]   5. [læːg]
       3. [ruːd]   6. [tuː]

6.16   1. [raɪs:up]
       2. [kaʔn̩:ɛɾɪŋ]
       3. [bɪg:ʌnz]
       4. [pætʃt:aɪəz]
       5. [teɪl:aɪt]

       6. [ka(l)m:ɔrnɪŋ]
       7. [bɑr:um]
       8. [rɑk:ændɪ]
       9. [lif:aɪə]
      10. [pʊʃ:ɛrɪ]

6.17   1. [I want hot dogs | ice cream | and cotton candy ‖]
       2. [They left | didn't they ‖]
       3. [The family | who lived next door | moved away ‖]
       4. [What is her problem ‖]
       5. [My uncle | the dentist | is 34 years old ‖]

Review Exercises

A.

1. [kæm meɪk]	m/n	bilabial
2. [haʊʒɚ mʌðɚ]	ʒ/z+j	palatal
3. [dʒɪŋ geɪm]	ŋ/n	velar
4. [lɛb paɪp]	b/d	bilabial
5. [hæʒ ʃeɪkn̩]	ʒ/z	palatal
6. [rɛg gaʊn]	g/d	velar

B.   1. /bɛnz/
       2. /wɪnɚ/
       3. /lænmaɪn/
       4. /kæn ə wɜmz/

       5. /kaʊnɚ/
       6. /twɛlfs/
       7. /wəts ɚ prɑbləm/
       8. /wɛp laʊdlɪ/

C.   1. /aɪ wɑnt tu goʊ hoʊm/
         /aɪwɑnəgohom/

       2. /lɛt mi si jɔr bʊk/
         /lɛmɪsijɚbʊk/

       3. /kʊd ju muv eɪ lɪɾl̩ tu ðə raɪt/
         /kʊdʒəmuvəlɪɾl̩təðəraɪt/

       4. /dɪd dʒan ɛvɚ gɛt peɪd/
         /dɪdʒanɛvɚgɛtpeɪd/

       5. /waɪ dɪd ʃi liv soʊ ɜlɪ/
         /waɪdʃilivsoɜlɪ/

       6. /ɪt ɪz reɪnɪŋ kæts ænd dɑgz/
         /ɪtsreɪnɪŋkætsn̩dɑgz/

       7. /wɛn ɑr ju goʊɪŋ tu liv/
         /wɛnɚjəgʊnəliv/

       8. /ju hæv gɑt tu bi kɪdɪŋ/
         /juvgɑɾəbikɪdɪŋ/

       9. /hu ɪz goʊɪŋ tu reɪk ðʌ livz tunaɪt/
         /huzgʊnərekðəlivztənaɪt/

     10. /aɪ wɑnt tu wæks maɪ trʌk tumaroʊ mɔrnɪŋ/
         /aɪwɑnəwæksmaɪtrʌktəmaromɔrnɪŋ/

D.   1. Did you ever go to the circus?
2. When did she leave Georgia?
3. My sister got a new boyfriend.
4. Give me a day to decide.
5. I am going to have to say "No" for now.
6. I think it is going to rain either today or tomorrow.
7. Would you ever think of doing that for me?
8. Do you think that Susan took enough of them?
9. I am sure that they are going to tell you what you need to do it.
10. Try as he might, he just could not do what she wanted.

E.   1. cour'ageous
2. 'terri ˌfied
3. ma'jestic
4. ˌasth'matic
5. 'Plexi ˌglas
6. plur'ality
7. 'manda ˌtory
8. ˌclan'destine
9. ˌflam'boyant
10. ˌcre'ation
11. ˌcompu'tation
12. 'cran ˌberry
13. 'bulletin
14. sur'rendered
15. se'mantics
16. co'lonial
17. 'mercen ˌary
18. inde'pendent
19. ˌOc'tober
20. ˌballer'ina

F.

		Reduced	Full
1. /ˈɔrɪʤɪn/	/əˈrɪʤɪnˌet/	X	
2. /ˈmaɪkrəˌskop/	/ˌmaɪˈkrɑskəpɪ/		X
3. /əˈrɪstəˌkræt/	/ˌɛrɪsˈtɑkrəsɪ/		X
4. /ˈstrærəʤɪ/	/strəˈtiʤɪk/		X
5. /ˈmeɪnɪˌæk/	/məˈnaɪəkḷ/	X	
6. /ˌhoˈmɑʤənəs/	/ˌhoməˈʤinɪəs/		X
7. /ˈpɛrəˌlaɪz/	/pəˈræləsɪs/		X
8. /ˈfɛlənɪ/	/fəˈlounɪəs/		X
9. /pəˈspaɪə/	/pəspəˈeɪʃn̩/	X	
10. /ˌriˈpit/	/ˌrɛpəˈtɪʃəs/	X	

G.

		Rising	Falling
1.	I got a sweater for my birthday.	___	X
2.	Are you happy?	X	___
3.	The girls had spaghetti for supper.	___	X
4.	Are you positive?	X	___
5.	When you're finished, go to bed.	___	X
6.	Were you late for work, today?	X	___
7.	Let me get back to you.	___	X
8.	Did you buy a new CD?	X	___
9.	What do you mean?	___	X
10.	Is that your idea of a joke?	X	___

H. 1. If I want your help | you'll be the first to know ||
2. Maybe I will | maybe I won't ||
3. They bought a new house | didn't they ||
4. The girls who went swimming | all got a cold ||
5. I can't really make up my mind ||
6. I scream | you scream | we all scream | for ice cream ||
7. When are you leaving on vacation ||
8. Are your cousins coming for a visit | or not ||
9. Do you have ants in your pants ||
10. I quit my job | but only when I was sure I could get another ||

I. 1. [aɪkɔtmaɪkæt:ɑm baɪðəteɪl ‖]
2. [wɪtʃ:æmpudɪʤubaɪætðəstɔr ‖]
3. [wuʤuputðəwaɪt:ebḷklɑθɑnðəteɪbḷ | pliz ‖]
4. [mɑm:aɪt:ekmɪʃɑpɪŋ ɪf aɪ gɛt gʊd gredz ‖]
5. [hævjəfɪnɪʃt:epɪŋ ðə ti vi spɛʃljɛt ‖]
6. [wɪθ:ɛm | ɪts hɑrdtətɛlwətðer θɪŋkɪŋ ‖]
7. [pliz | gɪmijəfon:ʌmbə bifɔr juliv ‖]
8. [klɛm:eɾə hoʊmrʌnætðəbɪg:emlæst:uzdeɪ ‖]
9. [tɛɾɪ n̩fɛrl̩:ʌv tuple aʊtsaɪd wɪð:əwɑɾəsprɪŋklə ‖]
10. [aɪwont:ekɛnɪmɔrəvðəʤʌŋk:ɛnhænzaʊt ‖]

J. 1. /waɪkænʧuɛvɚæktʃɚeɪʤ ‖/
/waɪkænʧuɛvɚæktjɚeɪʤ ‖/

2. /waɪ owaɪ | dɪdaɪɛvəlivaɪowə ‖/
/waɪ owaɪ dɪdaɪɛvəlivaɪowə ‖/

3. /wɛndðeseðɚflaɪtwʌz ‖/
/wɛndɪdðeseðɚflaɪtwʌz ‖/

4. /ɑlprabligohomtəmarou | ɔrðədeæftɚ ‖/
/aɪwɪlprabligohoumtəmarou | ɔrðədeæftɚ ‖/

5. /wɛrdʃiɛvɚgeʔn̩ aɪdiəlaɪkðæt ‖/
/wɛrdɪdʃiɛvɚgetænaɪdiəlaɪkðæt ‖/

6. /jugɑɾəbipʊlɪnmaɪlɛg ‖/
/juvgat təbipʊlɪŋmaɪlɛg ‖/

7. /maɪfrɛnz | ɛsbɪn̩deɪl | argunəpɪkmiəpətθri ‖/
/maɪfrɛnz | ɛsbɪn̩deɪl | argouɪŋtəpɪkmiəpætθri ‖/

8. /waɪʤu ripentðəbarnalrɛɹɪ ‖/
/waɪdɪʤu ripentðəbarnalrɛɹɪ ‖/

9. /ðɛrgunəteljuwəʧənid ‖/
/ðɛrgouɪŋtəteljuwətjunid ‖/

10. /dɪdʃitektuəvəm ‖ næ|ʃitʊkfɔr ‖/
/dɪdʃitektuəvðəm ‖ nɑːʃitʊkfɔr ‖/

Chapter 7

Chapter Exercises

7.1 1. nasals and stops
2. labial and alveolar
3. liquids, some fricatives, and affricates
4. stops

7.2 later developing phonemes (according to Smit et al.): /ŋ and r/
earlier developing phonemes: /t and v/ and /ð/ (for girls only)

7.3 ___ 1. yes   ___ 6. milk

  X 2. baby   X 7. mitten

  X 3. banana   ___ 8. lady

  ___ 4. mama   X 9. scissors

  X 5. today   ___ 10. juice

7.4 away   1. _____ _____   say   6. _____ _____

cup   2. X   /kʌ/   phone   7. X   /fou/

through 3. _____ _____   black   8. X   /blæ/

clown   4. X   /klaʊ/   stop   9. X   /stɑ/

bread   5. X   /brɛ/   go   10. _____ _____

7.5   ___ 1. wagon   X 4. pencil
     X 2. children   X 5. water
    ___ 3. jacket   ___ 6. yellow

7.6 X 1. blue   X 6. stop
    ___ 2. spot   X 7. crayon
     X 3. stripe   X 8. milk
    ___ 4. path   ___ 9. wish
     X 5. spring   X 10. grape

7.7 ___ 1. shoe   ___ 6. comb
     X 2. thank   X 7. summer
    ___ 3. raisin   ___ 8. yellow
     X 4. march   X 9. bath
    ___ 5. shave   X 10. shop

7.8 ___ 1. candy   X 6. ridge
     X 2. rake   ___ 7. fishing
     X 3. bring   ___ 8. paper
    ___ 4. clown   X 9. goose
     X 5. brush   ___ 10. sing

7.9 ___ 1. shake   ___ 6. gem
    ___ 2. choose   X 7. witch
    ___ 3. brush   X 8. chalk
     X 4. Jack   X 9. chase
    ___ 5. mesh   ___ 10. bridge

7.10 ___ 1. soap   ___ 6. yes
     X 2. leaf   X 7. loop
     X 3. ring   X 8. grow
     X 4. lazy   X 9. laugh
    ___ 5. rice   ___ 10. free

7.11 X 1. middle   X 6. belt
    ___ 2. lamp   X 7. bottle
     X 3. answer   X 8. curtain
     X 4. Kirk   ___ 9. bark
    ___ 5. could   X 10. fair

7.12 ___ 1. pie   X 6. boat

    X 2. tap   ___ 7. train

    ___ 3. frog   X 8. peg

    ___ 4. lip   ___ 9. cause

    X 5. numb   X 10. big

7.13 ___ 1. pig   X 6. knife

    X 2. pat   X 7. that

    X 3. short   X 8. phone

    ___ 4. Tom   ___ 9. vat

    ___ 5. tune   ___ 10. hard

7.14 X 1. turkey   ___ 6. ring

    ___ 2. kill   X 7. bang

    ___ 3. mouse   ___ 8. shook

    ___ 4. grass   X 9. cap

    X 5. fake   X 10. brag

7.15 P 1. pear   ___ 6. gone

    D 2. led   P 7. train

    P 3. fair   D 8. flag

    D 4. card   P 9. shoe

    ___ 5. high   ___ 10. chair

7.16
1. chairs   initial consonant deletion
2. letter   fricative replacing a stop
3. witch   stop replacing a glide
4. tape   backing
5. bunny   initial consonant deletion; glottal replacement
6. bad   backing; glottal replacement

7.17 1. ___ good   3. X drop   5. X keep

    2. X kiss   4. ___ clam   6. ___ comb

7.18 1. [ɛ̧] /ɔ/   5. [ɥ] /ʊ/

    2. [æ] /ɛ/   6. [ɛ̧] /æ/

    3. [o̧] /ɔ/   7. [ɹ] /ʊ/

    4. [o̧] /e/   8. [ɥ] /i/

7.19 1. [h̃ʊd]   4.   7. [s̃wit]
2.   5.   8. [d̃un]
3. [r̃uf]   6.

7.20 1. [ɪɱfɚɛntʃəl]   6. [kæɱfɚ]
2.   7. [sʌɱflaʊɚ]
3. [mɛɱfəs]   8.
4.   9.
5. [əɱfrɛndlɪ]   10. [kɪɱfo(l)k]

7.21 1. [æn̪θəm]   5. [mæθ̪taɪm]
2.   6. [wɛl̪θ]
3.   7.
4.   8. [pæn̪θɚ]

7.22 1. ___ lake   6. ___ liked
2. X mingle   7. X angle
3. ___ loop   8. X scald
4. X beagle   9. X ladle
5. X shoulder   10. X bile ___

7.23 1. ___ slack   5. X excuse
2. ___ praised   6. ___ surprise
3. X scorn   7. X stripe
4. X despite   8. ___ smooth

7.24 1. X skunk [sk⁼ʌŋkʰ]   _____
2. X snacked [snæk˺tʰ]   _____
3. ___ target [tɑrgət˺]   [tʰɑrgət˺]
4. ___ brave [bʰreɪv]   [breɪv]
5. ___ toga [tʰoʊgʰə]   [tʰoʊgə]
6. X guarded [gɑrdəd˺]   _____
7. ___ person [pɝsʰən]   [pʰɝsən]
8. X carefully [kʰɛrfʊlɪ]   _____
9. ___ slope [sl⁼oʊp˺]   [sloʊp˺]
10. ___ great [gʰreɪtʰ]   [greɪtʰ]

7.25 1. ___ mean [m̃in]   4. X string [strĩŋ]
2. X boon [bũn]   5. ___ slam [s̃læm]
3. ___ muddy [mʌdĩ]   6. X thong [θãŋ]

7.26 1. [kɛt̬l̩]   4.
      2.   5.
      3. [wɑt̬ɚ]   6. [bæt̬l̩d]

7.27 1. [pjuɾə]   5. [hi dʌz̥]
      2. [k̥ɪrlɪ]   6. [rɪd̥ʒ strit]
      3. [hiz̥ stʌbən]   7. [aɪ luz̥]
      4. [beɪd̥ pæm]   8. [ðeɪɣ pleɪd̥]

Review Exercises

A. 1. /teɪ/   6. /nis/
    2. /saɪd/   7. /tɝ/
    3. /kɛr/   8. /dɪn/
    4. /poʊ/   9. /kæn/
    5. /bæs/   10. /teɪ/

B. 1. d   6. d
    2. c   7. b
    3. a   8. c
    4. b   9. d
    5. a   10. a

C. 1. R   6. P
    2. R   7. P
    3. R   8. P
    4. P   9. R
    5. R   10. P

D. 1. c   6. d
    2. d   7. b
    3. a   8. c
    4. e   9. b
    5. a   10. e

E. 1. c   5. a,c
    2. a   6. a,c
    3. b   7. b
    4. b   8. a

F. 1. <u>a,b,c</u>   5. <u>b,d</u>

    2. <u>a,b</u>   6. <u>b,d</u>

    3. <u>a,c</u>   7. <u>a,d</u>

    4. <u>b,d</u>   8. <u>a,b,c</u>

G. 1. /sip/ or /lip/
    2. /græg/
    3. /dɑr/
    4. /wɛmən/ or /jɛmən/
    5. /beɪp/
    6. /ʒɛlɪ/
    7. /bʌv/
    8. /taɪn/
    9. /teɪm/
    10. /groʊ/

H. 1. No   7. No
    2. No   8. Yes
    3. Yes   9. Yes
    4. Yes   10. No
    5. Yes   11. Yes
    6. No   12. No

I. 1. wɑbstɚ   14. hæmɚ
    2. nɝs   15. wɑrm kwɑk
    3. souldʒɚ   16. vækjum kwinɚ
    4. æstrənat   17. ɛlfənt
    5. titʃɚ   18. taɪgɚ
    6. trʌk draɪvɚ   19. skwɝl
    7. dɛntɪst   20. paɪɾɚ
    8. frɪdʒɚɛɚ   21. jaɪən
    9. tɛləfon   22. dɑlfɪn
    10. wæmp   23. kæŋgru
    11. tusbwəʃ   24. ɑktəpʊs̠
    12. bæftəb   25. jɔɪjɚ
    13. tɔɪwət

J. 1. tʃɛrɪz̠   11. ɑktəpʊs̠
    2. s̠ɛləi   12. s̠kwɝl
    3. tʃiz̠   13. s̠neɪk
    4. s̠iriəl   14. s̠kʌŋk
    5. greɪps̠   15. dʒinz̠
    6. aɪs̠krim   16. s̠wɛɾɚ
    7. piz̠   17. pədʒæməz̠
    8. pænkeks̠   18. s̠ændl̩z̠
    9. ɛgz̠   19. mɪʔn̠z̠
    10. s̠paɪɾɚ   20. s̠lɪpɚz̠

21. We went to Ben Franklin's and looked at the toys.
/wiwɛnˀtubɛnfræŋklɪnz̪ | ænd lʊktætðətɔɪz‖/

22. I saw some dolls that I liked.
/aɪs̪as̪əmdɑlz̪ðætaɪlaɪkt ‖/

23. They traveled to Maine from Nebraska.
/ðeɪtrævl̪dtumeɪn| frʌmnəbras̪kə ‖/

24. We do spelling and math.
/widus̪pɛlɪŋænmæθ‖/

25. Sometimes we play mystery games.
/s̪ʌmtaɪmz̪wipleɪmɪs̪trigeɪmz̪ ‖/

K.
1. frɑg
2. z̪ibrə
3. kʊkɪz̪
4. hæmbəgə
5. skʌŋk
6. strɔbɛrɪz̪
7. pɛrəkit
8. kɛrəts̪
9. s̪ɪrɪəl
10. hɑtdɑg
11. pænkeks̪
12. s̪ɛləi
13. dʒɚæf
14. lamps̪tə
15. ɚæbɪt
16. s̪paɪdə
17. ɛləfənt
18. aɪs̪krim
19. bʌtʌ
20. tʃɛrɪz̪
21. skwʊl
22. ɑrəndʒ
23. hɔs̪
24. pəteɪtoʊ
25. tʌtʊl

L.
1. [pʰ]   aspirated /p/
2. [u̜]   lowered production of /u/; more like /ʊ/
3. [r̥]   devoiced /r/
4. [g̃]   labialized production of /g/ (with lip rounding)
5. [ɬ]   lateral plus central /s/
6. [õ]   /o/ produced with nasal emission
7. [z̤]   whistled /z/
8. [e̙]   backed production of /e/

M. Possible answers include:
1. [st̄ɔr]
2. [m̃aɪ]
3. [rʌb̚]
4. [hɛ̃n]
5. [bɛt̬ə]
6. [tɛn̪θ]
7. [d̬rɪŋk]
8. [kɑɫ]
9. [ɪɱfɔrm]
10. [kɪʔn̩]

N.
1. X   ʰ▢
2. X   ▢̃
3.   ▢̚
4. X   ▢⁺
5.   ▢̄
6.   ▢̬
7.   ▢̆
8. X   ▢̞

O. 1. clue   **[kʰlu]**   [k̥ɬu]   [kˈlu]
    2. lymph   **[lɪɱf]**   [ɬɪmf]   [lɪmpˈ f]
    3. money   [mʌ̃ni]   **[mʌ̃nɪ]**   [m̥ ʌnɪ]
    4. coop   [kˈupʰ]   **[kʰupʰ]**   [kʰupˈ⁼]
    5. trial   **[t̪ʰ ɹaɪɬ]**   [tʰɹaɪɬ]   [tʰɹaɪɬ]
    6. skunk   [skˈʌŋkʰ]   [skˈʌ̃ŋkʰ]   **[sk⁼ ʌ̃ŋkʰ]**
    7. menthol   **[mɛ̃ n̪ θaɬ]**   [mɛ̃ n θ ɑ l]   [mɛ̃ n θɑ ɬ]
    8. sweet   [s̥wit⁼]   [s̃ʍitˈ]   **[s̃ʍ̥itʰ]**

Chapter 8

Chapter Exercises

8.2 1. lid   /lɪd/   [lɪ̪d]   4. caught /kɔt/   [kɔ̪t] or /kɑt/ (if pronounced as /kɑt/)
     2. when   /wɛn/   [wɛ̪n] or [wɛ̪n]   5. left   /lɛft/ [lɛ̪ft]
     3. rub   /rʌb/   [rʌ̪b]

8.3 1. may   /mei/   /me̪ɪ/   4. like   /laɪk/   /la̪ɪk/
     2. lick   /lɪk/   /lɪ̪k/   5. weed   /wid/   /wɪ̪d/
     3. bone   /boʊn/   /bo̪ʊn/

8.4 These vowels will vary, based on your dialect.

8.5 1. ɝ → ʌ   6. ɔɪ → ɔː
     2. ɔ → ɑ   7. ɝ → ɜː
     3. r → ə   8. ʊ → u
     4. ar → ɑː   9. ɛ → eɪ
     5. aɪ → a   10. r → ə

8.6 1. ɑ → ɒ   6. ɛr → ær
     2. æ → a   7. ə → ɚ
     3. ɝ → ɜː   8. ɚ → ə
     4. ɔr → ɔ   9. ɝ → ʌ
     5. æ → ɑ   10. ar → ɑː

8.7 1. /ræ̃ː/   6. /jɛlɪn/
     2. /wɪf/   7. /blæs/
     3. /kɛəktɚ/   8. /haɪnd/
     4. /wiz/   9. /dɪnɪ/
     5. /hædn̩t/   10. /kæʔ/

8.8 1. z → s   6. æ → ɑ
     2. ʌ → ɑ   7. ɪ → i
     3. ɝ → ɛr   8. v → b
     4. j → dʒ   9. ʊ → u
     5. epenthesis of /ə/   10. dʒ → tʃ

8.9   Chinese
    1. /sɪŋk/   think
    2. /suz/   shoes
    3. /waɪn/   vine
    4. /bʌt/   bought

    Japanese
    5. /zɪs/   this
    6. /hri/   free
    7. /ʃip/   ship

    Pilipino
    8. /paɪn/   fine
    9. /tsɛk/   check
  10. /fit/   fit

8.10

X	1.	pack	/bæk/	
X	2.	very	/wɛrɪ/	v → w
___	3.	patch	/pæʃ/	
X	4.	think	/θɪnk/	ŋ → n
X	5.	candy	/kɛndɪ/	æ → ɛ
X	6.	written	/rɪtn̩/	ɪ → i
___	7.	meant	/mʌnt/	
X	8.	them	/dɛm/	ð → d

8.11

X	1.	pink	/pɪnk/
X	2.	Paul	/bɔl/
___	3.	thought	/dɔt/
X	4.	check	/ʃæk/
___	5.	reed	/ræd/
X	6.	vine	/faɪn/
___	7.	lucky	/loʊkɪ/

Review Exercises

A. 1. /raɪɾə/   6. /əpɪə/
    2. /klɑːk/   7. /deɪndʒə/
    3. /əwɛə/   8. /mɜːdə/
    4. /skɔ, skɔə, skoə/   9. /tʃɑːrə/
    5. /kɜːtɪnz/   10. /bɜːbən/

B. 1. lemon   9. result
    2. orange   10. flurry
    3. precious   11. worthy
    4. cushion   12. chair
    5. stew   13. sister
    6. various   14. pure
    7. watch   15. cart
    8. real   16. sport

C. 1. /biwɛə/   6. /stɔə/
    2. /stat/   7. /skwɜ:t/
    3. /hæŋgə/   8. /glɛə/
    4. /səvɪə/   9. /dɑktə/
    5. /klɜ:ʤɪ/   10. /kɑ:bən/

D. 1. clogged   9. coffee
    2. Tuesday   10. parrot
    3. can't   11. sorry
    4. broom   12. explore
    5. marrow   13. charter
    6. blurring   14. largest
    7. fawn   15. demand
    8. bath   16. conspire

E. 1. /mɑf/   6. /dɛm/
    2. /niθ/   7. /bəhand/
    3. /ðɪn/   8. /weɪsəz/
    4. /kæ:/   9. /əlɛbn̩/
    5. /potɛkʃn̩/   10. /draɪvɪn/

F. | X | 1. | bread | /brɛ/ | final stop deletion |
    | | 2. | | | |
    | X | 3. | suppose | /pouz/ | deletion of unstressed initial syllable |
    | | 4. | | | |
    | X | 5. | raced | /reɪs/ | word-final cluster reduction |
    | | 6. | | | |
    | X | 7. | when | /wɪn/ | ɛ → ɪ (vowel raising) |
    | X | 8. | light | /lat/ | diphthong simplification |
    | X | 9. | hold | /houd/ | /l/ (liquid) deletion |
    | | 10. | | | |
    | | 11. | | | |
    | X | 12. | washing | /wɑʃən/ | ŋ → n |
    | X | 13. | could | /kʊʔ/ | glottal stop replacement |
    | | 14. | | | |
    | X | 15. | corn | /koʊn/ | /r/ (liquid) deletion |

G.

X	1.	bath	/bæt/	stopping
X	2.	been	/bin/	ɪ → i
___	3.			
X	4.	oven	/avən/	ʌ → a
___	5.			
X	6.	Jimmy	/jɪmɪ/	deaffrication
___	7.			
X	8.	cushion	/kuʃən/	ʊ → u
___	9.			
___	10.	shallow	/ʧælou/	affrication
X	11.	vine	/baɪn/	stopping
___	12.			
X	13.	stood	/əstʊd/	epenthesis of /ə/
X	14.	zebra	/sibrə/	consonant devoicing
___	15.			

H.
1. Vietnamese
2. Cantonese and Mandarin
3. Korean, Japanese, and Pilipino
4. Cantonese, Vietnamese, Korean, and Pilipino
5. Cantonese
6. Cantonese, Mandarin, and Korean
7. Cantonese, Mandarin, Vietnamese, and Japanese
8. Pilipino
9. Japanese
10. Mandarin, Japanese

I.

	Russian	Arabic	Both
1. p → b	___	X	___
2. v → w	X	___	___
3. ð → d	X	___	___
4. ɔ → o	___	___	X
5. ʌ → u	___	X	___
6. dʒ → ʃ	___	X	___
7. θ → t	X	___	___
8. ŋ → n	___	___	X
9. æ → ɛ	X	___	___
10. θ → s	___	X	___

J. 1. /ma ǀ aɪ gaɾə goɾəðəstɔ: wɪθ pɔl tədeɪ ‖ /
    2. /wəɾəju tɔkɪŋ əbaʊt ‖ fəget əbaʊt ɪt ɔlɾɛdɪ ‖/
    3. /ka:lɪ ǀ waɪ dəju hæftə run ɛvɾɪθɪŋ ‖/
    4. /aɪ hævə dɛntɪst əpɔɪntmənt æt sɪks θɜɾɪ ‖/
    5. /rɔbət nidz təgoʊɾəðə bɔbə ǀ hɪz hɛrz tu lɔŋ ‖/
    6. /aɪ wɔkt ovətəðə mɔl jestədeɪ æftənun tə gɛtənu pɛɾəʃuz ‖/
    7. /maɪ dɔg laɪks təɾən ɔl əraʊnd ðə ja:d n̩ ba:k ‖/
    8. /wɛn aɪ wəz pleɪŋ bæskətbɔlǀ aɪ ræn ɔlovəðəkɔ:t ‖/
    9. /aɪ gaɾəgofudʃapən ‖ aɪ nid wɔɾəmɛlən ǀ kɔn ǀ n̩ soʊdə ‖/
    10. /maɪ frɛn mɛrɪzə wɪədoʊ ǀ ʃidontwanəlimɪəloʊn ‖/

K. 1. /pak ðə ka ɪnðə gəraʒ ‖/
    2. /əmgoʊənəðəmakət ɪn bɔstən ‖/
    3. /aɪ lʌvtə ʃɔp havəd skwɪə ‖/
    4. /hæv juz gaɪz bɪnəðəkeɪp ɔ maθədz vɪnjəd fəðəsʌmə ‖/
    5. /doʊnt fəgeɾəbrɪŋ jə pɔkətbuk ‖/
    6. /danə lʌvztə drɪŋk tɔnɪk ‖/
    7. /kɪn ju wɪə jə dʌŋgəriz n̩ snikəz ‖/
    8. /geɾəfak fəðæt judʒ hɛlpənə pastəŋgreɪvɪ ‖/
    9. /gəhedŋgɪvmʌmɪ səm dʒɪmɪz fəɚ bənænəɚ splɪt ‖/
    10. /dʒɔn mɪlə ɪzə disənt jumən bɪən ‖/

L. 1. /ʃiz dravɪn tu luzɪænə təmarə mɔrnɪn ‖/
    2. /əmgunə bɔ:l ədəzən ɛgz fɚ istɚ ‖/
    3. /læs naɪt ǀ aɪwəz takən təma frɛn mɛrɪlɪn ‖/
    4. /əmfɪksən təhævtə ba səm tɑrz fəməkar ‖/
    5. /əmlukənfəma blu bɑl pɔɪnt pɛn ‖/
    6. /ju bɛɾə kʌvɚ ðæt brɔ:lən pæn wɪθ əlumɪnəm fɔ:l ‖/
    7. /weɪɾəmɪnətleɪɪ ǀ a nid ənəðɚ mɪnət təmeɪkəpma mand ‖/
    8. /a lɛft ðə tʃɪkən aʊt ɑn ðə kaʊnɚ ænd ɪt spɔ:ld ‖/
    9. /ðə junɪvəɚsɪ əv tɛnəsi ɪz ɪn naksvəl ‖/
    10. /hɜɪkənz n̩ tɔrneɪɾəz arboθ lardʒ dæmədʒɪn wɪndstɔrmz ‖/

M. 1. /də bɔɪ nid moʊ mʌnɪ ‖/
    2. /wi fɪksəntə goʊtudə stoʊ ‖/
    3. /hi bi pleɪən bɑl ætdəpark ‖/
    4. /ðɛr ar foʊ nu kɪdz ɪn maɪ klæs/
    5. /maɪ sɪstɚ æn brʌvɚ wəzætdæt kansət ‖/
    6. /maɪ fæmlɪ goʊ tətʃɜtʃ ɛr: ɪ sʌndeɪ ‖/
    7. /joʊ maməkar ɪnə mɪl̩əðəʃtri:ʔ ‖/
    8. /ʃi faʊn faɪ: kwoʊɾəz ɪn hɚ pɜs ‖/
    9. /kwanzə gat hɚ hɛr dən ‖/
    10. /ðə studənts hɛlpt dɛmsɛlvz tu brɛkfəs ‖/

N. 1. /pliz pʊt ðəflaʊəz ɪndə beɪs ‖/
    2. /ɪt wəs ə bɛrɪ əspeʃɪəl okeɪzjən ‖/
    3. /ju sʊd kwɪt dʒɛlɪŋ æt jɔr mʌdɚ‖/
    4. /aɪ wəs nat suɚ aɪ wʊt bi eɪbl̩ tu hɛlp ‖/
    5. /maɪ feɪbəɾɪ:tʃɚs neɪmis mɪstɚ dʒons ‖/

6. /doʊnt lɛt jɔr dɑk pleɪ ɪn maɪ ʤɑrt ‖/
7. /waɪ dont ju pʊt dis kloʊðz ɪn də gʌrɑʒ ‖/
8. /jɛstədeɪ | aɪ wɛnt:u də su wiθdʌk ‖/
9. /sɛlɪ pʊt ðə poteɪtoʊ ʧips an ðə loʊə sɛlf ‖/
10. /aɪwəs bɛrɪ ɛksaɪtət əbaʊt winɪŋ ðə fʊtbɑl geɪm ‖/

O.
1. /aɪ hæv wʌn jʌŋgə brʌzə ɪn maɪ fæməɪ ‖/
2. /aɪwʊd raɪkə grɪld ʧiz sandwɪʧ fɔr:ʌnʧ priz ‖/
3. /ɪt ɪz səpoʊs tu reɪn hɛvrɪ fɔr mʌʧəvðəwik ‖/
4. /zə rɪvə ɪz hɛvrɪ pərutəd ‖/
5. /maɪ θɪstə kjoʊkoʊ wɪl bi twɛnɪsri jɪrzold nɛkstɜsdeɪ ‖/
6. /wʊd ju raɪk tu goʊ ʃapɪŋ wɪsmi æftəaɪ gɛt af wɜk ‖/
7. /wʊd jɔr ʌðə brʌzə hɛlp mi rɪft ðɪθ ‖ ɪts hɛvɪ ‖/
8. /sæŋk ju bɛrɪ mʌʧ fɔr zə bjutɪful fraʊəz ‖/
9. /aɪ hæv ə hard taɪm dɪstɪŋgwɪʃ bitwin zə sɪŋgjurə ænd prɜəl fɔrms ‖/
10. /ði oʊnrɪ konɛktɪŋ fraɪt ɪs: ru pɔrtrənd ɔrəgon ‖/

P.
1. /taɪpɪŋ imeɪl z hɛlps mi fɪŋk ɪn ɪŋgrɪʃ ‖/
2. /aɪ wɛnt tudə ʃu tu si də nu pændə bɪrs ‖/
3. /wʌt duju θɪŋkəvðə nu tɛrəvɪʒn̩ ʃoʊ ‖/
4. /aɪ hæb tu ɔr θri frɛnz hu ar goʊɪŋ tu də sakə geɪm ‖/
5. /juzəlɪ | si ɪs nat so fɔrgɛtful ‖/
6. /aɪ bɛt ju dæt aɪ wɪl wɪn də reɪs ‖/
7. /maɪ gɜlfrɛnd sɛnt mi fraʊəz last wik fɔr maɪ bɜfdeɪ ‖/
8. /dɛr ar sɛvrəl pipəl aɪ nid tu gɛt tu noʊ ‖/
9. /də leɪaʊt əv dis:ɪrɪ ɪs nat vɛrɪ kanvinɪənt ‖/
10. /aɪ præn tu goʊ tu pədu fɔr maɪ mæstəs digri ‖/

Q.
1. /aɪwʊd laɪk e wɔdkə ænd tɔnɪk pliz/
2. /pʊt de bʊks oʊə dɛr an də teɪbl̩/
3. /ɪt wʌz difikʊlt fɔr mi tu lɔrn də kərɛkt pronaʊnseɪʃən/
4. /aɪ hæv bɪn livɪŋ in də junaɪɾəd steɪts sins last ɔgʊst/
5. /xi xæz mɛni prabləmz wɪθ hɪz vokæbəlɛrɪ/
6. /də rʌʃən ikɔnəmi dipɛnz ɔn də karənt praɪs əv ɔil/
7. /maɪ jʌŋgə brʌdə aləgzandə ɪz stʌdɪŋ mɛtəlʊrdʒi æt mɔskoʊ steɪt junivɜsiti/
8. /di aʊtə əv də bʊk wʊz e feɪməs raɪtur/
9. /aɪ hɛd sɛvɔrəl wizɪtəz frəm vʊrdʒinɪə last mɑnθ/
10. /haʊ mɛni ʌðə pipʊl nidəd tu teɪk di klɛs/

R.
1. /bliz juz dæt wʊrd ɪn e sɛntəns/
2. /aɪ nid ʃugə səbɪstɪtut fɔr maɪ kɔfi/
3. /dʊktə kubə tɔld mi tu meɪk e kɔbi əv ðə hoʊmwək əsaɪnmənt/
4. /ðɛr frɛnd robɪn gat mɛrɪd tu fɪktɔr maɪ nɛkst dɔr neɪbɔr/
5. /aɪ wʌz diprɛst bikʊz wi hæv hæd soʊ mʌʧ bæd wɛdə/
6. /bit gɔt ə prɛzn̩ sɛntɪns bikʊz hi hɛd ðə polismɛn/
7. /maɪ feɪfərɪt kɔtən ʃɜt ʃrʌŋk ɪn ðə lɔndərɪ/
8. /bɛnɪ vizɪtəd hɜ fiɑnseɪ an fraɪdeɪ/
9. /aɪ nid tu stʌdɪ ɪŋgəlɪʃ fonəloʊdʒɪ tu ɪmbruv maɪ pronaʊnzɪeɪʃən/
10. /aɪ gru e bɪrd so ðæt aɪ wʊd əbɪr oʊldə/

Glossary

abduction   a movement of the vocal folds away from the midline (closed) position

accent reduction   therapy for a nonnative speaker of English, designed to increase speech intelligibility, without jeopardizing the integrity of the individual's first dialect

acoustic phonetics   the study of the auditory aspects of speech including frequency, intensity, and duration (length)

addition   the insertion of an extra phoneme in the production of a word, usually used in reference to disordered speech; epenthesis

adduction   a movement of the vocal folds toward the midline (closed) position

affricate   a consonant characterized as having both a fricative and a stop manner of production, e.g., /ʧ and ʤ/

African American Vernacular English (AAVE)   a dialect of English, spoken throughout the United States, thought to have originated as a pidgin of European and African languages; also referred to as Black English, Black English Vernacular, and Ebonics

allograph   differing letter sequences that represent the same phoneme, e.g., h<u>ea</u>t, k<u>ey</u>, and r<u>ee</u>d

allophone   variant production of a phoneme, e.g., [pʰ] and [p˺]

alveolar   referring to the alveolar ridge; a consonant produced with a constriction formed by the tongue apex or blade and the alveolar ridge, e.g., /t, d, n, s, z, and l/

alveolar assimilation   an assimilatory phonological process that occurs when a nonalveolar consonant is produced with an alveolar place of production due to the presence of an alveolar phoneme elsewhere in the word

alveolar ridge   the gum ridge of the maxilla located directly behind the upper front teeth

apex   the tip of the tongue

approximant   a consonant, such as a glide or liquid, produced with an obstruction in the vocal tract, less than that associated with the obstruents or nasals but greater than that associated with the vowels

articulation   modification of the airstream by the speech organs in production of spoken language

articulation disorder   difficulty in coordinating the articulators in production of a limited set of phonemes; difficulty with the motoric aspects of speech production

arytenoid cartilages   paired cartilages of the larynx that attach to the superior portion of the cricoid cartilage; each vocal fold attaches to one arytenoid cartilage

aspiration   the production of a frictional noise (similar to /h/) following the release of a voiceless stop consonant

assimilation   the process by which phonemes take on the phonetic character of neighboring sounds due to coarticulation; refers to articulatory changes that result in the production of an allophone, or of a completely different phoneme

assimilatory processes   phonological processes that involve an alteration in phoneme production due to phonetic environment

back (of the tongue)   the portion of the tongue body posterior to the front of the tongue; it lies inferior to the velum

Bernoulli effect   a drop in air pressure, created by an increase in airflow through a constriction; helps to explain, in part, vocal fold adduction

blade   the part of the tongue located just posterior to the tip

body (of the tongue)   the portion of the tongue posterior to the blade comprised of the front and the back of the tongue

bound morpheme   a morpheme that must be linked to another morpheme in order to convey meaning; e.g., <u>pre</u>date and think<u>ing</u>

bunched   one method of /r/ production in which the tongue apex is lowered as the tongue blade is raised to form one constriction with the palate, while the tongue root forms a second pharyngeal constriction; see retroflexed

central incisor   any of the four front teeth, located in both the upper and lower jaws

chain shift   a current dialectal modification in the pronunciation of English vowels, reflecting an alteration in their place of production; the change in the articulatory target for one vowel has a relative effect on the targets for other vowels, e.g., Northern Cities Shift and Southern Shift

citation form   the pronunciation of a word as a single, isolated item

clinical phonetics   the study of aberrant speech behaviors

closed syllable   a syllable with a consonant phoneme in the final position

close internal juncture   two syllables in the same tone group with no transitional pause between them, e.g., /aɪskrim/

cluster reduction   a syllable structure phonological process that results in the deletion of a consonant from a cluster

coarticulation   an articulatory process whereby individual phonemes overlap one another due to timing constraints and ease of production

coda   the consonants that follow a vowel in any syllable; not all syllables have a coda

cognates   phonemes that differ only in voicing, e.g., /t/ and /d/

complementary distribution   refers to allophone production that is tied to a particular phonetic environment

connected speech   an utterance consisting of two or more continuous words

consonant   a phoneme produced with a constriction in the vocal tract; consonants are usually found at the beginning and end of a syllable and generally have less sonority than vowels

consonant cluster   two or three contiguous consonants in a syllable, e.g., s<u>tr</u>ike, <u>pl</u>ease, and lea<u>pt</u>

content word a word that contains the most salient information in an utterance; e.g., noun, verb, adjective, and adverb

cricoid cartilage the posterior cartilage of the larynx, shaped like a signet ring

customary production the age at which a particular speech sound is produced with greater than 50 percent accuracy in at least two word positions

deaffrication a substitution phonological process that involves the replacement of a fricative for an affricate

denasality (hyponasality) production of nasal phonemes with raised velum

dental (interdental) referring to the teeth; a consonant produced with a constriction formed by the tongue apex and the teeth, e.g., /θ and ð/

dentalization production of an alveolar phoneme as linguadental, that is, with the tongue tip more forward than normal

devoicing an assimilatory phonological process (voicing assimilation) that involves the replacement of a voiceless phoneme for a normally voiced, syllable-final consonant preceding a pause or silence

diacritic a specialized phonetic symbol used in both systematic and impressionistic transcription to represent both allophone production as well as suprasegmental features of speech

dialect a variation in speech or language due to geographical area, social class, or ethnic group

diaphragm the major muscle that separates the abdomen from the thorax

digraph pair of letters that represent one sound; the letters may be the same or different, e.g., loo͟k, thi͟nk, and e͟ar

diphthong a single phoneme consisting of two vowel elements, the first termed the onglide and the second termed the offglide

distinctive feature a subphonemic property used in the classification of the sounds of the world's languages, e.g., voicing, consonantal, vocalic, etc.

distortion a characteristic of disordered speech involving the production of an allophone of an intended phoneme

dorsum the body of the tongue, comprised primarily of the front and back; also, the back of the tongue

Eastern American English a regional dialect of English spoken in the New England states and in New York, New Jersey, and Pennsylvania

elision the omission of a phoneme from a word as a result of a historical change, or from coarticulation associated with connected speech

epenthesis the addition of a phoneme to a word during speech production as a result of coarticulation, dialect, or a speech disorder

epiglottis a cartilaginous structure that protects the larynx from food and drink during swallowing

eustachian tube a tube, composed of cartilage and bone, which connects the nasopharynx with the middle ear; important for equalization of changes in air pressure and in drainage of middle ear fluids

experimental phonetics the laboratory study of physiologic, perceptual, and acoustic phonetics

external intercostal muscles muscles located between the ribs that aid in inhalation; the internal intercostals are deep to the external intercostals

external juncture a pause serving to connect two tone groups in connected speech

extIPA an extension to the IPA that has become the official diacritic set for the transcription of disordered speech; adopted by the International Clinical Phonetics and Linguistics Association in 1994

falling intonational phrase a fall, or declination, in the pitch of the voice across the length of an intonational phrase; usually associated with complete statements and commands, as well as wh-questions

final consonant deletion a syllable structure phonological process that involves the deletion of the final consonant in a syllable, resulting in an open syllable (CV)

formant a resonant frequency of the vocal tract

free morpheme a morpheme that can stand alone yet still carry meaning

free variation refers to allophone production that is not tied to a particular phonetic environment

fricative a consonant produced by forcing the breath stream through a narrow channel formed by two separate articulators in the vocal tract

front (of the tongue) the part of the tongue body anterior to the back of the tongue; it lies inferior to the (hard) palate

fronting a substitution phonological process that involves the replacement of an alveolar consonant for a velar or palatal consonant

function word a word that contributes little to the meaning of an utterance, e.g., pronoun, article, preposition, and conjunction

fundamental frequency the basic rate of vibration of the vocal folds

given information previous exchange of words, or shared world knowledge between two conversational participants

glide a consonant characterized by a continued, gliding motion of the articulators into the following vowel; also referred to as a semi-vowel, e.g., /j/ and /w/

gliding a substitution phonological process that involves the replacement of a glide for a liquid

glottal referring to the glottis; a phoneme produced with a constriction formed at the level of the vocal folds, e.g., /h/

glottal stop an allophonic variation of /t/ or /d/, produced when the release of the stop is at the level of the vocal folds instead of in the oral cavity, i.e., /ʔ/

glottis the space between the vocal folds

grapheme a printed alphabet letter used in the representation of an allograph

habitual pitch the inherent fundamental frequency of a given individual

hard palate the structure known as the "roof of the mouth" that separates the oral and nasal cavities

historical phonetics the study of sound changes in words over time

homorganic two consonants sharing the same place of articulation, e.g., ti͟me and ͟neck

hyoid bone a "floating bone" that provides structural support for the larynx; it attaches inferiorly to the larynx by a broad curtain-like ligament and superiorly to the tongue by muscle tissue

hypernasality the presence of excessive nasality accompanying the production of a non-nasal phoneme due to improper velopharyngeal closure

hyponasality (denasality) production of nasal phonemes with a raised velum

idiolect a speech pattern unique to an individual, based on dialect and personal speaking habit

idiosyncratic process a phonological process that is not typical of the speech behavior of a normally developing child

impressionistic transcription allophonic transcription of an unknown speaker or an unknown language

internal intercostal muscles muscles located between the ribs that aid in exhalation; the internal intercostals are deep to the external intercostals

International Phonetic Alphabet (IPA) an alphabet used to represent the sounds of the world's languages; created to promote a universal method of phonetic transcription

intervocalic a consonant located between two vowels, e.g., abo͟ve

intonation the modification of voice pitch associated with varying utterance types (such as a question or a statement), or associated with a speaker's particular mood

intonational phrase the changes in the fundamental frequency of the voice spanning the length of a meaningful utterance (a word, phrase, or sentence)

intraoral pressure the air pressure within the oral cavity, created by a constriction of the articulators during production of stop consonants

juncture the transitional pauses and breaks between syllables and words in speech production

labial (bilabial) referring to the lips; a consonant produced with a constriction formed at the lips, e.g., /p, b, m, and w/

labial assimilation an assimilatory phonological process that occurs when a nonlabial phoneme is produced with a labial place of articulation due to the presence of a labial phoneme elsewhere in the word

labialization addition of lip rounding to the articulation of a typically unrounded phoneme

labiodental a consonant produced with a constriction formed by the lower lip and upper central incisors, e.g., /f and v/

larynx cartilaginous and muscular structure that houses the vocal folds; responsible for phonation

lateral a manner of production in which the airstream is directed over the sides of the tongue, e.g., /l/

lax the description of a vowel produced with a reduction in muscular effort; a lax vowel does not appear in the final position of an open monosyllable, e.g., /ɪ, ɛ, æ, ʊ, ɚ, ʌ, and ə/

limited English proficiency (LEP) lack of familiarity of the English language by a nonnative speaker

lingual referring to the tongue; a consonant produced with the tongue as the major articulator

liquid a generic label used to classify two English approximant consonants, /r/ and /l/

Low Back Merger a dialectal variation reflecting a change in the articulatory targets for /ɑ and ɔ/, so that no differentiation occurs in their production; characteristic of certain Western, Midwestern, and New England speakers

mandible the lower jaw

manner of production the way in which the airstream is modified as it passes through the vocal tract in production of consonants; English manners of production include stop, fricative, affricate, nasal, glide, and liquid

mastery the age at which a particular speech sound is produced with some degree of accuracy, usually 75 to 100 percent

maxilla the upper jaw

mean length of utterance (MLU) a measure of language behavior that indicates the number of morphemes per utterance a child is capable of producing

metathesis the switching of two phonemes in a word due to a speech error, dialectal variation, or a speech disorder

minimal pair a pair of words that vary by only one phoneme, e.g., cook/book and passed/last; *minimal contrast*

misarticulation an articulatory error, classically categorized as an omission, substitution, distortion, or addition

monophthong a vowel phoneme consisting of one distinct articulatory element (as opposed to a diphthong, which has two elements)

morpheme the smallest unit of language capable of carrying meaning

nares the nostrils

nasal a consonant produced with complete closure in the oral cavity along with a lowered velum to allow airflow through the nasal cavity

nasal emission the audible escape of air through the nares due to improper velopharyngeal closure or to a cleft in the palate or the velum

nasalization production of an oral phoneme with accompanying nasal resonance, due to a lowered velum, e.g., [mẽn]

nasal plosion the release of a stop consonant through the nasal cavity, as opposed to the oral cavity, as in the word /sʌdn̩/

natural phonology Stampe's theory that supports the idea that young children are born with innate processes necessary for the development of speech

new information an exchange of words between two conversational participants that adds to the knowledge already shared

nonresonant consonants (nonresonants) a class of sounds characterized by a noise source that originates at a constriction in the vocal tract, as air flows through the supralaryngeal system; the nonresonant consonants include the stops, fricatives, and affricates

Northern Cities Shift an ongoing change in the production of vowels, causing a shift from their standard place of articulation in the vowel quadrilateral; this shift is seen in the northern tier of the United States in cities such as Cleveland, Detroit, and Buffalo

nucleus the part of a syllable with the greatest acoustic energy; usually, but not always, a vowel

obstruent a class of sounds (with a noise source) including the stops, fricatives and affricates; also referred to as nonresonant consonants

offglide the second element of a diphthong

omission the deletion of a phoneme in a word, usually related to disordered speech

onglide the first element of a diphthong

onset all consonants preceding a vowel in any syllable; not all syllables contain an onset

open internal juncture a transitional pause between two syllables within the same tone group, e.g., /aɪ + skrim/

open syllable a syllable with a vowel phoneme in the final position

oral sounds produced with a raised velum (velopharyngeal closure)

palatal referring to the hard palate; a consonant produced with a constriction formed by the tongue blade and the hard palate, e.g., /ʃ, ʒ, ʧ, ʤ, r, and j/

palatoalveolar a consonant produced with a constriction formed by the tongue blade and the hard palate, slightly posterior to the constriction formed during production of alveolar consonants; often used to describe the place of production of /ʃ and ʒ/; also referred to as postalveolar

perceptual phonetics the study of listeners' perception of speech sounds in terms of pitch, loudness, perceived length, and quality

pharynx a muscular tube-like structure that connects the larynx and the oral cavity; the throat

phonation the vibration of the vocal folds in creation of a voiced sound

phoneme a speech sound capable of differentiating morphemes

phonetic alphabet an alphabet that contains a separate letter for each individual sound in a language, e.g., the IPA

phonetics the study of the speech sounds of a language

phonological disorder a difficulty in speech sound production resulting in multiple speech sound errors ultimately involving the sound system of a language; also used to describe articulation disorder

phonological processes simplifications used by children not capable of producing adult speech patterns

phonology the systematic organization of speech sounds in the production of language; the study of the linguistic rules that specify the manner in which phonemes are organized and combined into syllables, words, and sentences

physiological phonetics the study of the function of the speech organs and their role in speech production

pidgin a language that results when individuals speaking two different languages begin to communicate; typically characterized as having a reduced vocabulary and grammar

place of articulation refers to the specific articulators employed in the production of a particular phoneme; the location of the constriction in the vocal tract in production of a consonant

point vowel one of four extreme corner vowels of the vowel quadrilateral, i.e., /i, æ, u, and ɑ/

postalveolar *see* palatoalveolar

postvocalic a consonant following a vowel, e.g., a<u>t</u>

prevocalic a consonant preceding a vowel, e.g., <u>m</u>e

prevocalic voicing an assimilatory phonological process (voicing assimilation) that involves the voicing of a normally unvoiced consonant preceding the nucleus of a syllable

progressive assimilation a modification in the identity of a phoneme due to a previously occurring phoneme; left-to-right or perseverative assimilation

quality the perceptual character of a sound based on its acoustic resonance patterns; timbre

r-colored vowel a speech sound consisting of the two elements: vowel + /r/. e.g., /ɪr, ɛr, ʊr, ɔr and ɑr/; rhotic diphthong

reduplication a syllable structure phonological process that involves the repetition of a syllable of a word

regressive assimilation a modification in the identity of a phoneme due to a later occurring phoneme; right-to-left or anticipatory assimilation

resonance the vibratory properties of any sound-producing body

resonant consonants (resonants) a class of sounds produced with a resonance throughout the entire vocal tract, e.g., the nasals, glides, and liquids

retracted a spread or unrounded lip position during vowel production, e.g., /i, ɪ, e, ɛ, æ, ɑ, ʌ, and ə/

retroflexed one method of /r/ production in which the tongue tip is raised and curled back toward the alveolar ridge, as the back of the tongue creates a second velar constriction; *see* bunched

rhotacization   the production of a phoneme with an /r/ quality, e.g., /ɝ/ and /ɚ/

rhotic diphthong   *see* r-colored vowel

rhyme   a syllable segment consisting of an obligatory nucleus (usually a vowel) and an optional coda

rising intonational phrase   a general rise in the pitch of the voice across the length of an intonational phrase; usually associated with yes/no questions, lists, and incomplete utterances

root   the portion of the tongue that attaches to the anterior wall of the pharynx and to the mandible

rounded   a rounded lip position during vowel production; the rounded English vowels include /u, ʊ, o, ɔ, ɝ, and ɚ/

sentence stress   added emphasis given to a specific word in a sentence due to the importance of that word in conveying meaning, or due to speaker intent; often found in association with the last word in a declarative utterance

sibilant   the alveolar and palatal fricatives /s, z, ʃ, and ʒ/, which are perceived as being louder than the other fricatives

Southern American English   a regional dialect spoken in the Southern and South Midland states

Southern Shift   an ongoing change in the production of vowels, causing a shift from their standard place of articulation in the vowel quadrilateral; this shift is seen in the southern, middle Atlantic, and southern mountain states

spectrum   the frequency array, or energy pattern, characteristic of any sound

Standard American English (SAE)   a form of English that is relatively devoid of regional characteristics; the English used in textbooks and by national broadcasters

sternum   the breast bone

stop   a consonant characterized by (1) a complete obstruction of the outgoing airstream by the articulators, (2) a build up of intraoral air pressure, and (3) a release

stopping   a substitution phonological process that involves the replacement of a stop for a fricative or an affricate

subglottal pressure   the air pressure applied to the inferior surface of the vocal folds (glottis); the air pressure (from the lungs) necessary to blow the vocal folds apart

substitution   the replacement of one phoneme by another in a syllable or word

substitution processes   a phonological processes involving the substitution of one phoneme class by another, e.g., gliding, deaffrication, fronting, etc.

suprasegmental   a feature of speech production, such as stress, intonation, and timing, which transcends the phonemic level

syllabic consonant   a consonant that serves as the nucleus of a syllable, e.g., /l, m, and n/

syllable   a basic unit of speech production and perception generally consisting of a segment of greatest acoustic energy (a peak, usually a vowel) and segments of lesser energy (troughs, usually consonants); a unit of speech consisting of an onset and/or a rhyme

syllable structure processes   phonological processes that generally simplify the production of syllables, creating a consonant-vowel (CV) pattern

systematic narrow transcription   allophonic transcription of an individual, used when the rules of the language are known; also referred to as *narrow transcription* or *allophonic transcription*

systematic phonemic transcription   phonemic transcription of an individual, used when the rules of a language are known; variant phoneme (i.e., allophone) production is not recorded; also referred to as *broad transcription* or *phonemic transcription*

tap   a manner of consonant production involving a rapid movement of the tongue tip against the alveolar ridge resulting in the creation of a very brief phoneme, i.e., /ɾ/

tempo   the timing, or durational aspect, of connected speech

tense   the description of a vowel produced with an increased muscular effort; a tense vowel can be located in the final position of an open monosyllable, e.g., /i, e, u, o, ɔ, ɑ, and ɝ/

thoracic cavity (thorax)   the part of the human body between the head/neck and the abdomen; the chest cavity

thyroid cartilage   the most anterior cartilage of the larynx to which the vocal folds attach; the notch of the thyroid cartilage forms the "Adam's apple"

timbre   sound quality

tongue advancement   a term used to classify vowel production in relation to tongue position along the front/back dimension in the oral cavity

tongue height   a term used to classify vowel production in relation to tongue position along the high/low dimension in the oral cavity

tonic (nuclear) accent   the emphasis given to the tonic (nuclear) syllable in any particular intonational phrase

tonic (nuclear) syllable   the syllable that contains the greatest pitch change in any particular intonational phrase

trachea   a tube, comprised of cartilaginous rings, embedded in muscle tissue, that connects the lungs with the larynx; windpipe

unreleased   a stop consonant produced with no audible release burst

uvula   the rounded, tablike structure located at the posterior tip of the velum

velar   referring to the soft palate (velum); a consonant produced with a constriction formed by the back of the tongue and the velum, e.g., /k, g, and ŋ/

velar assimilation   an assimilatory phonological process that occurs when a nonvelar phoneme is produced with a velar place of production due to the presence of a velar phoneme elsewhere in the word

velarization   the backed production of an alveolar phoneme (such as /l/) so that the tongue is more posterior than normal (in the velar region); e.g., [rigɫ]

velopharyngeal closure   a constriction formed by the velum and the rear wall of the pharynx, resulting in a diversion of the airstream into the oral cavity

velum   a muscular structure located directly posterior to the hard palate; the soft palate

vocal folds   elastic folds of tissue, primarily composed of muscle; the vocal cords

vocalization (vowelization)   a substitution phonological process that involves the replacement of vowel for postvocalic /l/ or /r/

vocal tract   the network consisting of the larynx, pharynx, and the oral and nasal cavities

voiced   a sound produced with vocal fold vibration

voiceless   a sound produced without vocal fold vibration

voicing   the participation of the vocal folds during phoneme production; all vowels are voiced, whereas only certain consonants are voiced

VoQS   the voice quality symbols diacritic set; designed to be used in the transcription of individuals with voice disorders

vowel   a phoneme produced without any appreciable blockage of air flow in the vocal tract

vowel merger   a current dialectal modification in which vowels with separate articulations fuse into one similar place of articulation, e.g., /ɑ/ and /ɔ/ both being produced as /ɑ/

vowel quadrilateral   a two-dimensional figure (representing tongue height and tongue advancement) that displays the relative position of the tongue during vowel production

vowel reduction   an articulatory process associated with connected speech whereby the full form of a vowel is produced with less weight due to a more central production in the oral cavity, often similar to a mid-central vowel

weak syllable deletion   a syllable structure phonological process that involves the omission of an unstressed (weak) syllable either preceding or following a stressed syllable

word class   also known as "part of speech," e.g., noun, verb, adjective

word stress (lexical stress)   the production of a syllable with increased force or muscular energy, resulting in a syllable that is perceived as being louder, longer in duration and higher in pitch; also known as word accent

Index

A

AAVE. *See* African American Vernacular English
Abduction, 41
Accent (dialect), 265–267
    reduction, 267, 286
Addition error, 211
Adduction, 41
Advancement (of tongue), 50
    diacritic for, 231
Affricate manner, 140–143
African American Vernacular English (AAVE), 58, 280–284
Allograph, 8, 70, 125, 274, 277–278
Allophone, 18–19, 59–60, 71–72, 78, 116, 211, 287
    complementary distribution, 19
    free variation, 19
Allophonic transcription, 20, 230–243
Alveolar place of articulation, 44, 111, 115
    fricative, 130, 133–134
    liquid, 147
    nasal, 122, 124
    stop, 112, 114
Alveolar assimilation, 114, 124, 223–224
Alveolar ridge, 40, 43–45, 115
Anticipatory assimilation, 171
Apex (tongue), 46, 115
Approximant manner, 143–147
Arabic-Influenced English, 294–295
Articulation, 42–46
Articulation disorder, 209–210
Articulators (speech organs), 21, 43
Arytenoid cartilages, 39–40

Asian/Pacific-Influenced English, 290–292
Aspiration of stops, 19
    diacritic for, 235
Assimilation, 170–172, 178
    progressive, 171–172, 222–224
    regressive, 171–172, 222–224, 293
Assimilatory processes, 215, 222–225
    alveolar assimilation, 223–224
    devoicing, 225
    labial assimilation, 222–223
    prevocalic voicing, 224–225
    velar assimilation, 224

B

Back of tongue, 43–46
Back tongue position (diacritic), 230–231
Back vowels, 66–77
    /u/, 66–69
    /ʊ/, 69–71
    /o/, 71–73
    /ɔ/, 74–75
    /ɑ/, 76–77
Bernoulli effect, 40
Bilabial place of articulation, 43, 111, 114, 124
    glide manner, 144–145
    nasal manner, 123–124
    stop manner, 113–114
Blade of tongue, 43, 46, 115
Body of tongue, 46, 54, 56, 231
Bound morpheme, 10
Braces (in transcription), 239–240
Brackets (in transcription), 20

Breathy voice (diacritic), 239
Broad transcription, 19
Bunched (articulation of /r/), 146

C

Casual speech (pronunciation), 2, 175, 178
Central incisors, 44
Central vowels, 77–86
    /ə/, 77–79
    /ɚ/, 82–83
    /ʌ/, 79–81
    /ɝ/, 83–86
Chain shift, 268–270
Citation form, 169–170, 175, 178
Cleft palate, 44
Clinical process, 209–212
Close internal juncture, 194
Closed syllable, 24, 52, 228
Cluster reduction, 218, 225–227, 288
Coarticulation, 170–171, 174
Coda, 22–23, 216, 229
Cognates, 111, 136
Complementary distribution, 19
Connected speech, 169–170, 177, 194
Consonants, 107–149
    definition, 107
    difference from vowels, 107–109
    non-pulmonic, 11, 13
    physical and acoustic characteristics, 108–109
    pulmonic, 11, 13
    sound source, 108, 112–113, 130, 140
    syllabic, 22, 109, 119, 123–125, 147
Consonant cluster, 21, 210, 228, 283, 290, 293